## AN OUNCE OF PREVENTION

The boundaries of psychology are expanding as growing numbers of psychological scientists, educators, and clinicians take a preventive approach to social and mental health challenges. Offering a broad introduction to prevention in psychology, this book provides readers with the tools, resources, and knowledge to develop and implement evidence-based prevention programs. Each chapter features key points, a list of helpful resources for creating successful intervention programs, and culturally informed case examples from across the lifespan, including childhood, school, college, family, adult, and community settings. It is also an important resource for students, researchers, and practitioners in counseling, clinical, health, and educational psychology, social justice and diversity, social work, and public health.

Sally M. Hage is Professor of Psychology at Springfield College, USA. She is an accomplished scholar in the fields of prevention and counseling psychology and has a range of clinical experiences with culturally diverse youth, college students, and adults. She is an APA fellow, co-author of *Best Practices in Prevention* (2013), and founding editor of the *Journal of Prevention and Health Promotion* (*JPHP*).

# An Ounce of Prevention

## EVIDENCE-BASED PREVENTION FOR COUNSELING AND PSYCHOLOGY

*Edited by*

**Sally M. Hage**

Springfield College

CAMBRIDGE
UNIVERSITY PRESS

CAMBRIDGE
UNIVERSITY PRESS

Shaftesbury Road, Cambridge CB2 8EA, United Kingdom

One Liberty Plaza, 20th Floor, New York, NY 10006, USA

477 Williamstown Road, Port Melbourne, VIC 3207, Australia

314–321, 3rd Floor, Plot 3, Splendor Forum, Jasola District Centre, New Delhi – 110025, India

103 Penang Road, #05–06/07, Visioncrest Commercial, Singapore 238467

Cambridge University Press is part of Cambridge University Press & Assessment, a department of the University of Cambridge.

We share the University's mission to contribute to society through the pursuit of education, learning and research at the highest international levels of excellence.

www.cambridge.org
Information on this title: www.cambridge.org/9781009244480

DOI: 10.1017/9781009244503



First published 2024

*A catalogue record for this publication is available from the British Library*

*Library of Congress Cataloging-in-Publication Data*
Names: Hage, Sally M., author.
Title: An ounce of prevention : evidence-based prevention for counseling and psychology / edited by Sally M. Hage, Springfield College.
Description: New York, NY : Cambridge University Press, 2024. |
Includes bibliographical references and index.
Identifiers: LCCN 2023059596 | ISBN 9781009244480 (hardback) |
ISBN 9781009244527 (paperback) | ISBN 9781009244503 (ebook)
Subjects: LCSH: Preventive mental health services. |
Child mental health. | Counseling psychology.
Classification: LCC RA790 .H27 2024 | DDC 362.2083–dc23/eng/20240207
LC record available at https://lccn.loc.gov/2023059596

ISBN 978-1-009-24448-0 Hardback
ISBN 978-1-009-24452-7 Paperback

*This book is dedicated to my son, Evan, with all my love.*

# Contents

# Figures

# Contributors


LAUREN E. ADAMS Indiana University

CONLIN BASS Yale School of Public Health

GENEVIEVE E. CHANDLER University of Massachusetts-Amherst

STEPHANIE IRBY COARD University of North Carolina – Greensboro

ROBERT K. CONYNE University of Cincinnati

PATRICIA COOK-CRAIG University of Nevada, Las Vegas

SEAN DEMARTINO Springfield College

DONNA DOWNING Maine Medical Center and Tufts University

ASHLEY G. EVANS University of North Carolina, Greensboro

CLAIRE FURTADO Loyola University Chicago

MICHEAL GARZA Indiana University

SANDRA A. GRAHAM-BERMANN University of Michigan

MALAÏKA GUTEKUNS Lehigh University

SALLY M. HAGE Springfield College

ANNA N. HAMILTON Boston College

JIM HELLING University of Massachusetts-Amherst

KEITH C. HERMAN University of Missouri

MARY IELLAMO Brattleboro Retreat

REBECCA JAYNES Maine Medical Center and Tufts University

YAT MING JUDE LEUNG Contra Costa County Behavioral Health Services

MAUREEN E. KENNY Boston College

KIRSTEN G. KLEIN University of Florida

BROOKE KOHLER Lehigh University

ALEXANDER KOPELOWICZ Maine Medical Center and Tufts University

LISA DE LA RUE University of San Francisco

CHRISTOPHER T. H. LIANG Lehigh University

SARAH LYNCH Maine Medical Center and Tufts University

WILLIAM R. MCFARLANE Maine Medical Center and Tufts University

WENDY M. REINKE University of Missouri

JULIA RONCORONI University of Denver

TERESA ROSENBERGER Lehigh University

JESSICA M. SAFI Lehigh University

LIISA SLOAT Maine Medical Center and Tufts University

BARBARA STUART Maine Medical Center and Tufts University

QUANG D. TRAN Boston College

CAROLYN M. TUCKER University of Florida

ELLEN L. VAUGHAN Indiana University

ELIZABETH VERA Loyola University Chicago

BARBARA C. WALSH Maine Medical Center and Tufts University

MARY E. WALSH Boston College

KEADIJA C. WILEY University of North Carolina, Greenboro

EVELYN CLAIRE WILLIAMS Indiana University

KEYA WILLIAMS Lehigh University

GUILLERMO WIPPOLD University of South Carolina

CHELSEA YANUARIA Loyola University Chicago

# Acknowledgments

The *Ounce of Prevention* book represents the culmination of more than two years of collaborative work among nearly 50 scholars from across the United States. I express my deepest gratitude to these contributing authors whose incredible work provides insightful evidence-based models to further the field of prevention and health promotion. These committed scholars donated their valuable time and shared their insights, wisdom, and experience, providing an extraordinary gift to the mental health professions, students, and researchers.

I also want to thank the highly professional editorial team at Cambridge University Press who provided support and vision throughout the process, in particular my Editor Stephen Acerra and his staff, including Rowan Groat and the production team. I am also indebted to my research assistants, Arianna Ciccarelli, Janna Grimsrud, Danielle A. Farrar-Noonan, Chen Liang, and Weston Sharpe, who provided support and assistance in the process of completing the project. Finally, I want to thank the six anonymous peer reviewers who provided tremendously helpful feedback on the book proposal that ultimately shaped the focus of the book.

# Acknowledgments

PART ONE

# A FOUNDATION IN PREVENTION

# 1 The Practice and Science of Prevention: Introduction and Overview

Sally M. Hage and Mary Iellamo

An ounce of prevention is worth a pound of cure.
—Benjamin Franklin, *Pennsylvania Gazette*, February 4, 1735

If you have come to help me you are wasting your time. But if you have come because your liberation is bound up with mine, then let us work together.
—Lilla Watson, 1985 United Nations Decade for Women Conference, Nairobi

## 1.1 Focus of This Book

This book fills an important gap in the growing field of prevention, that is, to provide training, resources, and exemplary illustrations of evidenced-based prevention programs for students, practitioners, researchers, educators, and policy makers to utilize in developing and implementing their own prevention initiatives. The specific aims of this book are twofold:

1. to provide training for students, educators, and practitioners in psychology, social work, human services, medicine, and public health in designing and implementing prevention, and
2. to highlight established and promising model programs in health promotion and prevention that may reduce the negative effects for people and communities struggling with psychological disorders, trauma, or mental distress.

## 1.2 Chapter Authors' Perspectives

One of my (Sally) favorite tasks as founding editor of the *Journal of Prevention and Health Promotion* (https://us.sagepub.com/en-us/nam/journal-of-prevention-and-health-promotion/journal203644, *JPHP*, Sage) is presenting the annual *JPHP* Best Paper Award to an author or set of authors whose work stands above the rest. In 2022, I presented this award to Dr. Richard Lee who, with his colleagues Xiaug Zhou and Judy Ohm, wrote an outstanding paper about the Incredible Years Attentive Parenting program (Zhou et al., 2021). When Dr. Lee accepted the award, he remarked that as mental health professionals, "prevention is in our bones, but it is not in our training" (R. Lee, personal communication, August 6, 2022). Long after hearing this remark, I pondered the meaning of these words and the larger context in which they were uttered. The majority of mental health professionals believe wholeheartedly in the importance of prevention, yet few of us engage in or purport to have the skills and knowledge to actually carry it out. This discrepancy – between our beliefs and our actions related to prevention– not only creates ethical dissonance but likely contributes to burnout among mental health professionals, many of whom indicate they feel overwhelmed by being unable to meet current demand for mental health services. Nearly half of psychologists report feeling burned out during the past year (APA, 2022).

As a practicing mental health professional, I (Mary) have been fortunate to work in fast-paced, acute settings providing care to a wide variety of presentations, demographics, and levels of need. It has been a privilege to be schooled in evidence-based practice in order to provide the most effective treatment possible to the people I serve. Throughout my training and practice, it has been astoundingly apparent that the need for prevention in the mental health setting is essential. While such a need is evident, what is less evident is the manner in which mental health professionals can actually implement preventative measures with clients, students, and communities. It is for this reason that this volume is of extreme interest to me as a provider. In an era in which we are seeing more attention given to the research–practice gap, this book is a welcome resource for taking the current research and offering practical, empirically supported recommendations for prevention in clinical practice.

## 1.3 How Clinical Experience Informs This Chapter

Well-intentioned clinicians are taught to look toward symptoms and diagnoses to guide treatment. In an era of increasing importance placed on evidence-based practice, such an approach allows practitioners to match a client's presentation with empirically supported treatments that literature tells us have the best chances of offering improvement. There is nothing inherently "wrong" with this approach; it is indeed the therapist's responsibility to provide care to a client using interventions grounded in scientific evidence. While not inherently "wrong," it is nonetheless an approach of omission. It omits an orientation toward prevention.

Post-pandemic times have revealed both an increase in demand for psychotherapeutic intervention and a shortage of available mental health professionals. Given substantial waiting lists and populations that remain chronically underserved, prevention allows practitioners the opportunity to intervene before the wait-list of need exceeds who the clinician can serve and before burnout impedes their work. The guidelines, recommendations, and interventions detailed in this book provide the practitioner with specific, culturally informed strategies for prevention-oriented practice. As trainees, mental health providers are presented with intensive theoretical knowledge intended to be implemented in field placements and entry-level positions. Novice practitioners develop applied skills under the supervision of more experienced professionals guiding their interventions. The normative process is to be handed a new client, conceptualize the case for presentation to the treatment team, and develop a treatment plan in response to "chief complaints" and "presenting problems." It is thus my (Mary's) fortune as an early career practitioner to be emerging in a time in which prevention is of increasing focus. I will provide anecdotes from my clinical practice in support of just how relevant preventive efforts are to the current field of health service psychology.

After several years providing care for individuals with eating disorders, the utility of prevention is evident. I have seen devastating consequences from these illnesses, ranging from severe medical complications to impaired mental health to families torn apart in the wake of a loved one's struggle to be nourished. The tragic state of eating disorder life, one cultivated in trauma and adversity, family and relational conflict, genetic vulnerability, and sociocultural pressures, is one pouring out a need for prevention. The National Eating Disorders Association (NEDA) recognizes the need for eating disorder prevention programs while describing modest benefits of existing programs (NEDA, n.d.). Many existing prevention efforts target sociocultural pressures (Ciao et al., 2014), including the Body Project (Stice et al., 2012). A widely implemented dissonance-based prevention initiative for adolescents and college students, the Body Project has been found to be moderately to highly effective in preventing eating disorder development among participants (Becker & Stice, 2017; Stice et al., 2012, 2017). Positive outcomes have also been observed when the Body Project has been implemented among diverse racial and ethnic groups (Stice et al., 2021).

Crucial research efforts, both recently completed and currently in progress, have targeted genetic vulnerability to better understand the biological susceptibility to eating disorders (e.g., ANGI study [Watson et al., 2019]; EDGI study [Bulik et al., 2021]). Within the growing field of eating disorder research, food insecurity is a risk factor of increasing awareness. Individuals who experience inconsistent access to nutritional intake are at elevated risk of developing eating disorder symptoms (Christensen et al., 2021; Hazzard et al., 2020). While the literature continues to unfold more evidence that food insecurity is a risk factor for eating pathology, an absence of prevention initiatives exists that are targeted directly at the relationship between food insecurity and eating disorders. The emerging literature on factors contributing to eating disorder development contains exciting implications for prevention; with enhanced understanding regarding disordered eating etiology, we can generate better-informed preventive efforts targeting vulnerable populations. Such efforts must involve community participation, address both eating disorder symptom severity *and* the very onset of these disorders, and receive more research attention to better understand their efficacy (Stice et al., 2013).

In addition to appreciating the role of prevention in eating disorder care, I am also reminded of the journeys of clients with whom I have worked in medical settings, pawns in the game of health-care chess; they are shuffled from one provider to the next in times of crisis. Consider the cardiac patient recovering from a myocardial infarction, pumped with new medications, adjusting to lifestyle and dietary changes, and living in the aftermath of a near-death experience. Consider the motor vehicle accident survivor who obtained a traumatic brain injury, plagued now with memory and concentration problems, left scrambling to recreate life as they navigate their injuries. They may receive state-of-the-art medical care, yet they remain left in a period of adjustment to new health-care regimens, new physiological processes, and new identities and health statuses.

I am optimistic upon consideration of emerging prevention trends in the field of health psychology. Going back to the example of the cardiac patient, it is imperative to consider the association between cardiovascular disease and mental health problems (Centers for Disease Control and Prevention, 2020; Chaddha et al., 2016; De Hert et al., 2018). While many bidirectional factors may be at play in the relationship between heart disease and mental health problems, the need for prevention is apparent. Cardiac rehabilitation programs offer a secondary prevention intervention for cardiovascular patients that includes psychological intervention as a component tantamount to other components such as regulating blood pressure, optimizing physical activity, and enhancing nutrition (Winnige et al., 2021). Research even suggests that cardiac rehabilitation participation is more common among people who experience mental health problems such as depression and posttraumatic stress disorder (Krishnamurthi et al., 2019). It is encouraging to see positive outcomes across health domains reported in studies on such cardiac rehabilitation programs (e.g., Listerman et al., 2011; Martin et al., 2012; Pintor Reverte et al., 2021; Taylor et al., 2022).

Ultimately, in this book, practitioners across settings are provided with a multitude of empirically supported, culturally informed, practical techniques for meaningful prevention. As a clinician, it is exciting and refreshing to see detailed discussion on prevention for individuals with psychosis in this book. Sadly, I have observed fatalistic, complacent, symptom-focused attitudes toward this population; I know I am far from unique with this observation. It is refreshing to read positive outcomes from a program designed to prevent increased problems in individuals with first-episode psychosis. The practitioner is offered prevention recommendations tailored for unique developmental, clinical, and other demographic populations. From individual therapy to system-oriented change, this book gives mental health practitioners valuable prevention strategies for applied practice. In Section 1.4, we offer strategies for applied practice to better face the mental health crisis we find ourselves in at that time.

## 1.4 The Mental Health Crisis in the United States

A recent snapshot of the state of mental health in the United States (Reinert et al., 2021) details an alarming array of statistics. In 2022 (pre-COVID), approximately 50 million or one in five adults had a mental illness. A 2023 report by Mental Health American (MHA) indicated that the prevalence of adults with mental illness ranged from 17.49% in Florida to 29.68% in Utah. More than half of adults with a mental illness (i.e., 27 million people) did not receive any treatment (Mental Health America, 2023). Further, over 60% of youth with major depression did not receive any treatment, and more than 11% of Americans with mental illness were uninsured (Reinert et al., 2021). These numbers point to the overwhelming inadequacy of our public mental health system as well as the critical need for mental health professionals to engage in prevention.

In comparison with other public health systems around the world, the United States ranks at the bottom in terms of universal health-care coverage, lagging far behind similarly wealthy nations that censure equitable access to medical services, reduce administrative inefficiencies, and invest in social programs. Limited access to health care and increases in poverty amid the COVID-19 pandemic have also exacerbated the problem, especially for marginalized groups, such as communities of color, people who identify as sexual and gender minorities, and people who are low income (Schneider et al., 2021).

Moreover, since 2020, the COVID-19 pandemic has presented a growing and unremitting threat to people's lives, their physical welfare, and their psychological and social well-being (Galea et al., 2020). Furthermore, killing of Black Americans, such as George Floyd and Tyre Nichols, and the Black Lives Matter movement have illuminated the persistent and tenacious health, social, and economic disparities that undermine the lives of entire communities and, in particular, marginalized communities in the United States. Finally, the advent of climate change and extreme weather events are causing extreme hardship in this country and throughout the world. In the context of these stress-inducing events, mental health has plummeted, with one in three Americans (32%) and nearly half of millennials (48%) indicating that they are sometimes so stressed that they struggle to make even basic decisions, such as what to wear and what to eat (APA, 2021).

Those of us working as health-care professionals discover, time and time again, when working with clients and communities that the mental health issues presented to us as individual "problems" began long before we ever see the client. The seeds of psychopathology and mental distress are often planted in the systemic challenges that people face – poverty, racism, sexism, homophobia, interpersonal abuse or family violence, discrimination, and lack of community or connectedness. A subtle but deep awareness of underlying reasons for mental health concerns truly is in our "bones," and it is our hope that the wisdom and practical training related to how to engage in prevention practice and research found in this book will fuel a passion in mental health professionals to create lasting mental health in our clients and communities. This introductory chapter will lay the groundwork for the chapters that follow. In this chapter, we provide a definition of prevention, a rationale for expanding prevention activities in mental health service and training, and an overview of the model prevention programs that will be presented in this book.

## 1.5 What Is Prevention?

The definition of prevention employed in this book is a broad-based framework to guide prevention activities, and it is taken from a seminal article I [Sally] co-authored more than 20 years ago (Romano & Hage, 2000). Prevention includes one or more of the following elements. First, it is targeted at stopping (preventing) a problem behavior from ever occurring, which historically has been called primary or universal prevention (Caplan, 1964; Gordon, 1983). Examples of primary prevention include a school-based bullying prevention or social and emotional learning program that is routinely presented to all students in a school. A second type of prevention, often called secondary or selective prevention (Caplan, 1964; Gordon, 1983), is aimed at early identification of symptoms of a mental health problem or disorder, so as to delay the onset or duration of a problem behavior. Examples of secondary prevention include screening days for depression on a college campus so as to prevent severe depression or suicidal risk or a dating violence prevention program for youth with a history of violence in their family.

A third type of prevention is called tertiary or indicated prevention (Caplan, 1964; Gordon, 1983) and is focused on reducing the impact of an existing mental health problem or behavior. An example of indicated or tertiary prevention includes a harm-reduction prevention program for college students who drink alcohol heavily or use drugs and have experienced or who are at risk for alcohol or substance-use-related problems. In sum, these first three types of prevention – primary, secondary, and tertiary – often apply to individual, group, or community interventions with individual clients. Working with individuals is the cornerstone of what mental health professionals, quite literally, the bread and butter of what we do. However, if we are *truly* going to make a difference in changing the widespread mental health problems in the United States, namely, the fact that at least 21% or 50 million adults and more than 15% of youth struggle with a mental illness (Reinert et al., 2021), then we need to broaden the focus of our professional efforts to add community-based, institutional, and policy-based health-promoting preventative interventions, which describe the final two types of prevention.

The next two types of prevention include environmental or systemic intervention that aims to create social and health equity. The goal of the first of these systemic interventions is to strengthen knowledge, attitudes, and behaviors that promote emotional, psychological, and physical well-being (Hage et al., 2007; Romano & Hage, 2000). Activities include those focused on health promotion, building strengths, and attending to wellness and resources in communities in which we work. One example of this type of prevention is the Fun for Wellness (FFW) Program, which is a global, online behavioral intervention that encourages growth in well-being by providing capability-enhancing learning opportunities to the participants. The FFW program utilizes self-efficacy theory to promote physical activity, and evaluations of FFW demonstrate that participation in the program produces significantly higher subjective well-being scores, as compared to a wait-list control group (Myers et al., 2019).

The final type of prevention is aimed at systemic policy change that promotes institutional, community, and government policies that further physical, social, psychological, and emotional well-being (Hage et al., 2007). One example of a governmental policy that promotes emotional and physical well-being and equity is New York State Education Law on bullying prevention (*The Dignity for All Students Act*, 2010). The goal of this act is to ensure a safe and supportive environment free from discrimination, intimidation, taunting, harassment, and bullying on school property, a school bus, and/or at a school event. In addition, this bullying prevention act also requires prevention education aimed at positively impacting school culture and climate, in order to reduce harassment and discriminatory behaviors. Further, a level of accountability exists as the act also requires school administrators to collect and report data regarding incidents of discrimination and harassment.

## 1.6 The Critical Need for Training in Prevention

The failure to incorporate prevention practice and research in the training of mental health professionals has been widely documented (Albee, 2000; Lichtenberg et al., 2018; Romano & Hage, 2000). For example, Matthews

(2003) surveyed training directors from APA-accredited counseling psychology programs and found that close to 75% of counseling psychology programs did not offer any prevention-specific courses. This void in prevention courses was in spite of the fact that 80 of respondents reported viewing prevention as important to the field of psychology, and 70% reported believing that prevention should receive increased attention in training. In a more recent national study, Lichtenberg et al. (2018) surveyed 799 psychologists about their professional activities, and the authors compared the results to an earlier survey completed in 2000. They found that the mean percentage of time mental health professionals devoted to prevention had actually declined over time, from spending about 10.5% to 9.2% of their time on prevention activities. This means that mental health professionals likely spend about 90% of their time in direct service, coined remedial work or research. In this same survey, prevention was identified as eighth in importance in terms of core values of these practitioners (only career and research were less valued). Further, mid- and late-career professionals placed higher value on preventative interventions that did early career professionals. A commitment to prevention work seems to be falling, despite the current mental health crisis, which follows the "unfathomable" stress of COVID-19 (APA, 2021; Office of the Surgeon General [OSG], 2021).

While the previous findings suggest a decline in prevention, they stand in stark contrast to recent advances in psychology-related policy initiatives on prevention. For example, APA endorsed a set of practice guidelines on prevention (APA, 2014), and Division 17 of APA started a new journal on prevention, namely, the *Journal of Prevention and Health Promotion* (Sage Publications). The *APA monitor* also recently released their top eleven trends of 2023, with four of these trends specifically targeted at prevention activities, including suicide prevention (Clay, 2023), social connectedness in schools to address "record high levels of anxiety and depression" (Abrams, 2023, p. 63), a focus on worker well-being (Stringer, 2023), and a call to "rebrand the field" of psychology to "take a more preventive approach" (Weir, 2023, p. 88). This inconsistency – between actual prevention happenings and a growing awareness of the critical need for prevention – points to the imperative of implementing training to prepare mental health professionals to do prevention work.

## 1.7 Why Current Approaches to Training Are Limited

One of the most significant arguments for a prevention focus is that it would address existing disparities in mental health care, which have been exacerbated by the recent mental health epidemic. Traditional psychological treatments are not only in short supply, but they are limited by their tendency to be reactionary and overly focused on symptoms, while ignoring systems such as oppression and institutional barriers. Racial/ethnic, gender, and sexual minorities often suffer from poorer mental health outcomes due to several factors, most notably, inaccessibility of high-quality mental health-care services, stigma surrounding mental health care, discrimination, and lack of awareness about mental health.

For example, American Indians and Alaska Natives males, aged 18–24, experienced the highest suicide rate in the United States during the pandemic. The higher rates have been associated with COVID-19, including negative social (e.g., community gatherings postponed), cultural (e.g., inability to gather for ceremonies), and economic (e.g., loss of tribal revenue to fund local services) consequences. Additional cited factors include lack of clinician cultural responsiveness, stigma, under resourced mental health care, and structural barriers to accessing services, which are related to mental health inequities (Bridget et al., 2023).

## 1.8 Why Mental Health Professionals Are Uniquely Poised to Include Prevention in Our Work

Despite a dearth of training opportunities in prevention, mental health professionals may be in the very best position to engage in prevention work. One major reason for this assertion is that accreditation requirements for mental health professions include knowledge and skill competency domains important in preparing mental health professionals to engage in prevention work (Conyne, 1997; Hage et al., 2007; O'Neil & Britner, 2009). These domains include: (a) understanding distinctions between preventive and remedial approaches; (b) designing and implementing educational programs; (c) assessing community needs; (d) understanding systemic approaches that incorporate cultural and contextual factors into preventive interventions; (e) collaborating with interdisciplinary teams that include professionals and community leaders; (f) promoting positive development across the lifespan; (g) empowering individuals and communities to work on their own behalf; (h) developing strength-based approaches that reduce risk and enhance resilience in individuals and communities; (i) influencing policy decisions and their impact on prevention efforts; and (j) evaluating prevention interventions. In sum, mental health professionals may be in the very best position, due to their training and credibility with community leaders, to engage in preventative work in their communities.

Similarly, a CDC report released in February 2023 indicates that nearly 3 in 5 (57%) teen girls in the United States in 2021 felt persistently sad or hopeless, and nearly 1 in 3 (30%) seriously considered attempting suicide – both statistics were double that of boys, representing a nearly 60% increase and the highest level reported over the past decade. Similarly, Hispanic and

Latina girls in grades 9–12 report almost twice as many suicide attempts as their non-Latinx White peers; yet both these groups have less access, quality, and overall mental health care (Center for Disease Control and Prevention, 2022; Schnitzer et al., 2023). It is clear that racial/ethnic health inequities exist and are tied to several factors, such as supply and demand related to mental health treatment services, stigma, and discrimination, as well as institutional barriers related to lack of access, systemic inequities, and deficits in cultural responsiveness among providers. These factors can only be addressed by reducing incident rates and instituting policy changes through prevention and health promotion interventions, including structural changes to expand access to health care and wellness-related practices.

In addition, while a dearth of prevention training exists in mental health training programs, a new focus on addressing social and contextual factors in mental health has emerged. Many of the prevention approaches described in this book may be conceptualized as largely synonymous with social justice (Coard et al., this volume; Liang et al., this volume; Tucker et al., this volume; Vera et al., this volume). These interventions align with emerging trends in critical and liberation psychology that calls upon mental health professionals to address environmental factors (not just individual or person-focused dimension) (Hage & Kenny, 2009; Kenny & Hage, 2009), "name oppressive structures and systems within our society," and "to communicate their commitment to countering injustices and how they wish to work alongside their client(s)" (Singh, 2020, p. 219).

Further, prevention efforts with marginalized communities are a positive step both in addressing health inequities while reducing the overall cost of health care (Maciosek et al., 2010; Tolan & Dodge, 2005). For example, the Washington State Institute for Public Policy's analysis of an elementary-school-based preventative intervention called the Good Behavior Game saved taxpayers $25.92 for each dollar invested. Similarly, an analysis of the Communities That Care prevention system, which helps communities utilize their resources most effectively to address identified risk factors for substance use, aggression, and other problems in youth, showed that an approximately $602 investment in each child yielded an estimated $7754 in savings by the time participants were aged 23 – a $12.88 return for each dollar invested (Volkow, 2022). In other cases, prevention programs may be deemed cost effective, meaning that they may not save money but rather they improve health at a price that is considered good value for the funds that are spent (Baid et al., 2021).

The positive impact of prevention interventions on increasing healthy functioning and decreasing psychological distress has been demonstrated across several studies (Catalano et al., 2002; Durlak et al., 2007; Evidence-Based Practices Resource Center, 2023; Greenberg et al., 2001; O'Connell et al., 2009). The integral components of successful prevention interventions include social and cultural relevance, a strong theoretical base, comprehensiveness (multicomponent interventions that address multiple ecological levels, such as individual, family, school, community, and of sufficient dosage), developmental appropriateness, and a focus on person- and environment-centered change (Nation et al., 2003; Walsh et al., 2009). Effective programs also have well-trained staff and support positive relationships with adults and peers (Durlak, 2003, Nation et al., 2003; Rotheram-Borus & Duan, 2003).

## 1.9 Theoretical Framework for This Book

This *Ounce of Prevention* book does not promote one particular theory, discipline, or research methodology. That said, this book includes an intentional integration of multicultural and social justice content throughout, recognizing the importance of addressing the social and cultural context and systems when engaging in prevention work (Hage et al., 2020). The prevention and health promotion programs highlighted in this book are evidenced-based and mirror recent developments in the field of prevention and health promotion related to optimizing the efficacy of preventative programming.

These developments include the critical importance of focusing on societal change (i.e., going beyond individual change), as long-term success requires also engaging in social and policy change efforts in systems and institutions (Banyard & Hamby, 2022; Prilleltensky, 2008). In addition, the highlighted programs are theory-based (Nation et al., 2003), and they address the importance of ongoing evaluation to improve outcomes (Maxwell et al., 2015), along with tailoring prevention interventions to be culturally responsive to the specific communities in which they are implemented (Jones & Neblett, 2016; Reese & Vera, 2007). This cultural responsiveness means direct collaboration with a target community in designing, implementing, and evaluating the program (Anyon et al., 2018; Gittelsohn et al., 2020). Further, the innovative prevention programs in this book reflect an approach that is strength-based (not just admonishment programs or those that focus on negative behaviors) and aim to measure concrete changes in behavior and/or behavioral intention, not just changes in knowledge or attitudes (Banyard & Hamby, 2022). Finally, the book has an explicit emphasis on tailoring prevention to developmental level of the target community in which it is implemented, and illustrations of model programs are presented across the lifespan.

A feature of this book is the strong integration of the practice and science of prevention, utilizing a multidisciplinary perspective, appealing to students, educators, practitioners, researchers, and policymakers from a diverse number of specialty areas in the mental health fields. The book is comprehensive, and topics address psychological practices and model interventions across the lifespan and include detailed discussion of program development and implementation, which is not typically taught in counseling and psychotherapy theory courses and other applied areas. Students and practicing psychologists often have interest in prevention, and they may be asked to engage in prevention activities during their career. However, until recently psychologists and counselors generally received little, if any, training during their academic programs in how to plan and implement prevention programming. The book fills a gap in providing training and exemplary prevention interventions and effective research strategies, aimed at addressing emerging trends in psychology, which include a focus on systems and social justice. Finally, the book reflects the application of the aspirational principles and guidelines APA's Professional Practice *Guidelines for Prevention in Psychology* (APA, 2014).

## 1.10 Organization of This Book

Each chapter illustrates the design and evaluation of an evidence-based program focused on a particular period in the lifespan. These developmental periods are broken up into (a) prevention with children and youth,(b) prevention with emerging adults, and (d) prevention with adults, including older adults, and families. The overall goal of each chapter is to provide readers with illustrations of model prevention programs, concrete tools, resources, and strategies to design and evaluate culturally specific prevention programs in their own communities.

The first section of the book lays for the foundational knowledge and skills for the remainder of the book. In the first chapter, a definition of prevention is presented along with a compelling rationale for the need for an expanded focus on prevention training, practice, and research. In addition, a theoretical framework for the book is presented along with an in-depth focus on clinical training and how mental health professionals are uniquely poised to engage in prevention work.

The second section of the book presents four evidenced-based, model prevention programs that address racial health disparities, discrimination, and the structural inequalities with children and youth. These interventions include the Black Parenting Strengths and Strategies (BPSS; Coard [this book]) program that promotes positive and culturally relevant parenting practices for fostering cultural, social, and behavioral competence in African American children. A second intervention, City Connects, has a 20-year track record of providing an evidence-based intervention that helps teachers and schools provide integrated supports to address the unique needs of students in schools serving underresourced neighborhoods and families. In their chapter, Walsh et al. detail how City Connects utilizes a public health/clinical model to intervene at individual, group, and school levels to ensure that each student is provided with a support plan tailored to their unique needs and strengths. The third chapter in this section provides impactful illustrations of school-based systems-centered interventions that focus on improving school climate and educational resources, particularly for BIPOC, immigrant, and refugee children and families. These interventions adopt Mahoney et al.'s (2021) systemic social-emotional learning framework and uniquely draw on the strengths of students' family systems and the broader community to promote well-being in BIPOC youth. The final chapter in this section presents a race-centered, trauma-responsive, transformative school approach that is responsive to family- and community-based trauma. This framework provides tools to reduce negative outcomes of child of the global majority (i.e., Black, Indigenous, Asian, Latinx, the Global South) and to interrupt the current prevailing school-to-prison pipeline (Liang et al., this volume).

The third section of the book centers on emerging adults, defined as people in the developmental period from the late teens through the 20s, with a particular focus on ages 18–25 years (Arnett, 2000). Arnett's research suggests that emerging adulthood is a distinct period demographically, subjectively, and finally, in terms of identity explorations. The first paper in this section, by Vaughan and colleagues, presents several examples of evidence-based prevention interventions to address problematic substance use and substance use disorders among emerging adults. The authors utilize an ecodevelopmental and multicultural framework to target risk and protective factors of substance use, with a focus on Latinx emerging adults. The next chapter is written by the founder of the Bandana Project (www.thebandanaproj.org), Conlin Bass, a nation-wide campaign to raise awareness of the importance of mental health and to reduce the risk of suicide by engaging supportive peers in facilitating the help-seeking behavior of those at risk. Bass (this volume), who was an undergraduate when he developed the Bandana Project, went on to earn a public health degree from Yale and aptly describes the context for this movement and how to start your own chapter. The third chapter details key strategies and evidence in developing an effective and comprehensive campus-based sexual violence prevention program (Cook-Craig, this volume). Cook-Craig adopts a public health model to effectually describe how to choose a prevention strategy and how to implement and evaluate a campus-based program.

The final chapter in this section details the development of an experiential learning curriculum, Changing Minds, Changing Lives, that aims at buffering stress, boosting adaptive resilience by fostering connections, and promoting healthy growth in college students, particularly in college athletes and first generation and BIPOC students and students from underresourced public schools. Outcomes of the program include social–emotional skill development and personal growth and transformation. The final section of the book aims at model prevention evidenced-based interventions with adults and families. The first of these programs, the Kid's Club and Mom's Empowerment Program that has been adopted both nationally and internationally, targets mothers and their children who have been exposed to intimate partner violence. The ten-week programs (one for children and one for moms) foster resilience, parenting emotional regulation, safety planning, stress management, and problem-solving skills (Graham, this volume). The next chapter describes two variations of an evidence-informed, culturally sensitive health promotion program for Black adults, the Health-Smart Holistic Health Program (for seniors) and the Health-Smart for Weight Loss (for Black women). What makes these grant-funded interventions especially noteworthy is that they were developed using a community-based participatory action research approach that works in partnership with community members/leaders who were involved in all aspects of the planning, implementation, and evaluation of the interventions.

The next chapter details a unique, innovative Psychosis Identification and Early Referral (PIER) program (McFarlane et al., this volume). This nationwide evidence-based, family- and community-aided program targets early intervention with youth at risk of psychosis, significantly minimizing the impact of mental illness (e.g., schizophrenia) in adolescents and young adults so they can live healthy, rewarding, and productive lives. The program incorporates best practices in adapting the program to fit a client's cultural background and urging cultural humility and competence of facilitators. The final chapter in this section focuses on older adults and in particular, aims at reducing the negative impact of the transition to retirement. In this chapter, Conyne (this volume) presents a five-phase Charting Your Personal Future intervention that draws on a person-centered enhancement approach, aimed at promoting well-being and resilience and aimed at buffering the losses and negative impact of the transition. The final chapter in the book synthesizes the lessons learned across the chapters and charts a course for future directions in the field of prevention and health promotion. We offer a blueprint for training, interdisciplinary community collaborations, evaluation and dissemination of evidence, and future practice. Each chapter also includes a detailed list of resources for readers who wish to delve further into the topic of the chapter. These resources provide further reading and sources of knowledge, skills, and strategies for the reader who is ready to further their learning beyond this book.

## 1.11 Conclusion

In our work as counselors, mental health professionals, psychologists, educators, and researchers, we often feel powerless to prevent human suffering, and yet, we may yearn, deep in our hearts, for a way to intervene earlier so as to prevent or reduce the pain and distress in our communities, intuitively aware that a way to make our clients' lives easier and our work more impactful exists. This book is about giving mental health professionals the knowledge, resources, and tools to engage in "before the fact" intervention, to apply an ounce of prevention to the work we do, knowing that, ultimately, it will be worth a "pound of cure," while also better aligning our deepest hearts with our work and significantly expanding the depth and breadth of our impact. The model programs in this book illustrate strength-based, culturally informed efforts to work with families and communities instead of around public health problems. This approach, as noted in the quote by Lila Watson at the beginning of this chapter, is by necessity collaborative and ties the liberation of an individual with that of the entire community.

## References


Abrams, Z. (2023, January). Kids' mental health is in crisis. Here's what psychologists are doing to help. *APA Monitor*, *54*(1), 63. www.apa.org/monitor/2023/01/trends-improving-youth-mental-health

Albee, G. W. (2000). Commentary on prevention and counseling psychology. *The Counseling Psychologist*, 28(6), 845–853. doi.org/10.1177/0011000000286006

American Psychological Association. (2014). Guidelines for prevention in psychology. *American Psychologist*, *69*(3), 285–296. doi.org/10.1037/a0034569

American Psychological Association. (2021). *Stress in America: Stress and decision-making during the pandemic*. www.apa.org/news/press/releases/stress/2021/decision-making-october-2021.pdf

American Psychological Association. (2022). *Psychologists struggle to meet demand amid mental health crisis*. www.apa.org/pubs/reports/practitioner/2022-covid-psychologist-workload.

Anyon, Y., Bender, K., Kennedy, H., & Dechants, J. (2018). A systematic review of youth participatory action research (YPAR) in the United States: Methodologies, youth outcomes, and future directions. *Health Education & Behavior*, *45*(6), 865–878.

Arnett, J. J. (2000). Emerging adulthood: A theory of development from the late teens through the twenties. *American Psychologist*, *55*(5), 469–480.

Baid, D., Hayles, E., & Finkelstein, E.A. (2021). Return on investment of workplace wellness programs for chronic disease prevention: A systematic review. *American Journal of Preventive Medicine*. *61*(2), 256–266. doi.org/10.1016/j.amepre.2021.02.002

Banyard, V. L., & Hamby, S. L. (2022). *Strengths-based prevention: Reducing violence and other public health problems*. American Psychological Association.

Becker, C. B., & Stice, E. (2017). From efficacy to effectiveness to broad implementation: Evolution of the body project. *Journal of Consulting and Clinical Psychology*, *85*(8), 767–782. doi.org/10.1037/ccp0000204

Bridge, J. A., Ruch, D. A., Sheftall, A. H., Hahm, H. C., O'Keefe, V. M., Fontanella, C. A., Brock, G., Campo, J. V., & Horowitz, L. M. (2023). Youth suicide during the first year of the COVID-19 pandemic. *Pediatrics*, e2022058375. Advance online publication. doi.org/10.1542/peds.2022-058375

Bulik, C. M., Thornton, L. M., Parker, R., Kennedy, H., Baker, J. H., MacDermod, C., Guintivano, J., Cleland, L., Miller, A. L., Harper, L., Larsen, J. T., Yilmaz, Z., Grove, J., Sullivan, P. F., Petersen, L. V., Jordan, J., Kennedy, M. A., & Martin, N. G. (2021). The Eating Disorders Genetics Initiative (EDGI): Study protocol. *BMC Psychiatry*, *21*(1), 234. doi.org/10.1186/s12888-021-03212-3

Caplan G. (1964). *Principles of preventive psychiatry*. Basic Books.

Catalano, R. F., Berglund, M. L., Ryan, J. A. M., Lonczak, H. S., & Hawkins, J. D. (2002). Positive youth development in the United States: Research findings on evaluations of positive youth development programs. *Prevention & Treatment*, *5*(1), Article 15. doi.org/10.1037/1522-3736.5.1.515a

Centers for Disease Control. (2022). *Suicide prevention resource for action*. US Department of Health and Human Services. www.cdc.gov/suicide/resources/prevention.html

Centers for Disease Control and Prevention. (2020). Heart disease and mental health disorders. www.cdc.gov/heartdisease/mentalhealth.htm

Chaddha, A., Robinson, E. A., Kline-Rogers, E., Alexandris-Souphis, T., & Rubenfire, M. (2016). Mental health and cardiovascular disease. *The American Journal of Medicine*, *129*(11), 1145–1148. doi.org/10.1016/j.amjmed.2016.05.018

Christensen, K. A., Forbush, K. T., Richson, B. N., Thomeczek, M. L., Perko, V. L., Bjorlie, K., Christian, K., Ayres, J., Wildes, J. E., & Mildrum Chana, S. (2021). Food insecurity associated with elevated eating disorder symptoms, impairment, and eating disorder diagnoses in an American University student sample before and during the beginning of the COVID-19 pandemic. *The International Journal of Eating Disorders*, *54*(7), 1213–1223. doi.org/10.1002/eat.23517

Ciao, A. C., Loth, K., & Neumark-Sztainer, D. (2014). Preventing eating disorder pathology: Common and unique features of successful eating disorders prevention programs. *Current Psychiatry Reports*, *16*(7), 453. doi.org/10.1007/s11920-014-0453-0

Clay, R. (2023, January). Suicide prevention gets a new lifeline. *APA Monitor*, *54*(1), 73. www.apa.org/monitor/2023/01/trends-suicide-prevention-lifeline

Conyne, R. (1997). Educating students in preventive counseling. *Counselor Education and Supervision*, *36*, 259–269.

De Hert, M., Detraux, J., & Vancampfort, D. (2018). The intriguing relationship between coronary heart disease and mental disorders. *Dialogues in Clinical Neuroscience*, *20*(1), 31–40. doi.org/10.31887/DCNS.2018.20.1/mdehert

Durlak, J.A. (2003). Effective prevention and health promotion programming. In T. Gullotta (Ed.), *Encyclopedia of primary prevention and health promotion* (pp. 61–69). Springer. doi.org/10.1007/978-1-4615-0195-4_6

Durlak, J. A., Taylor, R. D., Kawashima, K., Pachan, M. K., DuPre, E. P., Celio, C. I., Berger, S. R., Dymnicki, A. B., & Weissberg, R. P. (2007). Effects of positive youth development programs on school, family, and community systems. *American Journal of Community Psychology*, *39*(3–4), 269–286. doi.org/10.1007/s10464-007-9112-5

Evidence-Based Practices Resource Center. (n.d.). www.samhsa.gov/resource-search/ebp

Galea, S., Merchant, R. M., & Lurie, N. (2020). The mental health consequences of COVID-19 and physical distancing – The need for prevention and early intervention. *JAMA Internal Medicine*, *180*(6), 817–818.

Gittelsohn, J., Belcourt, A., Magarati, M., Booth-LaForce, C., Duran, B., Mishra, S. I., Belone, L., & Jernigan, V. B. B. (2020). Building capacity for productive indigenous community-university partnerships. *Prevention Science*, *21*(1), 22–32.

Gordon, R. S. Jr. (1983). An operational classification of disease prevention. *Public Health Reports*, *98*(2), 107–109.

Greenberg, M. T., Domitrovich, C., & Bumbarger, B. (2001). The prevention of mental disorders in school-aged children: Current state of the field. *Prevention & Treatment*, *4*(1), Article 1a. doi.org/10.1037/1522-3736.4.1.41a

Hage, S. M., & Kenny, M. E. (2009). Promoting a social justice approach to prevention: future directions for training, practice, and research. *The Journal of Primary Prevention*, *30*(1), 75–87. doi.org/10.1007/s10935-008-0165-5

Hage, S. M., Miles, J. R., Lewis, J. A., Grzanka, P. R., & Goodman, L. A. (2020). The social justice practicum in counseling psychology training. *Training and Education in Professional Psychology*, *14*(2), 156–166. doi.org/10.1037/tep0000299

Hage, S. M., Romano, J. L., Conyne, R. K., Kenny, M., Matthews, C., Schwartz, J. P., & Waldo, M. (2007). Best practice guidelines on prevention practice, research, training, and social advocacy for psychologists. *The Counseling Psychologist*, *35*(4), 493–566. doi.org/10.1177/0011000006291411

Hazzard, V. M., Loth, K. A., Hooper, L., & Becker, C. B. (2020). Food insecurity and eating disorders: A review of emerging evidence. *Current Psychiatry Reports*, *22*(12), 74. doi.org/10.1007/s11920-020-01200-0

Jones, S. C. T., & Neblett, E. W. (2016). Racial–ethnic protective factors and mechanisms in psychosocial prevention and intervention programs for black youth. *Clinical Child and Family Psychology Review*, *19*(2), 134–161. doi.org/10.1007/s10567-016-0201-6

Kenny, M. E., & Hage, S. M. (2009). The next frontier: Prevention as an instrument of social justice. *Journal of Primary Prevention*, *30*, 1–10.

Krishnamurthi, N., Schopfer, D. W., Shen, H., & Whooley, M. A. (2019). Association of mental health conditions with participation in cardiac rehabilitation. *Journal of the American Heart Association*, *8*(11), e011639. doi.org/10.1161/JAHA.118.011639

Lichtenberg, J. W., Hutman, H., & Goodyear, R. K. (2018). Portrait of counseling psychology: Demographics, roles, activities, and values across three decades. *The Counseling Psychologist*, *46*(1), 50–76. doi.org/10.1177/0011000018754532

Listerman, J., Bittner, V., Sanderson, B. K., & Brown, T. M. (2011). Cardiac rehabilitation outcomes: Impact of comorbidities and age. *Journal of Cardiopulmonary Rehabilitation and Prevention*, *31*(6), 342–348. doi.org/10.1097/HCR.0b013e31822f189c

Maciosek, M. V., Coffield, A. B., Flottemesch, T. J., Edwards, N. M., & Solberg, L. I. (2010). Greater use of preventive services in U.S. health care could save lives at little or no cost. *Health Affairs (Project Hope)*, *29*(9), 1656–1660. doi.org/10.1377/hlthaff.2008.070

Mahoney, J. L., Weissberg, R. P., Greenberg, M. T., Dusenbury, L., Jagers, R. J., Niemi, K., Schlinger, M., Schlund, J., Shriver, T. P., VanAusdal, K., & Yoder, N. (2021). Systemic social and emotional learning: Promoting educational success for all preschool to high school students. *The American Psychologist*, *76*(7), 1128–1142. doi.org/10.1037/amp0000701

Martin, B. J., Hauer, T., Arena, R., Austford, L. D., Galbraith, P. D., Lewin, A. M., Knudtson, M. L., Ghali, W. A., Stone, J. A., & Aggarwal, S. G. (2012). Cardiac rehabilitation attendance and outcomes in coronary artery disease patients. *Circulation*, *126*(6), 677–687. doi.org/10.1161/CIRCULATIONAHA.111.066738

Maslow, G. R., & Chung, R. J. (2013). Systematic review of positive youth development programs for adolescents with chronic illness. *Pediatrics*, *131*(5), e1605–e1618. doi.org/10.1542/peds.2012-1615

Matthews, C. R. (2003, August). Training for prevention competency in counseling psychology. In M. Kenny (Chair), Competencies for prevention training in counseling psychology. *Symposium presented at the 111th Annual Convention of the American Psychological Association*, Toronto, ON, Canada

Matthews, C. R. (2013). Teaching prevention: Preparing the next generation of psychologists. In E. M. Vera (Ed.), *The Oxford handbook of prevention in counseling psychology* (pp. 76–90). Oxford University Press

Maxwell, S. E., Lau, M. Y., & Howard, G. S. (2015). Is psychology suffering from a replication crisis? What does "failure to replicate" really mean? *American Psychologist*, *70*(6), 487–498. doi.org/10.1037/a0039400

Mental Health America. (n.d.). *Prevalence data 2023*. www.mhanational.org/issues/2023/mental-health-america-prevalence-data#two

Myers, N.D., Prilleltensky, I., Lee, S., Dietz, S., Prilleltensky, O., McMachon, A., Pfeiffer, K. A., Ellithorpe, M. E., & Brincks, A. M. (2019). Effectiveness of the fun for wellness online behavioral intervention to promote well-being and physical activity: Protocol for a randomized controlled trial. *BMC Public Health*, *19*(1), 737

Nation, M., Crusto, C., Wandersman, A., Kumpfer, K., Seybolt, D., & Morrissey-Kane, E., et al. (2003). What works in prevention: Principles and effective prevention programs. *American Psychologist*, *58*(6–7), 449–456. doi.org/10.1037/0003-066X.58.6-7.449

National Eating Disorders Association [NEDA] (n.d.). *Prevention*. www.nationaleatingdisorders.org/learn/general-information/prevention

O'Connell, M. E., Boat, T. & Warner, K. E. (2009). *Preventing mental, emotional, and behavioral disorders among young people: Progress and possibilities*. The National Academies Press.

Office of the Surgeon General (OSG). (2021). *Protecting youth mental health: The U.S. surgeon general's advisory*. U.S. Department of Health and Human Services.

O'Neil, J. M. & Britner, P.A. (2009) Training primary preventionists to make a difference in people's lives. In M. E. Kenny, L. E. Reese, A. Horne, & P. Orpinas (Eds.), *Handbook of prevention: Promoting positive development and social justice* (pp. 141–162). American Psychological Association Books.

Pintor Reverte, R., Chabbar Boudet, M. C., Valls Lázaro, E., Albarrán Martín, C., Untoria Agustín, C., & Garza Benito, F. (2021). Evaluation of the efficacy of a psychological intervention program in a cardiac rehabilitation unit after acute coronary syndrome. *Journal of Healthcare Quality Research*, 36(5), 286–293. doi.org/10.1016/j.jhqr.2021.04.001

Prilleltensky, I. (2008). The role of power in wellness, oppression, and liberation: The promise of psychopolitical validity. *Journal of Community Psychology*, *36*(2), 116–136. doi.org/10.1002/jcop.20225

Reese, L. E., & Vera, E. M. (2007). Culturally relevant prevention: The scientific and practical considerations of community-based programs. *The Counseling Psychologist*, *35*(6), 763–778. doi.org/10.1177%2F0011000007304588

Reinert, M., Fritze, D., & Nguyen, T. (October 2021). The state of mental health in America 2022. *Mental Health America*. http://hdl.handle.net/10713/17070

Romano, J. R., & Hage, S. M. (2000). Prevention and counseling psychology: Revitalizing commitments for the 21st century. *The Counseling Psychologist*, *28*(6), 733–763. dx.doi.org/10.1177/0011000000286001

Rotheram-Borus, M. J., & Duan, N. (2003). Next generation of preventive interventions. *Journal of the American Academy of Child & Adolescent Psychiatry*, *42*(5), 518–526. doi.org/10.1097/01.CHI.0000046836.90931.E9

Schneider, E. C., Shah, A., Doty, M. M., Tikkanen, R., Fields, K., & Williams II, R. D. (2021). *Mirror, mirror 2021: Reflecting poorly. Health care in the U.S. compared to other high-income countries.* www.commonwealthfund.org/publications/fund-reports/2021/aug/mirror-mirror-2021-reflecting-poorly

Schnitzer, P. G., Dykstra, H., & Collier, A. (2023). The COVID-19 pandemic and youth suicide: 2020–2021. *Pediatrics*, e2022058716. Advance online publication. doi.org/10.1542/peds.2022-058716

Singh, A. (2020). Building a counseling psychology of liberation: The path behind us, under us, and before us. *The Counseling Psychologist*, *48*(8), 1109–1130. doi.org/10.1177/0011000020959007

Stice, E., Becker, C. B., & Yokum, S. (2013). Eating disorder prevention: Current evidence-base and future directions. *The International Journal of Eating Disorders*, *46*(5), 478–485. doi.org/10.1002/eat.22105

Stice, E., Onipede, Z. A., Shaw, H., Rohde, P., & Gau, J. M. (2021). Effectiveness of the Body Project eating disorder prevention program for different racial and ethnic groups and an evaluation of the potential benefits of ethnic matching. *Journal of Consulting and Clinical Psychology*, *89*(12), 1007–1019. doi.org/10.1037/ccp0000697

Stice, E., Rohde, P., & Shaw, H. (2012). *The body project: A dissonance-based eating disorder prevention intervention* (2nd ed.). Oxford University Press. doi.org/10.1093/med:psych/9780199859245.001.0001

Stice, E., Rohde, P., Shaw, H., & Gau, J. M. (2017). Clinician-led, peer-led, and internet-delivered dissonance-based eating disorder prevention programs: Acute effectiveness of these delivery modalities. *Journal of Consulting and Clinical Psychology*, *85*(9), 883–895. doi.org/10.1037/ccp0000211

Stringer, H. (2023, January). Worker well-being is in demand as organizational culture shifts. *APA Monitor*, *54*(1), 58. www.apa.org/monitor/2023/01/trends-worker-well-being

Taylor, R. S., Dalal, H. M., & McDonagh, S. T. J. (2022). The role of cardiac rehabilitation in improving cardiovascular outcomes. *Nature Reviews Cardiology*, *19*, 180–194. doi.org/10.1038/s41569-021-00611-7

Tolan, P. H., & Dodge, K. A. (2005). Children's mental health as a primary care and concern: A system for comprehensive support and service. *American Psychologist*, *60*(6), 601–614. doi.org/10.1037/0003-066X.60.6.601

Volkow, N. (2022, April 28). *Investing in prevention makes good financial sense.* National Institute on Drug Abuse. https://nida.nih.gov/about-nida/noras-blog/2022/04/investing-in-prevention-makes-good-financial-sense

Walsh, M. E., DePaul, J., & Park-Taylor, J. (2009). Prevention as a mechanism for promoting positive development in the context of risk: Addressing the risk and protective factors of our cultures. In M. Kenny, L. E. Reese, A. Horne, & P. Opinas (Eds.), *Realizing social justice: The challenge of preventative interventions* (pp. 57–78). American Psychological Association.

Watson, H. J., Yilmaz, Z., Thornton, L. M., Hübel, C., Coleman, J., Gaspar, H. A., Bryois, J., Hinney, A., Leppä, V. M., Mattheisen, M., Medland, S. E., Ripke, S., Yao, S., Giusti-Rodríguez, P., Anorexia Nervosa Genetics Initiative, Hanscombe, K. B., Purves, K. L., Eating Disorders Working Group of the Psychiatric Genomics Consortium, Adan, R., … Bulik, C. M. (2019). Genome-wide association study identifies eight risk loci and implicates metabo-psychiatric origins for anorexia nervosa. *Nature Genetics*, *51*(8), 1207–1214. doi.org/10.1038/s41588-019-0439-2

Weir, K. (2023, January). Psychologists are rebranding the field, expanding the one-to-one therapy approach. *APA Monitor*, *54*(1), 87. www.apa.org/monitor/2023/01/trends-rebranding-psychology

Winnige, P., Vysoky, R., Dosbaba, F., & Batalik, L. (2021). Cardiac rehabilitation and its essential role in the secondary prevention of cardiovascular diseases. *World Journal of Clinical Cases*, *9*(8), 1761–1784.

Zhou, X., Lee, R. M., & Ohm, J. (2021). Evaluating the feasibility of the incredible years attentive parenting program as universal prevention for racially diverse populations. *Journal of Prevention and Health Promotion*, 2(1), 32–56. doi.org/10.1177/2632077020976401

# 2 Best Practices for the Evaluation of Prevention Programs

Lisa De La Rue and Maureen E. Kenny

> Simply put, when we heal individuals, we are healing the world.
>
> —Lillian Comas-Díaz (Comas-Díaz & Rivers, 2020)

Prevention efforts have been shown to enhance the well-being and development of people across the lifespan and in their broader communities. The concept of prevention can be defined as an effort to enhance the personal and collective well-being of people and communities, including programs that seek to create social and political changes that aim to improve the environments in which people live, work, and are generally engaged (Hage et al., 2007; Romano & Hage, 2000). The American Psychological Association's (APA, 2014) aspirational "Guidelines for Prevention in Psychology" encourage psychologists to select and implement prevention programs that are culturally relevant and are theory- and evidenced-based. Fortunately for practitioners selecting programs, there is a rich scholarship demonstrating the effectiveness of prevention programs in mitigating the effects of a broad range of adverse health outcomes and in promoting well-being. This literature includes interventions to reduce substance misuse (Spoth et al., 2022), support mental health (Werner-Seidler et al., 2017), and improve physical health outcomes (Wang, 2021). Nevertheless, an ongoing need exists for prevention scientists to incorporate assessment and evaluation across all stages of planning, implementation, and the application and expansion of programs to new settings. Such research is needed to add to the evidence base for prevention programs, especially as they are developed and applied in new settings.

While many prevention programs have demonstrated significant and clear impacts, many questions remain about the specific mechanisms of change which drive the desired outcomes. Additionally, there are times when programs may not achieve the high level of impact that was expected or desired. In these instances, programs may require adaptations or tweaks in order to fully realize their potential. In some cases, even well-grounded prevention programs will fall short in meeting their aims and will not be able to improve the prognosis or well-being of the targeted community. As such, in order to fully realize the potential of prevention science in reducing the incidence of distress and advancing well-being, it is important to increase the use of a variety of types of program evaluation across early, intermediate, and later phases of intervention and to assess a variety of outcomes.

The key questions being explored in prevention program evaluation are how effective is the program, for whom, and under what circumstances. Depending on program goals, this work may include an evaluation of whether new cases of a disorder have been reduced or eliminated, whether risk factors were reduced, whether the environment was improved, and whether individual strengths or natural supports increased (Conyne, 2013). Program evaluation is a specific methodology in which the researcher will systematically collect information about the program, including all the activities, their implementation, and the outcomes, in order to evaluate the program's effectiveness and efficiency (Davis et al., 2013). This process and its findings can help inform decisions about future programming and modifications that may be helpful in improving program efficiency or effectiveness. Evaluation should be an intentional part of our prevention program work, especially as part of critical efforts to determine program effectiveness.

Although the process of program evaluation is complex and varied, we seek to present some key best practices to guide the culturally responsive evaluation of prevention programs. We discuss the process of evaluation, types of evaluations, considerations in designing evaluations that are culturally responsive and that promote social justice, and concerns for grant funding. We seek to provide some practical examples to illustrate these practices and to offer additional resources that might be helpful in moving forward in program evaluation.

## 2.1 Theory Development and Logic Models

A meaningful evaluation plan starts with clarifying the components of the program, diagraming the theory of change, and then constructing a logic model (Davis et al., 2013). Effective prevention programs need to be anchored in a theory that identifies the leverage points that can move people to change and that creates an environment that makes people more willing, ready, and able to make these changes (Herman et al., 2020). Assessing these leverage points as part of the program evaluation will help in understanding whether and how a program produces the expected changes required to realize its stated goals. For example, if a teen dating violence prevention program is implemented in high schools, a hoped-for outcome may be a corresponding reduction in rates of sexual harassment and coercion. The theoretical model should consider, however, not only the desired outcomes but also possible shortcomings that could limit the chance of realizing these goals. For instance, what is the role of school climate and how might that inhibit or promote dismissive attitudes about harassing or demeaning types of behaviors? The theory of change model should be developed based on prior research and practice and will need to include consultation with relevant stakeholders.

Common sources of information that are used in formulating a theory of change model include gathering input from key stakeholders, review of program documentation, interviews and observations, and previous research and theories related to the prevention topic (Rosas, 2005). Stakeholders are an important source of expertise for the program, as they hold crucial knowledge about the community that is of interest. These stakeholders will also provide insight related to the specific problems the community is trying to manage. A community needs assessment may also be carried out to obtain a broader understanding of what the community views as salient needs, desired outcomes, and the possible barriers that may impede the realization of desired outcomes. Consultation with local stakeholders and community assessments are integral and a necessary part of any efforts to carry out a culturally responsive evaluation. Discussion of program assumptions, desired outcomes, potential obstacles, and possible actions among all stakeholders and the evaluation team will help clarify the theoretical model and possible levers or sources of change.

Concept mapping is a way to facilitate theory development. Many stakeholders and other key program members will have "mental maps" about their programs, and these maps partly determine their behavior (Yampolskaya et al., 2004). The information gathered from these individuals can be used to develop concept mapping or mental models of the theory of change. Concept mapping is useful in explicating program theory and identifying the key elements of a program and then portraying the relationship between these elements (Yampolskaya et al., 2004). This multistep process can help to articulate and to delineate the key components of the model and the interrelationships that are believed to be important for change (Rosas, 2005). Concept mapping has been shown to improve program evaluation because of the systematic process that supports the articulation and visual representation of the key concepts and how they are interrelated (Caracelli & Riggin, 1994).

With the increased expectation of accountability, including from funding agencies, programs are more often required to demonstrate that specific interventions result in the expected outcomes (Yampolskaya et al., 2004). As part of the evaluation process, and especially when expected outcomes are not observed, it is important to reflect on whether the assumptions made about the program being addressed are valid. It can be helpful to ask very specific questions related to whether something is lacking in the theory-of-change or the implementation process and whether this missing piece is the reason the desired outcomes are not being fully realized. For instance, this process may include considering the qualifications of staff or individuals who implemented the program curriculum, how many hours were spent on a specific activity, and so on. Considering a theory with "if-then" statements can allow some additional insights, which can then guide program refinement and improvement.

In sum, the most effective prevention programs work from a theory that identifies the leverage points that will lead to behavior change or action. They also consider what contextual factors make people more willing or able to engage in behavior change or action. Only through this process of theory development and the design of logic models can an evaluator truly design an evaluation that will reveal whether and how the program works both theoretically and logistically (Davis et al., 2013).

## 2.2 Types of Evaluations

Once the theory of change and logical model have been developed, the evaluation team can identify the type of evaluation in which they will engage: formative, process, or outcome. Each of these forms of evaluation will be important at various stages of a prevention program's development.

### 2.2.1 Formative Evaluations

Formative evaluations are concerned with the development of program materials and strategies related to delivery of the program (Davis et al., 2013). This type of evaluation will require input from the target population in order to increase the likelihood of success. For example, Moore and colleagues (2019) developed an interactive drug abuse prevention program focused on inhibiting the use of nonprescription drugs among youths. They conducted focus groups, used writing sessions, and utilized feedback sessions (on specific program modules) with young people with varied levels of exposure to prescription opioids (PO). They then used the information they learned to inform the development of their web-based PO prevention program.

By taking these initial steps, Moore and colleagues (2019) were able to make adaptations to the program content and delivery format before widely implementing it. For example, from the focus groups that included youth who had legitimate prescriptions for an opioid, the researchers learned that responses to if/when a friend requested to use the medication need to include indignation and affront. The youth in these groups made it clear that a simple "no" was not enough and that friends often persisted in their pressure to divert medication. As a result of learning this information, the researchers developed the skill-based video component on this topic with this reality in mind. They tailored the skill-based module to have a stronger refusal tactic in an effort to increase the likelihood that the young person would resist pressure to give their medication to a friend.

The time spent getting an in-depth assessment from the youth allowed the researchers to develop a program that reflected the perspective of the youth, who were the target of the prevention program. This process also contributed to the goal of maximizing acceptance of the program and increasing usability, credibility, and ultimately effectiveness (Moore et al., 2019). In formative evaluations, the focus is on understanding how to format and deliver the program in a way that increases participation from the targeted population and that makes the program more credible.

### 2.2.2 Process Evaluations

Process evaluations focus on assessing how and why a program is successful or, alternatively, unsuccessful. Here, the research question is focused on gathering information that will allow one to judge the operational performance of the program and provide insight into areas of needed change in the day-to-day activities or implementation of the program (Davis et al., 2013). This can include documenting the recruitment of participants and the quality of program implementation. Process evaluations are a helpful tool in identifying the specific components of a program that can be leveraged to achieve the desired changes and also to better understand factors that undermined or limit the desired outcomes.

Waterman and colleagues (2021) describe a process evaluation of a youth-led sexual violence prevention initiative. The authors used multiple data sources (survey questions, open-ended survey items, and interviews) from multiple youth to examine the timing of events and what the young people perceived as the benefits and drawbacks of participating in the program. Given the dearth of youth-led sexual violence prevention initiatives, the process evaluation allowed the researchers to understand what features of the program were helpful and what needed to be improved (Waterman et al., 2021). For example, they learned it was important to make use of pre-assessments to determine the current knowledge level of participants. They then tailored the curriculum so that youth were not bored or, alternatively, that the program was not too advanced. Waterman and colleagues also found it would be necessary to balance adult support in youth-led initiates, including making sure adults prevent negative youth behavior during program events. This type of evaluation is very much focused on the way the program is delivered and what components would support effective implementation.

### 2.2.3 Outcome Evaluations

Outcome evaluation seeks to assess whether an intervention has achieved the desired short-term and longer term benefits. The purpose is to determine the level of change in the hypothesized direction, for example, short-term changes in attitudes, beliefs, immediate changes in behaviors, or longer term outcomes like trends in morbidity or mortality (Davis et al., 2013). Long-term evaluation may also include an economic evaluation that seeks to assess the cost-effectiveness of the program.

Cost-effectiveness and cost-benefit analyses assess the benefits of a program in relation to the financial costs and any negative consequences or side effects (Raczynski et al., 2013). In this type of analysis, one is concerned with putting a value on changes in outcomes (e.g., recidivism, depression) that are produced by the program and comparing this to the cost of providing the program. Health promotion programs in the community and in the workplace have been shown to save large sums in health-care costs and avert human suffering, which constitutes strong evidence for prevention approaches (Romano, 2015).

Outcome evaluations are also interested in whether the program has made gains on the expected outcomes. Evaluators need to identify the outcomes they want to assess as connected to both short-term and longer term prevention goals. They also must consider for whom they want to assess outcomes and the conditions under which the evaluation will be conducted. The logic model that was developed as part of the program design, specifying desired outcomes and how they are expected to be related, should be reviewed in making these evaluation decisions (Davis et al., 2013).

While establishing the effectiveness of an intervention is of critical importance, the task is complicated. Evaluators are often in a position of making judgments about the level of scientific rigor that is possible in applied settings and how the constraints of research design can be applied in ways that are culturally responsive. In alignment with principles of research design, evaluators need to be attentive to issues of internal and external validity, including concerns for the reliability and validity of outcome measures. Internal validity relates to confidence that the observed outcomes were the result of the intervention being assessed. Alternative explanations for changes, such as participant maturation, participant selection or dropouts, the impact of participating in an assessment, and the use of measures that are not reliable or valid need to be taken into account in the program design and evaluation (Raczynski et al., 2013). External validity relates to whether the program being evaluated generalizes for use in the real world and across different groups of people, in different settings, and at different times. Evaluators also need to be aware of threats to external validity, such as the selection of participants to be assessed and the choice of settings where the assessment will take place, in the design of the evaluation.

Despite the value of random assignment and the use of no-treatment or waiting list control groups as important in a scientifically rigorous process, these practices are not always possible and may conflict with the priorities of community members (Vera & Kenny, 2013). Delaying or withholding treatment for instance might be viewed as not prioritizing the needs of the community and allowing the evaluators' goals to override the human need. As a result, flexible evaluation approaches that consider the local culture and context in an in-depth way are vital for effective and sustainable evaluation efforts.

Applying rigorous scientific methods means that prevention evaluation includes a series of studies with evidence accumulating over time. Pilot studies and formative evaluations, as described earlier, are used to examine the feasibility and likely efficacy of an intervention and can be used to modify or improve the intervention. Process evaluations, also described earlier, can be included to assess whether the intervention is being delivered as planned and to identify barriers to implementation. Outcome evaluation often proceeds from an efficacy phase to an effectiveness evaluation. Efficacy evaluations seek to control maximally for threats to internal validity and are carried out under relatively controlled circumstances to assess whether an intervention demonstrates benefits that can be clearly attributed to the theory that guided its development, while limiting the many factors that exist in natural settings. Effectiveness evaluation focuses on external validity and assesses outcomes under real-world conditions. The Society for Prevention Research, an international organization of prevention researchers, practitioners, and policymakers, has established standards for efficacy and effectiveness research (and for scale-up research that is discussed later; Gottfredson et al., 2015). We provide the link to learn more about these standards in the resource section of this chapter.

Prilleltensky and colleagues (2020) report on the evaluation of an online intervention, Fun for Wellness (FFW), designed to promote wellness in adults with obesity, which was assessed through programmatic evaluation. An efficacy evaluation (Myers et al., 2017) was initially carried out in a relatively controlled setting with adults at a university. Findings showed enhancements in well-being across multiple domains. Building on those positive findings, Prilleltensky and colleagues (2020) sought to assess the effectiveness of FFW beyond the university setting, using the intervention with a large national sample recruited through the general panel of SurveyHealth. This phase of the study was also designed with attention to rigorous scientific methods. For example, participants were randomly assigned into two conditions: (a) to engage in the FFW intervention and (b) to proceed with their lives as usual while being put on a wait-list for later participation. The study design was prospective with both intervention and the wait-list participants completing reliable and valid measures at baseline, 30 days, and 60 days. While this phase of the evaluation supported the effectiveness of FFW, continued evaluation, recruiting a more diverse socioeconomic sample than available through SurveyHealth, and including physiological measures that go beyond participant self-report are needed to address study limitations. Prilleltensky and colleagues (2020) also note the need for systemic change in health policy, as well as interventions such as FWW that focus on the individual.

### 2.3 Scaling Up

Relatively less rigorous research exists related to the process and systems through which evidenced-based prevention programs are then adopted, implemented, and sustained on a larger scale (Gottfredson et al., 2015). It is important to consider questions of scalability conjointly with effectiveness evaluations in order to proactively think about how to guide later scale-up efforts of the program (Spoth et al., 2013). This scaling-up process involves moving interventions that have been demonstrated to be effective when evaluated on a more limited degree to being able to be implemented on a broader (population-level) dimension (Gottfredson et al., 2015). Despite the importance of scaling up as a way to reach maximum benefit to a population, the realization of this goal remains a challenge. To address this complex need, the Society for Prevention Research formed a task force to identify specific ways to scale up evidenced-based interventions (EBIs; Fagan et al., 2019). The authors of the report identified specific actions that were needed:

> (1) provide more public policies and funding to support the creation, testing, and scaling up of EBIs; (2) develop and evaluate specific frameworks that address systems-level barriers impeding EBI scale-up; and (3) promote public support for EBIs, community capacity to implement EBIs at scale, and partnerships between community stakeholders, policymakers, practitioners, and scientists within and across systems.

More details about scale-up research can be found in the resource section of this chapter.

### 2.4 Dissemination

The dissemination or communication of evaluation findings is also an important part of the evaluation process (Conyne, 2013). Dissemination includes communication of findings to the local community and all stakeholders. The communication of positive effects through multiple sources (e.g., community presentations, government bodies, local new outlets) can help increase support and resources for the program. Less than desirable outcomes also need to be shared so that the design or delivery of the program can be improved or so that time and funds can be invested in more effective programs. Knowledge regarding what works in prevention and the advancement of prevention science can only occur when findings are shared and built upon. Dissemination to the scientific community through publications, conference presentations, and online clearinghouses is vital in advancing the scientific knowledge base for prevention. The prevention program should be described in sufficient detail so that it can be replicated if desired and its appropriateness for a particular setting can be judged.

While knowing whether a program works is critical, an exclusive focus on efficacy and effectiveness is not the only aspect of an evaluation. Questions of participant satisfaction, social utility, and other justice-oriented outcomes are equally vital. Conyne (2013) describes some general evaluation criteria that should be kept in mind across all phases of evaluation, from formative through outcome and in scaling up. These include looking at the adequacy or strength of the critical program components to effect desired change, the appropriateness of the program for the values and culture of the population and the context (e.g., history, economics, geography) in which it is being used, the existence of any unintended negative outcomes or side effects, the degree to which desired outcomes are observed, the cost or efficiency of the program in attaining desired outcomes, and the sustainability or stability of desired outcomes.

## 2.5 Culturally Responsive Evaluations

As referenced earlier, evaluation should be designed and carried out with consideration of the sociopolitical context within which the prevention effort is situated. Liberation theory that is grounded in cultural, historical, and sociopolitical contexts, offers a theoretical framework from which to approach this work (Comas-Díaz & Rivera, 2020). Liberation psychology centers on the struggle of people who are oppressed in society and gives focus to the way people thrive and become whole, despite these multiple oppressions (French et al., 2020). Goodman et al. (2004) identified several principles, consistent with a liberation psychology and social justice perspective, that are integral to culturally responsive evaluation. These include ongoing self-examination, sharing power with stakeholders, giving voice to the oppressed, consciousness raising, promoting strengths, and leaving participants and community members with tools.

The Centers for Disease Control (n.d.) provides guiding questions that reflect the abovementioned principles and integrate cultural competence into an evaluation process. Key components include engaging stakeholders and examining if stakeholders' perspectives are appropriately reflected in the program description and design. This includes self-reflection on the part of the evaluator to understand their own system of values, worldviews, and possible areas of bias. It is then important to specifically consider if the strengths, assets, challenges, and barriers of the identified community are included in the program model. Evaluators also need to gather credible evidence using culturally appropriate methods and instruments, involve stakeholders in the analysis and interpretation of data, and generate recommendations and a shared understanding of the conclusions with the stakeholders (Centers for Disease Control, n.d.).

A liberation psychology perspective highlights the importance of integrating alternative forms of knowledge in prevention program design and evaluation so as to nurture peoples' survival, cultural resilience, healing, and optimal development (Comas-Díaz & Rivera, 2020). In the context of evaluation, this includes the importance of looking at a variety of methods for gauging the effectiveness of any prevention program, including using quantitative, qualitative, mixed methods approaches, and participatory action research (PAR). Additional epistemologies, such as Indigenous ways of knowing and storytelling, might also be utilized (Smith, 2012).

PAR represents an approach that involves community members or intended recipients of the prevention program in the evaluation process. Community members or the participants are involved at all stages of evaluation, from identifying the problem(s) to be addressed, to data collection, data analysis, and then social action (Abraczinskas et al., 2022). The process begins with program recipients being active in identifying the problems or concerns that impact their lives. Thus, PAR has the potential to address gaps in implementation by working to make the program more aligned with the target population. Abraczinskas and colleagues (2022) demonstrated how youth PAR can improve a school-wide-positive behavioral intervention by increasing youth engagement in the program planning and implementation. They found that PAR allowed for increased equality of youth and adult voice, where each perspective was equally valued. This resulted in an increase in the balance of power. As a result of this increased power balance, there were more opportunities for clearer dialogue between youth and adults in the school system. Through evaluation of the interviews and archival data, the researchers were able to see how these improved relationships between students and teachers impacted power-sharing partnerships, contributed to reductions in bullying, and improved school climate. The power-sharing relationship in the youth and adult partnerships was also shown to support an effective intervention following a tragedy and helped set positive school norms related to empathy (Abraczinskas et al., 2022). Following the traumatic death of a student, students worked with the wellness center to create different levels of support for students, which included peer support and triaging students with higher needs to school counselors. PAR was helpful not only in more closely targeting the program to student needs but also in promoting equity by supporting changes in school policies, practices, and programming that benefitted traditionally marginalized students (Abraczinskas et al., 2022).

## 2.6 Person- and System-Focused Evaluation

Prevention has traditionally focused on work with individuals to achieve person-centered outcomes. System or environmental-focused interventions are also essential to address health disparities and foster equity through broader social change. George Albee, a pioneer in prevention and social justice, recognized the simultaneous need for person-level and systems intervention in order for deep change to be realized (Albee, 1986.) Vera (2020), for example, asserts that interventions that target systems, organizations, public policies, and natural ecologies are critical for addressing urgent health threats and disparities. These interventions required different types of evaluations that assess systemic change and structural or environment-centered outcomes. Because the results of systemic prevention efforts may not be observable in the short term, evaluation also needs to simultaneously monitor and document process-level factors that impact outcomes, in addition to short-term and long-term assessments. To ensure that programs are meeting the needs of People of Color and Indigenous individuals, French and colleagues (2020) emphasize the importance of including measures of structural racism in the evaluation process. As an example, French and colleagues (2020) suggest that prevention researchers assessing the engagement of Latino/a/x individuals in healing practices would want to understand and assess the level of discrimination, which might be experienced at the local level, and the role of larger intuitional policies like the ruling on Deferred Action for Childhood Arrivals (Singer & Svajlenka, 2013) or other recent restrictive immigration policies. These factors may not be the direct focus of the intervention, but they may affect program implementation and outcomes.

System-focused prevention may bring attention to effecting policy changes through advocacy outreach or alleviating disparities in neighborhoods or school settings, which have a direct impact on the well-being of individuals (Vera, 2020). Gay–Straight Alliances (GSAs) or genders and sexualities alliances, which aim to promote social inclusion and justice for sexual and gender minority youth [e.g., lesbian, gay, bisexual, transgender, or questioning youth (LGBTQ); Poteat et al., 2017], are an example of an intervention that seeks systemic change at the community level, in this case, the school being the community of focus. GSAs strive to provide support and resources, not just for their group members, but also seek to improve the experiences of the whole school through advocacy and awareness efforts (Poteat et al., 2017). Prevention research and program evaluation that examine the effectiveness of these programs for LGBTQ youth should include multiple methods and stakeholders over multiple years. Vera (2020) suggests that such evaluation might include a long-term goal to assess changes in student mental health in schools with and without GSAs. Short-term assessments might focus on changes in the number of students involved in GSAs and changes among teachers and school administrators in understanding the needs of LGBTQ+ students. Process evaluation might seek to identify the density of student participation in GSAs that is needed to improve school climate or reduce incidents of harassment.

Structural racism represents a pernicious societal problem that perpetuates health inequities and presents an ongoing barrier to social justice. While efforts to address racism can be directed at interpersonal racism, systemic change is ultimately needed. At the interpersonal level, primary prevention interventions may seek to prevent racist attitudes before they are learned or seek to empower people to examine their own as well as society's racism so that they do not engage in behaviors that perpetuate the harmful effects of racism (Buhin & Vera, 2009). The logic models for such programs need to be informed by an understanding of the critical ingredients that are most closely tied to the transformation of attitudes and behaviors (Buhin & Vera, 2009), with evaluation focusing on changes in attitudes as assessed by quantitative measures, qualitative interviews, or behavioral observations in school or other social settings. Efforts to dismantle racism at the systemic level may include interventions with political and legislative bodies. Community members may be involved in identifying change agents, leveraging pertinent data to influence policymakers, and crafting a message. The evaluation may look at short-term changes in funding or policy priorities and longer term changes, such as resource allocations, representation in leadership, and the creation of task forces or other structures to advance anti-racist policies and practices (Vera, 2020). Buhin and Vera (2009) describe their efforts in systemic prevention through political action, by presenting data-based testimony on high school dropouts to their state legislative assembly. Evaluation tracked the actions of the educational subcommittee of the assembly and found promising evidence that several policy changes were implemented that were consistent with their data and recommendations.

## 2.7 Funding Evaluation Research

For prevention specialists, the need to fund the delivery and evaluation of prevention programs can be a challenge. Prevention may be a priority in many community mental health, health care, and educational settings, such that a portion of the operating budget is allocated for prevention. However, more often direct care providers may encounter financial barriers to engagement in prevention work as prevention has not traditionally been covered through health insurance, despite evidence documenting the effectiveness of prevention initiatives and their cost-effectiveness in relation to treatment. Prevention efforts in all settings, including hospitals, universities, and community agencies, are often reliant on external grants for fundings. Grants are often critical in funding all phases of prevention, and evaluations often determine next step efforts.

To document the power of prevention science and intervention, evaluation needs to be a standard part of all prevention grant applications. Grant-funded research of prevention programs, including longitudinal studies, is an important part of building a strong knowledge base about what works in prevention science. Consequently, a portion of every prevention grant budget (for instance, between 7% and 8%) should be specifically devoted to evaluation. The cost of the evaluation should be a part of the design and implementation of the program operation, as this is a critical component to demonstrate program efficacy and effectiveness (Davis et al., 2013).

Many examples of grant-funded prevention research that includes an evaluation component can be found in the literature. The PROmoting School-Community University Partnerships to Enhance Resilience (https://helpingkidsprosper.org/) universal prevention delivery system (Spoth et al., 2022) is one strong example that incorporated evaluation across many phases of the program. This program was implemented in middle schools and sought to prevent or reduce the onset of substance misuse and conduct problem behaviors. The research, which was funded by the National Institute on Drug Abuse (DA013709) and the National Institute on Alcohol Abuse and Alcoholism, demonstrated the importance of looking at both feasibility of the program and effectiveness across all stages of the project. The specific component of interest was whether a hybrid model of participant recruitment would increase participant retention (Spoth et al., 2007). The hybrid model included community-led recruitment efforts heavily supported by tangible assistance from the university partner. By examining the recruitment efforts, the authors were able to evaluate how to keep participants engaged in the program, a necessary first step before evaluating if desired outcomes were even met (e.g., no substance use concerns).

The authors found that higher recruitment of participants could be gained through a strong university–community partnership. Specifically, if the community-led recruitment efforts were supported by technical assistance (TA) from the university partner (e.g., effective collaboration with TA, frequency of TA requests), higher rates of participant recruitment and engagement were found to exist (Spoth et al., 2007). Identifying the specific components that made this hybrid recruitment model effective led to the maintenance of high-quality implementation and sustained intervention delivery (Spoth et al., 2022). Overall, the focus on the evaluation and the specific components, which can lead to higher impact, led to stronger program delivery. Rigorous and systematic evaluation of this type can help ensure prevention science is reaching a wider touchpoint. Investment in prevention program evaluation is a wise investment in the continuation of a program and in future funding of programs, as the evaluation can help determine the overall efficiency and effectiveness of the invested resources (Davis et al., 2013).

## 2.8 Summary of Key Recommendations

Prevention science offers a powerful framework to help improve the human condition and make strides in solving some of the world's most difficult problems (Herman et al., 2020). Effective and culturally responsive program evaluation, including both process and outcome evaluations, is essential for realizing the potential of prevention science. In order to provide the most effective and culturally responsive interventions for individuals and communities, a variety of program evaluations, using diverse methodologies, and assessing varied short-term and long-term outcomes, are needed. Prevention evaluation needs to begin with attention to the theory and corresponding logic model that inform the program. Formative evaluation is particularly helpful as part of a process of piloting and refining the program to enhance its ultimate effectiveness. Process evaluation is integral in tracking factors that occur during the implementation of a program that may affect the outcomes. These data can be vital in making sense of program findings and understanding changes that may be needed to enhance effectiveness. Outcome evaluation may proceed through a series of stages for establishing efficacy and effectiveness. Cost-effectiveness may also be part of the evaluation, with dissemination of findings being a final stage. Program evaluation can be a recursive process with the findings from one evaluation informing program modifications and further evaluations.

Attention to rigor in program evaluation cannot overlook the importance of cultural responsiveness. Program stakeholders and community members must be involved and listened to across all phases of evaluation to enhance cultural responsiveness. Their voices can help inform decisions about evaluation design and how best to respond when scientific standards conflict with practical needs and cultural norms. Theoretical models, such as liberation psychology, can inform culturally responsive program evaluations, and research methods, such as PAR, which are useful for fully engaging the community in the evaluation process. In order to realize its potential and to advance equity and social justice, prevention needs to focus on environmental and societal level change, as well as individual change. Program evaluation focused on systemic change needs to specifically assess systemic outcomes. From a practical perspective, evaluators often need to seek external grant funding that can also include resources for the dissemination of findings and their modification or replication in new settings and with new populations. In this way, grant funding can contribute to the advancement of prevention science and enhance its benefits for varied communities and broader segments of the population.

## Resources

### Journals and Professional Organizations

The following organizations and journals are helpful resources to learn more about prevention evaluation and to find examples of prevention evaluation.

- American Psychological Association, Society of Counseling Psychology, Prevention Section: www.div17.org/resources-prevention-section
- *Journal of Prevention and Health Promotion*: https://journals.sagepub.com/home/prv
- *Journal of Prevention*: www.springer.com/journal/10935/
- Society for Prevention Research: www.preventionresearch.org/
- *Prevention Science*: www.springer.com/journal/11121
- Society for Prevention Research Standards of evidence for efficacy, effectiveness, and scale-up research: www.preventionresearch.org/wp-content/uploads/2011/12/Standards-of-Evidence_2015.pdf and www.preventionresearch.org/advocacy/standards-of-evidence/
- *American Journal of Preventive Medicine*: www.acpm.org/news-publications/american-journal-of-preventive-medicine/

### CDC: Program Evaluation Resources

The Centers for Disease Control offers many free resources related to program evaluation. Peruse the links in these varied resources:

www.cdc.gov/healthyyouth/evaluation/pdf/brief4.pdf
www.cdc.gov/evaluation/
www.cdc.gov/evaluation/approach/index.htm
www.cdc.gov/evaluation/framework/index.htm
www.cdc.gov/evaluation/guidelines/index.htm
www.cdc.gov/dhdsp/docs/cultural_competence_tip_sheet.pdf

### Grant Sources

Many sources for prevention funding can be identified through the following websites of these and other federal agencies and private foundations.

Substance Abuse and Mental Health Services Administration: www.samhsa.gov/grants

National Institute on Alcohol Abuse and Alcoholism: www.niaaa.nih.gov/grant-funding

National Institute of Health: www.nih.gov/grants-funding

National Institute of Mental Health: www.nimh.nih.gov/funding

Office of Juvenile Justice and Delinquency Prevention: https://ojjdp.ojp.gov/funding

U. S. Department of Education, Office of Safe and Healthy Students: https://oese.ed.gov/offices/office-of-formula-grants/safe-supportive-schools/

W. T. Grant Foundation: https://wtgrantfoundation.org/grants

W. K. Kellogg Foundation: www.wkkf.org/

### Evidenced-Based Practices

The following are examples of websites that disseminate evidence on effective programs.

Evidenced-based Practices Resources Center: www.samhsa.gov/ebp-resource-center/about

What Works Clearinghouse: https://ies.ed.gov/ncee/WWC

Social Programs that Work: https://evidencebasedprograms.org/

Washington State Institute for Public Policy – Benefits-Cost Information: www.wsipp.wa.gov/BenefitCost

### Further Reading

The following books and book chapters are also helpful in amplifying topics covered in this chapter.

Davis, M., Orpinas, P., & Horne, A. M. (2013). Design and evaluation of prevention programs. In E. M. Vera (Ed.), *The Oxford handbook of prevention in counseling psychology* (pp. 91–108). Oxford University Press.

Schwandt, T. A., & Gates, E. F. (2021, in press). *Evaluating and valuing in social research*. Guilford Press.

Romano, J. (2015). *Prevention psychology: Enhancing personal and social well-being*. American Psychological Association.

The following books are part of the Prevention Practice Kit published by Sage in 2013.

Conyne, R. K. (2013). *Program development and evaluation in prevention*. Sage.

Raczynski, K., Waldo, M., Schwartz, J., & Horne, A. (2013). *Evidenced-based prevention*. Sage.

Vera, E., & Kenny, M. E. (2013). *Social justice and culturally relevant prevention*. Sage.

## References

Abraczinskas, M., Kornbluh, M., Golden, A. R., Glende, J., Velez, V., Vines, E., & Ozer, E. J. (2022). Preventing bullying and improving school climate through integrating youth participatory action research into school-wide positive behavioral interventions and supports: An illustration using a multiple case study approach. *Journal of Prevention and Health Promotion*, *3*(2), 166–194. doi.org/10.1177/26320770221092148

Albee, G. W. (1986). Toward a just society: Lessons from observations on the primary prevention of psychopathology. *American Psychologist, 41*(8), 891–898. doi.org/10.1037/0003-066X.41.8.891

American Psychological Association. (2014). Guidelines for prevention in psychology. *American Psychologist, 69*(3), 285–296. doi.org/10.1037/a0034569

Buhin, L., & Vera, E. M. (2009). Preventing racism and promoting social justice: Person-centered and environment-centered interventions. *The Journal of Primary Prevention, 30*(1), 43–59. doi.org/10.1007/s10935-008-0161-9

Caracelli, V. J., & Riggin, L. J. C. (1994). Mixed-method evaluation: Developing quality criteria through concept mapping. *Evaluation Practice, 15*(2), 139–152. doi.org/10.1016/0886-1633(94)90005-1

Centers for Disease Control (n.d.). *Program evaluation tip sheet: Integrating cultural competence into evaluation.* www.cdc.gov/dhdsp/docs/cultural_competence_tip_sheet.pdf

Comas-Díaz, L. & Rivera, E. T. (2020). *Liberation psychology: Theory, method, practice, and social justice.* American Psychological Association.

Conyne, R. K. (2013). *Program development and evaluation in prevention.* Sage.

Davis, M., Orpinas, P., & Horne, A. M. (2013). Design and evaluation of prevention programs. In E. M. Vera (Ed.), *The Oxford handbook of prevention in counseling psychology* (pp. 91–108). Oxford University Press.

Fagan, A. A., Bumbarger, B. K., Barth, R. P., Bradshaw, C. P., Cooper, B. R., Supplee, L. H., & Walker, D. K. (2019). Scaling up evidence-based interventions in US public systems to prevent behavioral health problems: Challenges and opportunities. *Prevention Science, 20*, 1147–1168. doi.org/10.1007/s11121-019-01048-8

French, B. H., Lewis, J. A., Mosley, D. V., Adames, H. Y., Chavez-Dueñas, N. Y., Chen, G. A., & Neville, H. A. (2020). Toward a psychological framework of radical healing in communities of color. *The Counseling Psychologist, 48*(1), 14–46. doi.org/10.1177/0011000019843506

Gottfredson, D. C., Cook, T. D., Gardner, F. E. M., Gorman-Smith, D., Howe, G. W., Sandler, I. N., & Zafft, K. M. (2015). Standards of evidence for efficacy, effectiveness, and scale-up research in prevention science: Next generation. *Prevention Science, 16*(7), 893–926. doi.org/10.1007/s11121-015-0555-x

Goodman, L. A., Liang, B., Helms, J. E., Latta, R. E., Sparks, E., & Weintraub, S. R. (2004). Training counseling psychologists as social justice agents: Feminist and multicultural principles in action. *The Counseling Psychologist, 32*(6), 793–836. doi.org/10.1177/0011000004268802

Hage, S. M., Romano, J. L., Conyne, R. K., Kenny, M., Matthews, C., Schwartz, J. P., Waldo, M. (2007). Best practice guidelines on prevention practice, research, training, and social advocacy for psychologists. *The Counseling Psychologists, 35*(4), 493–566. doi.org/10.1177/0011000006291411

Herman, K. C., Reinke, W. M., Thompson, A. M. (2020). Prevention science as a platform for solving major societal problems and improving population health. *Journal of Prevention and Health Promotion, 1*(1), 131–151. doi.org/10.1177/2632077020948786

Moore, S. K., Grabinski, M., Bessen, S., Borodovsky, J. T., & Marsch, L. A. (2019). Web-based prescription opioid abuse prevention for adolescents: Program development and formative evaluation. *JMIR Formative Research, 3*(3). http://formative.jmir.org/2019/3/e12389/

Myers N. D., Prilleltensky I., Hill C. R., & Feltz D. L. (2017). Well-being self-efficacy and complier average causal effect modeling: A substantive-methodological synergy. *Psychology of Sport & Exercise*, *30*, 135–144. doi.org/10.1016/j.psychsport.2017.02.010

Poteat, V. P., Yoshikawa, H., Calzo, J. P., Russell, S. T., & Horn, S. (2017). Gay-straight alliances as settings for youth inclusion and development: Future conceptual and methodological directions for research on these and other student groups in schools. *Educational Researcher*, *46*(9), 508–516. doi.org/10.3102/0013189X17738760

Prilleltensky, I., McMahon, A., Myers, N. D., Prilleltensky, O., Dietz, S., Scarpa, M. P., Lee, S., Pfeiffer, K. A., Bateman, A. G., & Brincks, A. M. (2020). An exploration of the effectiveness of the fun for wellness online intervention to promote health in adults with obesity: A randomized controlled trial. *Journal of Prevention and Health Promotion*, *1*(2), 212–239. doi.org/10.1177/2632077020968737

Raczynski, K., Waldo, M., Schwartz, J., & Horne, A. (2013). *Evidenced-based prevention* (Vol. 6). Sage.

Romano, J. (2015). *Prevention psychology: Enhancing personal and social well-being*. American Psychological Association.

Romano, J. L., & Hage, S. M. (2000). Prevention and counseling psychology: Revitalizing commitments for the twenty-first century. *The Counseling Psychologist*, *28*(6), 733–763. doi.org/10.1177/0011000000286001

Rosas, S. R. (2005). Concept mapping as a technique for program theory development: An illustration using family support programs. *American Journal of Evaluation*, *26*(3), 389–401. doi.org/10.1177/1098214005278760

Singer, A., & Svajlenka, N. P. (2013). Immigration facts: Deferred action for childhood arrivals (DACA). *The Brookings Institution*. www.brookings.edu/wp-content/uploads/2016/06/DACA_singer_svajlenka_FINAL.pdf

Smith, L. T. (2012). *Decolonizing methodologies: Research and indigenous peoples* (2nd ed.). Zed Books.

Spoth, R., Clair, S., Greenberg, M., Redmond, C., & Shin, C. (2007). Toward dissemination of evidence-based family interventions: Maintenance of community-based partnership recruitment results and associated factors. *Journal of Family Psychology*, *21*(2), 137. doi.10.1037/0893-3200.21.2.137

Spoth, R., Redmond, C., Shin, C., Trudeau, L., Greenberg, M. T., Feinberg, M. E., & Welsh, J. (2022). Applying the PROSPER prevention delivery system with middle schools: Emerging adulthood effects on substance misuse and conduct problem behaviors through 14 years past baseline. *Child Development*, *93*(4), 925–940. doi.org/10.1111/cdev.13746

Spoth, R., Rohrbach, L. A., Greenberg, M., Leaf, P., Brown, C. H., Fagan, A., Catalano, R. F., Pentz, M. A., Sloboda, Z., Hawkins, J. D., & Society for Prevention Research Type 2 Translational Task Force Members and Contributing Authors. (2013). Addressing core challenges for the next generation of type 2 translation research and systems: The translation science to population impact (TSci Impact) framework. *Prevention Science*, *14*(4), 319–351. doi.org/10.1007/s11121-012-0362-6

Vera, E. (2020). A prevention agenda for 2020 and beyond: Why environmental interventions matter now more than ever. *Journal of Prevention and Health Promotion*, *1*(1), 5–33. doi.org/10.1177/2632077020937690

Vera, E., & Kenny, M. E. (2013). *Social justice and culturally relevant prevention*. Sage.

Wang, X. (2021). The role of perceived susceptibility and collectivist values in support for using social distancing to prevent COVID-19 in the United States. *Journal of Prevention and Health Promotion*, *2*(2), 268–293. doi.org.10.1177/26320770211015434

Waterman, E. A., Hutchison, C. A., Edwards, K. M., Hopfauf, S. L., Simon, B., & Banyard, V. L. (2021). A process evaluation of a youth-led sexual violence prevention initiative. *Journal of Prevention and Health Promotion*, *2*(2), 163–190. doi .org/10.1177/26320770211010817

Werner-Seidler, A., Perry, Y., Calear, A. L., Newby, J. M., & Christensen, H. (2017). School-based depression and anxiety prevention programs for young people: A systematic review and meta-analysis. *Clinical Psychology Review*, *51*, 30–47. dx.doi .org/10.1016/j.cpr.2016.10.005

Yampolskaya, S., Nesman, T. M., Hernandez, M., & Koch, D. (2004). Using concept mapping to develop a logic model and articulate a program theory: A case example. *American Journal of Evaluation*, *25*(2), 191–207. doi.org/10.1177/109821400402500204

# 3 Critical Features of Prevention Practice: Implementing Prevention That Works

Wendy M. Reinke and Keith C. Herman

Intellectuals solve problems, geniuses prevent them.

—Albert Einstein

In this chapter, we will discuss critical features of effective prevention practices. These include (a) using data to inform prevention efforts, (b) using a problem-solving approach to identify the problem to be prevented and the steps needed for effective implementation, (c) monitoring fidelity to prevention practices, and (d) using data to determine if prevention practices are working and for whom. In addition, we will discuss the need for collaborative relationships and using culturally responsive practices when determining and implementing prevention practices. Several school-based prevention examples will be provided throughout to add context. Lastly, we will discuss implications for practice.

## 3.1 Prevention and Implementation Science

Before jumping into the critical features of prevention practice, it is important to understand the theories behind these practices. In the early 1990s, a new field known as *prevention science* emerged (Kellam et al., 1999). Prevention science has been defined as the scientific study of systematic efforts to reduce the incidence of unhealthy or maladaptive behavior and to promote health and adaptive behavior across the lifespan through designing and evaluating interventions and utilizing knowledge about them (Herman, Reinke, & Thompson, 2019; Herman et al., 2020; Kellam et al., 1999). As an interdisciplinary field, prevention science provides a model for solving large-scale societal problems. Specifically, prevention science is a systematic method for identifying, monitoring, and altering meaningful malleable targets (risk factors) that have been demonstrated to be associated with significant negative outcomes (Kellam et al., 1999).

Stormont, Reinke, and Herman (2010) outlined critical aspects of successful prevention programming, including (a) articulating and refining a comprehensive conceptual model to identify the etiology of the targeted problem and malleable risk and protective factors contributing to this problem across development, (b) developing contextually relevant interventions that target the hypothesized risk and protective factors, (c) designing and implementing intervention trials to manipulate hypothesized risk and protective factors to determine their causal role, (d) implementing large field trials to determine the effectiveness of a promising intervention, and (e) disseminating and ensuring the sustainability of successful programs (Kellam et al., 1999).

As a result of prevention science, policies, programs, and practices have been generated that have shown to reduce the incidence and prevalence of individual and community vulnerabilities as well as to promote healthy lifestyles. Some of these accomplishments include (a) promoting daily physical activity and good nutrition to protect against chronic disease; (b) disrupting pathways to substance use disorder across the lifespan; (c) improving academic and behavioral outcomes with the expansion of high-quality childcare, early learning, and promoting positive and supportive school environments; (d) enhancing community-wide capacity to increase access to supportive services; (e) increasing resilience, social competency, and self-regulation to reduce impulsive, aggressive, and off-task behavior; (f) supporting the development of healthy relationships to reduce interpersonal and domestic violence; and (g) the use of evidence-based strategies to address systemic and structural inequities in neighborhoods, as well as educational and criminal justice practices, to name a few (see Fishbein, 2021; National Research Council and Institute of Medicine [NRC & IOM], 2009; National Prevention Science Coalition, 2019).

Adopting a prevention approach requires that psychologists and counselors reconceptualize their roles and responsibilities through a public health lens that moves beyond the "client" being an individual to the "client" being larger populations (e.g., communities, schools; Herman et al., 2019; Herman et al., 2020). While individualized interventions should be delivered when warranted, focusing on prevention will help decrease the number of individuals needing more intensive services in the long run. Understanding the critical features of effective prevention practices will put into context the need for this broader more inclusive vision of how a problem is determined and prevented.

Over the past 50 years, the field of prevention science has developed a large number of evidence-based interventions and practices that are known to improve the outcomes that individuals experience. More recently, at least in the area of psychology and education, the study of how these practices are adopted and implemented has emerged. *Implementation science* is the study of how evidence-based programs can be effectively implemented to maximize successful outcomes (Kelly & Perkins, 2012). We know that if evidence-based intervention and practices are not implemented with fidelity or are not adopted and utilized, the associated positive outcomes will not materialize. Implementation science works to bridge the gap between research and practice by understanding the barriers and facilitators to adoption and implementation of interventions with fidelity (Wiltsey & Beidas, 2020).

As a field, implementation science emphasizes the importance of understanding the context in which individuals will implement evidence-based practices and how these contextual factors, such as knowledge, skills, beliefs, and attitudes of those implementing, contribute to implementation success or failure. In addition, implementation science focuses on developing implementation approaches that target the factors that may accelerate or hinder implementation and examines the effectiveness of these approaches, intending to improve adoption and implementation of what we know works (Kelly & Perkins, 2012).

Thus, as you begin to incorporate prevention into practice it is important to give attention to the science behind the programs and practices that you select, ensuring that you are adopting and implementing only practices that have strong evidence for the likelihood of success with the targeted population. Also, it is critical to confirm that the evidence-based programs you decide to adopt are aligned with the problem area you are planning to prevent (e.g., adopting an evidence-based bully prevention curriculum to reduce and prevent bullying behaviors in schools). Lastly, poorly implemented programs, regardless of the evidence of their impact, will not produce successful outcomes. Often, when a preventive program or practice is not implemented as intended, stakeholders may determine that it was unhelpful or did not produce desired outcomes, but it is impossible to determine whether the program or practice was successful because it did not occur. Low fidelity to implementation can lead stakeholders or individuals to discontinue what might have been highly effective practices if implemented as intended. Thus, as you set out to employ prevention practices, it is important to give attention to the contextual barriers to implementation and work to overcome these barriers before and during implementation.

## 3.2 Public Health Three-Tiered Model of Prevention and Intervention

In addition to understanding the science behind prevention and implementation practices, it is important to be familiar with public health-tiered approaches to prevention. These models often utilize three tiers of prevention which include universal, selective, and indicated supports (Tiers 1, 2, and 3, respectively) for the delivery of research-based, evidence-based interventions and practices that increase in intensity at each level (Herman, Reinke, Huang et al., 2021; Stormont et al., 2012). This tiered system ensures a comprehensive and fluid process in which individuals receive various levels of care, dependent upon their need for more or fewer supports, as identified through the use of valid and reliable assessments.

Universal preventive interventions that are provided to all individuals within a selected population or setting serve as proactive and preventative measures. Universal preventive interventions reach a large number of people, are relatively inexpensive in comparison with more individualized supports, and can impact multiple risk factors that could lead to a host of poor outcomes. Examples of universal prevention efforts include school-wide implementation of a social–emotional learning curriculum, mandatory use of seat belts while driving, and mandatory social distancing during the COVID-19 pandemic. The expectation is that these universal supports will effectively support about 80% of the targeted population.

In the second tier, selective interventions are designed to meet the needs of a smaller group of individuals who require additional support beyond those received universally. Selective interventions offer more precision or focus on the area of risk and greater intensity than universal interventions. Theoretically, approximately 5–10% of individuals can benefit from selective interventions (Herman et al., 2020; Herman, Reinke, Thompson, et al., 2021). Selective interventions are specialized programs or services delivered to a subgroup of children, families, or communities with demographic characteristics or life experiences that place them at risk for later poor outcomes. Examples of selective interventions include small group prevention interventions for depression targeting adolescent female youth and permitting elderly individuals or individuals with autoimmune difficulties, which place them at risk for developing COVID-19, to enter grocery stores before the general population to reduce their exposure to the virus.

Indicated preventive interventions are more intensive and individualized than selective interventions. The preventive interventions are reserved for about 1–5% of the target population who are demonstrating early signs of risk for specific difficulty related to the development of disease, mental disorders, or other significant risks (Herman et al., 2020; Herman, Reinke, Thompson, et al., 2021). Such services and programs are more intensive and expensive but given the high cost and long-term effects of the problems they target, they can be cost-effective. The fluidity of this public health-tiered model of support allows for seamless service delivery, in which all individuals receive a universal prevention intervention, and those identified as individuals who would benefit from selective or indicated intervention services receive these services until they demonstrate that supports are no longer needed (Stormont et al., 2012).

### 3.3 Prevention Paradox

Prevention efforts should utilize all levels of intervention if we hope to prevent problems on a large-scale. A comprehensive public health model that offers a carefully coordinated sequence of universal, selective, and indicated preventive strategies, followed by treatment, is ultimately most likely to be effective and cost-efficient (Le et al., 2021; Offord et al., 1998). The fundamental importance of a universal approach to prevention can be illustrated through what is called the "prevention paradox." Geoffrey Rose, the British epidemiologist who coined the term prevention paradox more than 30 years ago, had the insight that "a large number of people exposed to a small risk may generate many more cases than a small number exposed to a high-risk" (Rose, 1992, p. 24). Rose highlights that while targeted high-risk populations for preventive interventions are useful, they will only impact a small number of individuals identified as having some risk to develop the problem being targeted. Some of these individuals who are identified may never develop the problem, whereas, in the larger population of individuals who are not identified as being at risk (i.e., 80%), there will be a subset who will develop the problem regardless of not having known risk factors.

Greenberg and colleagues (2017) applied the logic to adopting universal SEL curriculums in schools and offered the following example of the prevention paradox concerning school dropout. They provided a scenario in which 100 ninth-grade students are screened for risk of dropping out of school. Twenty percent of students at high risk for dropping out are identified. The screening is fairly accurate in that 75% of these students (i.e., 15 out of 20) drop out of school. However, another 20% of students from the low-risk group also drop out of school (i.e., 20 out of 80). In this scenario, 57% of all students who drop out of school come from the low-risk population (e.g., more than half). Given the high societal and individual cost of not finishing high school, a relatively low-cost universal intervention (e.g., universal SEL) that reduces the dropout rate among this low-risk group even by as little as 25%, or 5 students, could produce dramatic cost savings. In other words, although we can screen, identify, and provide interventions to some individuals who are at risk for later problems, we can markedly reduce the problem's prevalence in the long run by first using effective universal interventions.

Furthermore, recent studies demonstrate that not only does the "low-risk" population benefit from universal prevention efforts, but also individuals receiving other support benefit as well. For instance, a universal classroom management intervention that trained teachers in effective universal practices demonstrated behavioral benefits for students receiving additional support through special education in comparison with peers receiving special education services in classrooms that did not receive the intervention (Reinke, Herman, Stormont, & Dong, 2021). Thus, universal prevention efforts can be considered relevant to the full spectrum of risk, while also benefiting the population by reducing the overall prevalence of future problems.

In the following sections, critical features that constitute effective prevention practices and that will enhance the capacity of individual psychologists and counselors, as well as larger systems, to effectively employ evidence-based prevention are discussed.

## 3.4 Critical Features of Prevention Practice

### 3.4.1 Use Data to Inform Prevention Efforts

An important first step when planning prevention efforts is using data to inform decisions. Prevention that focuses on risk and protective factors is grounded in the public health approach, which relies on data-based predictors of problem behaviors and positive outcomes (Herman et al., 2020). These include the risk and protective factors that present themselves across the course of human development and make individuals and groups either more or less prone to a particular problem in certain social contexts. Further, conditions or environmental factors (e.g., living in poverty, systemic inequities, and racism) that are implicated in the development or consequences of the problem are identified (NRC & IOM, 2009). These data are then used to determine the problem to be prevented and guide what evidence-based preventive intervention should be selected. Larger entities, such as states or communities, often gather epidemiological data that can be used to determine funding for prevention, policies, and practices in efforts to reduce risk factors and increase protective factors associated with a problem, in order to prevent it (Purtle et al., 2020; Substance Abuse and Mental Health Services Administration, 2012).

An example of a community initiative to decrease mental health concerns for youth is school-based prevention and an early intervention model that utilizes universal social–emotional screening to gather data and make decisions about prevention efforts. Schools are an optimal setting to provide prevention and early intervention services to children and youth. Not only do youth spend a considerable portion of their day in schools, but schools are typically staffed with professionals that have the expertise and training necessary to support these efforts. Students are more likely to seek mental health services when they are available in schools (National Association of School Psychologists [NASP], 2021). Universal screening assists school decision-makers in efficiently identifying at-risk students and placing them in appropriate interventions as well as identifying areas to target universal interventions (Herman, Reinke, Thompson, et al., 2021; Reinke, Thompson, et al., 2018).

**The Early Identification System (EIS;** Herman et al., 2021; Reinke et al., 2022; Thompson et al., 2021) was developed to assist schools in their capacity to identify students who are experiencing social, behavioral, and emotional problems, in order to offer data to inform professional development and prevention activities within the schools. The screener provides data on several indicators that have been linked to serious future mental health and behavior problems. These include externalizing and internalizing problems, attention and academic competence issues, emotional dysregulation, peer relationship problems, bullying behaviors, and school disengagement.

Using the EIS universal screening system, students in grades 3 through 12 complete an assessment about themselves and teachers complete a brief checklist of risk indicators for each student in their classroom, grades kindergarten through 12th grade. These data are collected via a web-based system two to three times per year (fall, winter, and spring). Once a cycle of data collection closes, the system populates a series of reports that schools can use to determine areas of concern that may benefit from prevention or intervention efforts (Reinke, Thompson, et al., 2018). First, schools review school-level reports in which the data are aggregated and presented as the percentage of youth in a building reported to be experiencing a risk indicator (e.g., 28% of youth do not complete their assignments). Using a public health framework, the reports indicate risk by turning red (i.e., high risk) if 20% or more of students are experiencing the problem, meaning that it is an area that would benefit from a universal, evidence-based prevention intervention. When a larger portion of students in a building are reporting or exhibiting risk (i.e., 20% or greater), the use of universal supports is warranted rather than intervening one student at a time. Intervening one student at a time is not an effective use of resources if 20% or more would benefit from supports. If 15–19% of students experience risk, the report turns yellow (some risk), indicating that this area may benefit from prevention efforts. If less than 15% of students experience a risk indicator it turns green (no risk), meaning that is an area of strength for the school. The EIS system was built to make data easy to understand and is linked to an intervention hub that quickly informs schools of readily available, evidence-based interventions that are known to improve outcomes in the specific areas of risk.

In addition to school-level reports that help to guide universal prevention efforts in schools, individual data reports are generated. Similarly, a red, yellow, green system helps school personnel determine who would benefit from selective interventions or indicated interventions. For instance, if several students are yellow, meaning they have some risk but not a high level of risk (red), a school may choose to implement an evidence-based group intervention (e.g., an anger control skills group for externalizing problems), whereas students who are red may be provided with individualized supports such as individual therapy or behavior intervention planning (Reinke, Thompson, et al., 2018). These universal screening data are integral to schools identifying areas of need in order to design effective prevention efforts. When students are exposed to supports that are tied directly to targeted areas of need, significant improvements can be made in their social, emotional, behavioral, and academic functioning (Taylor et al., 2017).

## 3.5 Use a Problem-Solving Approach

Another critical feature of effective prevention practice is the use of a problem-solving approach (Reinke, Sims, et al., 2018). A problem-solving approach first identifies a problem. Data, as described in the prior section, are used to inform what problem(s) to target. Next, once the problem is determined, possible evidence-based interventions are identified. It is imperative that the intervention selected maps directly onto the problem, meaning the intended target problem is the one in which the intervention was developed to prevent. This seems obvious, but this is often where the first mistake is made in prevention efforts – selecting the wrong intervention to prevent the problem. Be sure to investigate evidence-based interventions to ensure they have evidence of preventing the problem in need of targeting. For instance, if universal social behavioral screening data indicate that large numbers of youth in a school are experiencing peer relationship problems and/or emotion dysregulation, a school may decide to implement a universal SEL curriculum that teaches social skills and strategies for understanding and regulating emotions, taught to all students by teachers once a week.

Once an appropriate prevention intervention is identified, the problems-solving approach necessitates that the process by which the intervention will be implemented is determined. Again, using the school-based SEL curriculum as an example, school-based teams would need to determine (a) how to train teachers in using the curriculum, (b) when teachers will teach the curriculum during the school days, (c) how fidelity to the curriculum will be assessed, (d) how teachers who are struggling to implement the curriculum will be supported (i.e., ongoing coaching to teachers to support high fidelity), and (e) how the effectiveness of the intervention will be determined.

It is important, before diving into a new intervention, that the implementation context is considered. For instance, with the example of using a universal SEL curriculum in which teachers are the implementers, it would be important to assess the level of buy-in from teachers in a school building, meaning, are teachers willing to implement the intervention, and do they find the idea of using an SEL curriculum important? Often an intervention can fail if the implementer does not find the need for the intervention important or if they feel like implementing an intervention is not part of their job.

Any barriers to implementation should be determined, and possible solutions for overcoming these barriers should be considered before deploying prevention efforts. This is the often hidden second layer in the problems-solving approach. First, the problem is found, and potential solutions are identified. Then, you determine what will impede the solution from occurring in the intervention context and a solution to these problems is found. For instance, if schools find that teachers feel they do not have time to implement a new SEL curriculum, school administrators may designate a specific time each day for doing so (e.g., 30 minutes first thing after morning announcements, with the school announcements indicating the lesson). If schools find that teachers are unwilling to implement an SEL curriculum because they feel it is not part of their job, they might utilize key stakeholders such as senior teachers respected by other teachers who are willing to implement and promote the idea, or they might instead use school counselors to teach the curriculum as potential solutions. With any intervention, it is important to find issues that might impede implementation with high fidelity, because as noted earlier, interventions that are not implemented with high fidelity may appear to fail, not because the intervention does not work, but because the intervention was simply not implemented.

### 3.6 Monitor Fidelity to Prevention Practices

Several studies suggest that implementing interventions as intended by developers, thereby with fidelity, is associated with better outcomes and increased chances of mirroring efficacy trial results (Durlak & DuPre, 2008). Therefore, in order to make valid decisions about the effects of an intervention, it is necessary to know the fidelity with which it was implemented. Fidelity was once thought of as simply making sure the steps of an intervention were administered, but a more nuanced approach to monitoring fidelity is needed (Reinke et al., 2013). For instance, Dane and Schneider (1998) examined fidelity levels on program outcomes across 162 studies that targeted social, emotional, and behavioral interventions, and delineated the following dimensions as essential to intervention implementation: dosage, adherence, quality of delivery, and participant responsiveness. *Dosage* refers to "how much" of an intervention an individual receives. In skill-based prevention programming, variability can result from the number of total sessions, time spent with the implementer, and duration of the intervention over time. *Adherence* refers to the completion of the required steps involved in the intervention. For example, in skill-based prevention programming, this could include completing the multiple steps it takes to build a skill (e.g., defining the different steps of using the skill, modeling the skill, and providing opportunities to practice the skill). *Quality of delivery* refers to how well the implementer delivers the intervention, which can be associated with *participant responsiveness* or how well the individual engages with the intervention. Quality and participant responsiveness can influence how well individuals acquire and become fluent in the skills being taught.

Each dimension of fidelity may contribute to overall intervention effectiveness (Dane & Schneider, 1998; Reinke et al., 2013).

Strategies for measuring these multifaceted dimensions of fidelity should be developed prior to implementation of a prevention intervention. For instance, dosage can be easily measured by having the interventionist complete an attendance sheet that indicates who attended each time and if they attended for the full session. Adherence is the more typical form of fidelity measured. The interventionist could check off whether they completed each component of an intervention per session. It is often a good idea to have a second person familiar with the intervention to also observe a few sessions to determine whether the intervention is occurring as intended from an outside perspective. To measure quality, the interventionist can ask the participants to complete an evaluation of each session (or overall intervention at the end) of whether they felt the intervention was well delivered, important, and if the skills learned were useful. Lastly, participant responsiveness can be gauged by having the interventionist indicate how engaged each participant was after each session. For instance, if a participant is not engaged (e.g., using phone during session, talking to others), they are unlikely to be receiving the content and therefore unlikely to benefit from the intervention. In fact, research has found that when a participant is more engaged in an intervention, they are more likely to use the skills later (Holmes et al., 2021).

Importantly, the purpose of measuring fidelity is to inform whether the intervention is being implemented as intended and if not, using these data to determine how to improve fidelity. Thus, fidelity checks should occur regularly. For instance, if individuals are missing sessions of an intervention, ensuring that these sessions are made up will be important. If the interventionist is missing a key component of the intervention during sessions or doing so with low quality, providing performance feedback and possibly ongoing coaching to help improve their implementation may be necessary. Coaching is an effective way to support and improve implementation of effective practices (Reinke, Thompson, et al., 2008, 2011; Stormont et al., 2015). Lastly, if participant responsiveness is low, strategies for improving engagement in the intervention should be considered (i.e., adding an incentive program for active participation). Being mindful of fidelity and monitoring it with the intent of improving implementation can increase the likelihood that a prevention intervention is effective.

## 3.7 Use Data to Determine if Prevention Practices Are Working and for Whom

Once an evidence-based intervention that targets the problem in need of prevention has been selected and implementation has begun, in addition to monitoring fidelity, gathering data on whether the intervention is impacting the intended outcome is a critical feature of effective prevention practices. Although many interventions have evidence that they are helpful, it is possible that the intervention may not produce positive outcomes. Gathering data on indicators that are expected to improve is needed to determine whether the intervention is helpful and with whom. Thus, monitoring whether the intervention is improving outcomes is useful.

There are several methods for determining the impact of an intervention, depending on the level of preventive intervention being applied. For instance, if a community-level preventive intervention is being implemented, higher level surveillance data can be used to monitor the impact. As an example, Biglan and colleagues (2000) implemented a community-level youth smoking prevention program. They used school-based surveys of adolescents from the targeted community to monitor the prevalence and reduction in tobacco use over time. The primary expected outcome was that youth would reduce their use of tobacco and/or not initiate smoking. Thus, the surveys asked youth about their use of cigarettes, including how often they smoked (i.e., *never, not even a puff,* up to *daily*) and how many cigarettes they smoked each day, week, and month. These data then provided evidence of whether the intervention was impacting the larger population as intended (i.e., reducing the prevalence of adolescent smoking).

Another example would be using universal screening data over time to determine if prevention efforts are effective. In a recent study (Reinke et al., 2021), the use of social–emotional and behavioral data was used to determine whether a tiered model of support to improve youth mental health was effective. In addition to looking at the overall impact, this study investigated patterns of improvement for youth and whether fidelity to implementation was associated with these patterns. Overall, they found the intervention was improving outcomes for youth over time; that is, on average, students in intervention schools experienced a significant decreasing slope in their self-reported emotional and behavioral symptoms over a three-year period which counters the escalating trends observed for youth across the nation over the same time period (Hellebuyck et al., 2019). The researchers also found that schools that implemented the full model with high fidelity were more likely to have students who demonstrated improvement in their total emotional and behavioral symptoms, whereas schools with lower fidelity were more likely to have students in their school who had increasing symptoms over time (Reinke, Herman, Thompson et al., 2021). This example demonstrates the intersection between fidelity and using data to monitor effectiveness over time and for whom.

When measuring the effectiveness of a preventive intervention on a smaller scale (e.g., an anger control training intervention group with eight children for reducing youth aggression and improving prosocial behaviors), it is important to select measures that will reliably and validly assess the behaviors that the intervention should reduce and/or increase. Determining what measures to utilize, which map onto the appropriate outcomes, should be done prior to the intervention. This way baseline data, or data prior to an intervention occurring, can be gathered. These baseline data provide information about the behavior of the individual prior to receiving a preventive intervention. For instance, if a school-based universal screener identified a student as being at risk for internalizing problems and it was determined that an evidence-based indicated depression prevention intervention was warranted, the implementer would first determine the outcome being prevented or improved. In this case, the implementer would be aiming to reduce symptoms of depression, improve mood, and prevent the onset of a major depressive episode. Furthermore, the implementer could have the youth report on their current depressive symptoms prior to the intervention using a valid measure such as the Patient Health Questionnaire (PHQ)-9 (Kroenke et al., 2001). The PHQ-9 would (a) confirm that depression symptoms are at a level that warrants a preventive intervention and (b) give an initial measure of the student's level of depressive symptoms prior to implementing the individualized intervention. In addition, the implementer may also want to ask questions related to whether the participant meets the clinical criteria for major depression or other depressive disorders prior to beginning the intervention. Next, the youth could progress monitor their mood on a daily basis. These mood ratings would allow for determining whether, over time, the preventive intervention is helping support a more positive mood for the youth. These mood ratings would also be an indicator of whether or not the youth is benefiting session by session. If it is found that the youth is reporting low mood with little change, this report may be an indication that the intervention needs to be modified in some way (e.g., adding more time to sessions to review and practice skills being taught). Importantly, interventions should not be adapted in a way that changes the content or activities critical to the underlying theory of why the intervention works. The implementers could also consider adding another or a more intensive intervention if the youth does not seem to be progressing as intended. Additionally, at the end of the intervention, a post-assessment of the same baseline measures (e.g., PHQ-9 and diagnostic assessment) could be administered. These measures assess whether the full intervention was helpful to the youth. Should it be found that the youth did not benefit from the intervention, a problem-solving approach to determine the next steps can be used. As with fidelity data, progress monitoring data and pre–post data can be used to determine what is working or not working and utilized to determine when modification or additional supports are needed.

In summary, data are a critical feature of effective prevention. Fidelity data tell us if a prevention intervention is being implemented as intended. Baseline data provides the starting point from where we hope to see improvement as a result of an intervention implemented with fidelity. Progress monitoring data give us information that can be used in a problem-solving format and guide whether an intervention needs to be intensified or if additional strategies are needed. Post-assessment data taken after an intervention is completed gives information about whether the intervention worked. If the intervention does not resolve the intended issue, problem-solving teams can use these data to determine (a) was fidelity monitored and demonstrated to be high, (b) would starting a different evidence-based intervention benefit the individual, and/or (c) would extending the intervention along with progress monitoring benefit the individual. Data really guide all aspects of prevention interventions, including identifying the problem to prevent, determining the appropriate preventive intervention, knowing whether the intervention was implemented, and determining whether it worked or needs adjustments.

## 3.8 Build Collaborative Relationships and Use Culturally Responsive Practices

One critically important feature of employing effective prevention practices is building collaborative relationships and using culturally responsive practices. When planning to implement preventive practices, it is imperative that the individuals or communities involved are collaborative partners. Collaboration increases buy-in from key stakeholders, which then improves the likelihood that the preventive efforts are considered important and necessary. These collaborations also make it more likely that the preventive intervention identified and implemented will be relevant to the cultural context of those being impacted. Preventive interventions sought out by stakeholders, which will benefit the population in ways that are seen as both important and relevant, are more likely to be implemented. These interventions, if successfully applied and invested in, will produce positive outcomes.

In particular, large-scale preventive initiatives can easily fail if those who are involved in implementing and monitoring are not full partners in the process. As a psychologist or counselor, it would be challenging to start something like a school-based multitiered model of prevention and intervention for youth mental health without having school administration, teachers, and even students on board. As an example, seven years ago we began working in partnership with six school districts in our community to implement such a model (Reinke, Thompson, et al., 2018). The first step in this process was conducting a needs assessment with the schools to identify the problem by talking with stakeholders, students, and parents. These data indicated that schools wanted and needed a systematic process for identifying youth who would benefit from mental health supports, professional development for school personnel in supporting mental health, a coordinated effort across school districts to communicate student needs when students transferred between schools, and, lastly, universal prevention efforts to reduce the number of students in need of supports. These data were reviewed by all partners, and next steps were developed to begin creating a comprehensive model to identify, prevent, and intervene in youth mental health. As a result, the EIS screener was developed and piloted in partnership with the schools. We wanted to develop a screener that was free to the schools, that did not overidentify youth in schools with low resources, and that captured a broad range of risk. Due to working alongside our school partners, we were able to develop procedures and processes that would be accepted by a large portion of the implementers (e.g., schools and school personnel).

Initially, we had upper school administration commitment and had many technical assistance resources in place to support schools, but not every school building was on board. We needed to constantly evaluate who was more or less willing to implement and why. Twice a year, we asked for stakeholder feedback. These data are important for ongoing quality improvement in the approach. We noticed that teachers and students provided feedback that they did not understand how the data from the universal screener were being used. This was a clear area for improvement. In response, we conducted focus groups with students and teachers to help us understand their perspective of the screener, data reports, and methods currently used, and to ask for ideas for improvement. In addition, we are currently forming student advisory groups, with whom we will meet with a minimum of three times a year to get their input on all aspects of the model. We are also in the process of recruiting teachers and students to develop social marking materials for their peers about the universal screener and how it is used to help with understanding and reduce distrust. These are just some of our initial ideas for building stronger partnerships among those involved in this school-based prevention initiative.

In addition, we found that Black students were reporting higher levels of mental health stigma compared to peers from other racial backgrounds. As a result, we conducted focus groups with Black high school students who offered important perspectives and ideas for improving our approach in schools. We also hired a group of these Black students as members of our research team to develop culturally responsive social media materials to reach more students who may otherwise not participate in the preventive intervention. Importantly, ensuring that the preventive intervention fits the context and culture of those receiving the intervention will increase the likelihood of success. In sum, actions that can carry prevention efforts forward in a sustainable manner consist of (a) working with the community to identify problems, rather than telling them what they are; (b) working alongside the key stakeholders and implementers; (c) soliciting feedback; (d) gathering data along the way to ensure ongoing quality improvement; and (e) being transparent and open to making needed changes. Further, in our research efforts to disseminate the model, we have counselors, psychologists, and other key stakeholders (i.e., students) present alongside us at local, state, and national conferences presenting findings from our research partnerships. We authentically view those with whom we work alongside in schools as partners in all aspects of the prevention cycle.

## 3.9 Conclusion

In this chapter, critical features of effective prevention practices were reviewed. By understanding the science behind prevention, including the evidence of prevention interventions and the importance of implementation in the overall process of prevention efforts, you have a grounding in how to be a prevention scientist and practitioner. Using data to identify the problem, determine the appropriate interventions, monitor fidelity of implementation, and progress monitor and determine effectiveness of intervention is key. Data help determine what intervention, with whom, and how well an intervention is working. Understanding the multitiered, public health approach to prevention also allows you to think about how societal problems can be conquered on a larger scale, rather than one person at a time. As psychologists and counselors, we have the ability to work across systems and settings. The skills we bring to the prevention effort are crucial. Finding ways to contribute to universal efforts, perhaps through indirect work such as providing professional development and coaching other implementers, may be one way to expand your current work. Learning about and implementing selective and indicative preventive interventions and/ or supporting others to do so with fidelity are other avenues for delving into preventive efforts. Preventing the next generation from some of the current problems faced in our society is an important endeavor that we can all embrace.

## References

Biglan, A, Ary, D., Smolkowski, K., Duncan, T., Black, C. (2000). A randomized controlled trial of a community intervention to prevent adolescent tobacco use. *Tobacco Control*, 24–32. doi.org/10.1136/tc.9.1.24

Dane, A. V., & Schneider, B. H. (1998). Program integrity in primary and early secondary prevention: Are implementation effects out of control? *Clinical Psychology Review*, *18*(1), 23–45. doi.org/10.1016/S0272-7358(97)00043-3

Durlak, J. A., & DuPre, E. P. (2008). Implementation matters: A review of research on the influence of implementation on program outcomes and the factors affecting implementation. *American Journal of Community Psychology*, *41*(3), 327–350. doi .org/10.1007/s10464-008-9165-0

Fishbein, D. (2021). The pivotal role of prevention science in this syndemic. *Prevention Science*, *22*(1), 94–99. doi.org/10.1007/s11121-020-01180-w

Greenberg, M., Domitrovich, C., Weissberg, R., & Durlak, J. (2017). Social and emotional learning as a public health approach to education. *The Future of Children*, *27*(1), 13–32.

Hellebuyck, M., Halpern, M., Nguyen, T., & Fritze, D. (2019). *The state of mental health in America 2019*. Mental Health America. Retrieved from https://mhanational.org/sites/default/files/2019-09/2019%20MH%20in%20America%20Final.pdf

Herman, K. C., Reinke, W. M., Huang, F. L., Thompson, A. M., & Doyle-Baker, L. (2021). Investigating the psychometric properties of the Early Identification System – Student report in a middle school sample. *School Psychology*, *36*(1), 34–46. doi.org/10.1037/spq0000414

Herman, K. C., Reinke, W. M., & Thompson, A. (2019). Prevention science: An approach to inform the future of school psychology. In M. Burns (Ed.), *Introduction to school psychology: Controversies and current practice* (pp. 195–213). Oxford University Press.

Herman, K. C., Reinke, W. M., & Thompson, A. (2020). Prevention science as a platform for solving major societal problems and improving population health. *Journal of Prevention and Health Promotion*, *1*(1), 131–151. doi.org/10.1177/2632077020948786

Herman, K. C., Reinke, W. M., Thompson, A., & Hawley, K. (2019). The Missouri Prevention Center: A multidisciplinary approach to reducing the societal prevalence and burden of youth mental health problems. *American Psychologist*, *74*(3), 315–328. doi.org/10.1037/amp0000433

Herman, K. C., Reinke, W. M., Thompson, A., Hawley, K., Wallis, K., Stormont, M., & Peters, C. (2021). A public health approach to reducing the societal prevalence and burden of youth mental health problems: Introduction to the special issue. *School Psychology Review*, *50*(1), 8–16. doi.org/10.1080/2372966X.2020.1827682

Holmes, S. R., Reinke, W. M., Herman, K. C., & David, K. B. (2021). An examination of teacher engagement in intervention training and sustained intervention implementation. *School Mental Health*, *14*, 63–72.

Kellam, S. G., Koretz, D., & Mościcki, E. K. (1999). Core elements of developmental epidemiologically based prevention research. *American Journal of Community Psychology*, *27*(4), 463–482. doi.org/10.1023/A:1022129127298

Kelly, B., & Perkins, D. F. (2012). *Handbook of implementation science for psychology in education*. Cambridge University Press.

Kroenke, K., Spitzer, R. L., Williams, J. B. (2001). The PHQ-9: Validity of a brief depression severity measure. *Journal of General Internal Medicine*, *16*(9), 606–13. doi.org/10.1046/j.1525-1497.2001.016009606.x. PMID: 11556941; PMCID: PMC1495268.

Le, L., Esturas, A. C., Mihalopoulos, C., Chiotelis, O., Bucholc, J., et al. (2021). Cost-effectiveness evidence of mental health prevention and promotion interventions: A systematic review of economic evaluations. *PLOS Medicine*, *18*(5), e1003606. doi.org/10.1371/journal.pmed.1003606

National Association of School Psychologists. (2021). Comprehensive School-Based Mental and Behavioral Health Services and School Psychologists [handout]. Author.

National Prevention Science Coalition. (2019). *What is prevention science?* www.npscoalition.org/_files/ugd/773dc1_0a8e24aa6e794231adce127ee935379e.pdf

National Research Council and Institute of Medicine. (2009). *Preventing mental, emotional, and behavioral disorders among young people: Progress and possibilities*. Washington, DC: National Academies Press.

Offord, D. R., Kraemer, H. C., Kazdin, A. E., Jensen, P. S., & Harrington, R. (1998). Lowering the burden of suffering from child psychiatric disorder: trade-offs among clinical, targeted, and universal interventions. *Journal of the American Academy of Child and Adolescent Psychiatry*, *37*(7), 686–694. doi.org/10.1097/00004583-199807000-00007

Purtle, J., Nelson, K. L., Counts, N. Z., & Yudell, M. (2020). Population-based approaches to mental health: History, strategies, and evidence. *Annual Review of Public Health*, *41*, 201–221. doi.org/10.1146/annurev-publhealth-040119-094247

Reinke, W. M., Herman, K. C., Huang, F., McCall, C., Holmes, S., Thompson, A., & Owens, S. (2022). Examining the factor structure and concurrent and predictive validity of the Early Identification System – Student Report in an elementary school sample. *Journal of School Psychology*, *90*(1), 114–134. doi.org/10.1016/j.jsp.2021.10.001

Reinke, W. M., Herman, K. C., & Sprick, R. (2011). *Motivational interviewing for effective classroom management: The classroom check-up*. New York: Guilford Press.

Reinke, W. M., Herman, K. C., Stormont, M., & Dong, N. (2021). Effects of the Incredible Years Teacher Classroom Management Training Program on elementary students with disabilities. *Remedial and Special Education*, *42*(1), 7–17. doi.org/10.1177/0741932520937442

Reinke, W. M., Herman, K. C., Stormont, M., Newcomer, L., & David, K. (2013). Illustrating the multiple facets and levels of fidelity of implementation to a teacher classroom management intervention. *Administration and Policy in Mental Health and Mental Health Services Research*, *40*(6), 494–506. doi.org/10.1007/s10488-013-0496-2

Reinke, W. M., Herman, K. C., Thompson, A., McCall, C., Copeland, C., Holmes, S., & Owens, S., (2021). Investigating the longitudinal association between fidelity to a large-scale comprehensive school mental health prevention and intervention model and student outcomes. *School Psychology Review*, *50*(1), 17–29. doi.org/10.1080/2372966X.2020.1870869

Reinke, W. M., Lewis-Palmer, T., & Merrell, K. (2008). The classroom check-up: A class-wide consultation model for increasing praise and decreasing disruptive behavior. *School Psychology Review*, *37*(3), 315–332. doi.org/10.1080/02796015.2008.12087879

Reinke, W. M., Sims, W. Cohen, D., & Herman, K. C. (2018). Problem-solving within an RTI framework: Roles and functions of effective teams. In Paige C. Pullen & Michael J. Kennedy (Eds.), *Handbook of response to intervention and multi-tiered systems of support* (pp. 80–103). Routledge.

Reinke, W. M., Thompson, A. Herman, K. C., Holmes, S., Owens, S., Cohen, D., Tanner-Jones, L., Henry, L., Green, A., Copeland, C., & County Schools Mental Health Coalition (2018). The County Schools Mental Health Coalition: A model for community-level impact. *School Mental Health*, *10*(2), 173–180. doi.org/10.1007/s12310-017-9227-2

Rose, G. (1992). *The strategy of preventive medicine*. Oxford University Press.

Stormont, M., Reinke, W. M., & Herman, K. C. (2010). Using prevention science to address mental health issues in schools. *Psychology in the Schools*, 47, 1–4.

Stormont, M., Reinke, W. M., Herman, K. C., & Lemke, E. (2012). *Academic and Behavior Supports for At-Risk Students: Tier 2 Interventions*. New York: Guilford Press.

Stormont, M., Reinke, W. M., Newcomer, L., Marchese, D., & Lewis, C. (2015). Coaching teachers' use of social behavior interventions to improve children's outcomes: A review of the literature. *Journal of Positive Behavior Interventions, 17*(2), 69–82. doi.org/10.1177/1098300714550657

Substance Abuse and Mental Health Services Administration. (2012), *Data-based planning for effective prevention: State epidemiological outcomes workgroups, HHS Publication No. (SMA) 12–4724*. Substance Abuse and Mental Health Services Administration.

Taylor, R. D., Oberle, E., Durlak, J. A., & Weissberg, R. P. (2017). Promoting positive youth development through school-based social and emotional learning interventions: A meta-analysis of follow-up effects. *Child Development, 88*(4), 1156–1171. doi .org/10.1111/cdev.12864

Thompson, A., Huang, F., Smith, T., Reinke, W. M., & Herman, K. C. (2021). Confirmatory factor structure and predictive validity of the Early Identification System-Student Report in a community sample of high school students. *School Mental Health, 13*(1), 28–40. doi.org/10.1007/s12310-020-09396-5

Wiltsey, Stirman, S., & Beidas, R. S. (2020). Expanding the reach of psychological science through implementation science: Introduction to the special issue. *American Psychologist, 75*(8), 1033–1037. doi.org/.1037/amp0000774. PMID: 33252942; PMCID: PMC8543736

PART TWO

# PREVENTION WITH CHILDREN AND YOUTH

# 4 Culturally Relevant Prevention Interventions for African American Children and Families: Lessons Learned from "Real-World" Implementation of the Black Parenting Strengths and Strategies – Racialized Short (BPSS-RS) Program

Stephanie Irby Coard, Ashley G. Evans, and Keadija C. Wiley

> May you find pride in knowing that you bear the image of your Creator. May you stand tall and strong against the winds of injustice when they blow with threats of inferiority.
>
> —Charlotte Betts, Dear Black Child … *A Love Letter from Your Parents*

In recent decades, research on racial discrimination and mental health has been a rapidly growing area of scientific investigation. We live in a racialized society plagued with an overarching racial bias and inequality system. Racism is a core determinant of health and well-being and has a profound impact on youth and families. Multiple comorbid negative psychological and physical health outcomes, both short and long-term, are well documented (Heard-Garris, 2018; Neblett, 2019; Pachter & Coll, 2009; Priest et al., 2013; Trent et al., 2019; U.S. Department of Health and Human Services, 2001). Models of health disparities have specifically highlighted the role that rumination and anticipation of future discrimination have in exerting a toxic effect on mental health, including racial vigilance, race rejection sensitivity, and imposter syndrome (Harrell et al., 2011; Mendoza-Denton et al., 2002). African Americans bear the brunt of these effects (Lloyd et al., 2021).

Given this reality, African American parents understand the overall influence that racism has on their family functioning, the importance of racial-ethnic socialization (RES), and engagement in developmentally appropriate race-related discussions with children. A significant body of research demonstrates that African American youth benefit from parental RES messages that aim to foster a strong, positive racial-ethnic identity and prepare youth to cope with experiences of racism and discrimination (Umaña-Taylor & Hill, 2020). According to recent meta-analyses, RES messages are associated with a stronger sense of commitment to and pride in one's group (Huguley et al., 2019), greater academic motivation, performance, and engagement (Wang et al., 2020b), and improved psychosocial outcomes (Wang et al., 2020a). Further, parental RES messages can prepare youth to cope with experiences of discrimination and buffer the damaging effects of these experiences on health and well-being (Brown & Tylka, 2011).

The negative impacts of racism and discrimination on African American youth and families are important social issues that speak to specific needs and concerns that warrant attention in designing interventions targeting this group. It is argued that programs targeting African American youth and families must be both culturally responsive (i.e., responsive to the realities of racism and the socio political realities and obstacles linked to its existence) and culturally relevant (i.e., attend to specific parenting strategies that African Americans use to navigate, insulate, and lessen the negative and often deleterious consequences that accompany racial group status). For African American parents, raising children to be socially, emotionally, and behaviorally competent and thrive in a society plagued by racial barriers and inequities is a parental priority. A key need is to intervene with African American parents to build their efficacy in engaging in effective RES with their youth with the goal of disrupting the harmful effects of discrimination and fostering youth well-being. The prevention field can do more to address these inequities by creating and providing high-quality and culturally appropriate programming and services to specific racial and ethnic groups, while also demonstrating effectiveness in improving targeted outcomes.

This chapter focuses on the Black Parenting Strengths and Strategies (BPSS) program. BPSS is a parenting intervention developed to incorporate the most successful strategies used by parenting and child development specialists, while drawing on the strengths, unique parental strategies, and processes inherent in Black families (e.g., racial ethnic socialization). BPSS was initially developed in response to the lack of evidence-based interventions that attend to the promotion of social, behavioral, and cultural competence through the lived experiences of Black/African American families. The *efficacy* (highly controlled lab setting) for BPSS has been previously established (Coard et al., 2007), and a description of the initial development, added value, challenges, and lessons learned in addressing racial, ethnic, and cultural factors, nuances, and competencies in both content and delivery adaptations has also been published (Coard et al., 2013). Interested in how BPSS fares when implemented in less controlled settings (real-world contexts), BPSS was subsequently evaluated via an *effectiveness* study (Coard et al., 2021), which provided additional support for the feasibility and receptibility of the BPSS program and highlighted its potential effectiveness.

We describe the process undertaken as part of the *effectiveness* study to evaluate BPSS. That is, we describe its "real world" implementation across multiple community centers/settings servicing Black/African American families. Informed by a community-based participatory approach (i.e., the process for collaborative research between a team of academic researchers and established community centers), the objectives are to (a) provide the rationale for and an overview of the BPSS and its warranted modification; (b) describe the translational process (efficacy to effectiveness) in implementing BPSS; (c) outline lessons learned and the challenges of research carried out in established community centers; and (d) summarize the recommendations for practitioners' use of BPSS.

## 4.1 The Rationale for the Black Parenting Strengths and Strategies (BPSS) Program

### 4.1.1 Racial-Ethnic Socialization and Efficacy among African American Families

As a result of racism, ethnic-racial discrimination, and structural inequalities in the United States, African Americans face the risk of negative emotional, psychological, and physical ramifications of mistreatment and racism (Neblett, 2019). This reality prompts African American families to find ways to support their youth to thrive in the racialized context of the United States. Further, families endeavor to teach their children about the cultural realms in which they find themselves. Boykin (1986) conceptualized the triple quandary theory including (a) "mainstream" experience that refers to individualistic and competitive beliefs and values common to the majority culture within the United States; (b) the "minority" experience that refers to coping strategies and defense mechanisms developed in response to oppression and social stratification, and (c) the "Afro-cultural experience" that refers to cultural aspects such as a value for kinship and extended family ties.

Boykin's classic theory lays the foundation for what we now refer to as RES. That is, families of color tend to engage in *cultural socialization*, whereby they provide children with messages about their cultural histories, traditions, legacies, beliefs, customs, and practices as well as instill pride in their heritage (Hughes et al., 2016). These messages typically begin in early childhood and persist throughout development as parents lay the foundation for a strong racial-ethnic identification and knowledge of cultural practices. Given the marginalization of African Americans, African American parents frequently deliver *preparation for bias* messages, that is, messages warning their children about potential discrimination and arming them with coping skills to confront this discrimination (Priest et al., 2014). Due to their complexity, these messages may be initiated later in development, typically in early adolescence (Priest et al., 2014), as parents attempt to wait until they perceive their child as cognitively ready to process race, understand racism, and as resilient enough to cope with the emotional ramifications that come with living in a racist society.

While the goal is to impart messages that are consistent with a child's emotional readiness and cognitive abilities, the racist, discriminatory, and structural inequalities that African American youth face are not developmental in nature. That is, African American youth are frequently the direct or observed target of racially discriminatory experiences that warrant immediate attention and preparation in a manner that African American parents do not have the luxury of ignoring. Black parents are more likely to deliver *preparation for bias* messages relative to other racial groups (Hughes et al., 2006; Priest et al., 2014) These realities place the perception of urgency in the minds of African American parents, and they strive to rapidly establish resilience and strength in their child(ren). This perceived resilience stems from fostering cognitive and emotional development and foundational racial identity development instilled through cultural pride socialization.

Although other types of racial-ethnic messages have also been examined (e.g., *egalitarian* messages that focus on shared humanity across groups and treating everyone equally), the BPSS intervention targeted *cultural socialization* and *preparation for bias* messages, due to their racial-ethnic salience and empirical support for the role they play in promoting positive youth outcomes. For *cultural socialization*, it is evident that messages aimed at strengthening racial identity, teaching about cultural beliefs and practices, and focusing on self-worth and pride support positive adaptation (e.g., Wang et al., 2020a) can buffer against the negative effect of racial discrimination on psychosocial outcomes in youth (e.g., Cheeks et al., 2020; Dotterer & James, 2018; Harris-Britt et al., 2007; Neblett et al., 2008). However, while *preparation for bias* messages may be crucial in arming youth with skills to deal with experiences of discrimination (Harris-Britt et al., 2007), these messages do not consistently predict adaptive functioning (Huguley et al., 2019; Wang, Smith, et al., 2020a). While there is not substantial literature examining the moderating effect of *preparation for bias* messages on the impact of racial discrimination, studies point to a nuanced relationship. For example, Dotterer and James (2018) showed that *preparation for bias* messages exacerbated the relationship between discrimination and depressive symptoms in a sample of African American middle school youth. On the other hand, in a daily diary study, Cheeks et al. (2020) found that *preparation for bias* messages mitigated the impact of discrimination on negative affect on the following day (although not concurrently) in a different sample of African American adolescents. Other work points to moderate amounts of *preparation for bias* messages being optimal in protecting youth when facing discrimination (Harris-Britt et al., 2007). Further, how *preparation for bias* messages mitigates risk may be dependent on other parenting processes, like parental warmth and child-focused parenting (Smalls, 2010). *Preparation for bias* messages may also be the most protective when delivered in conjunction with messages instilling pride and self-worth (cultural socialization), as profiles that consisted of a balance of these types of messages buffered the relation of discrimination to negative outcomes in African American youth when faced with greater discrimination (Neblett et al., 2008). Taken together, this literature suggests that *preparation for bias* messages has the potential to mitigate the relationship between discrimination and negative outcomes in African American youth, but these messages must be delivered in the context of a warm relationship and along with *cultural socialization* messages.

The differential outcomes in the *preparation for bias* literature may potentially be a result of the fact that these messages are more complex and require more parental skills and regulation of emotions (e.g., management of cultural pride and preparation of bias messages while simultaneously managing their own race-related stress and potential racial trauma). *Preparation for bias* messages is contingent upon parents' own experiences with racism (Osborne et al., 2020). Parents struggle with how to provide balanced messages that attend to developmental readiness, build skills to cope with discrimination, and not overinflate distrust for other groups (Hughes et al., 2006). Further, the emotional tone and delivery of parental racial socialization may also influence how youth make sense of these messages and whether these conversations ultimately strengthen the parent–child relationship (Anderson et al., 2018; Dotterer & James, 2018; Smalls, 2009).

## 4.2 Racial-Ethnic Socialization Interventions

Considering the importance of racial socialization, there is value in considering culturally based parenting practices and incorporating RES in interventions targeting African American families. Currently, the number of interventions that successfully include culturally relevant parenting practices within the curriculum is few (SAAF, Brody et al., 2004; BPSS, Coard et al., 2007; EMBRace, Anderson et al., 2018). To our knowledge, there are only three interventions that have focused on facilitating and supporting parents' use of RES. All three focus on Black families and view the use of RES as an essential and protective aspect of parenting children of color. *The Strong African American Families (SAAF) prevention program* was developed for rural African American families with middle school-aged youth (Murry et al., 2007). The seven-session family prevention program targeted decreasing engagement in substance use and sexual risk behaviors in African American youth by supporting positive parenting practices with a specific focus on racial socialization through the promotion of racial pride and coping with discrimination. In a randomized control longitudinal trial, improvement in parenting processes led to significant decreases in substance use, conduct problems, and sexual risk-taking (Brody et al., 2006a, 2006b; Murry et al., 2007). Socialization messages were linked to better academic outcomes through youth's increases in self-esteem and racial pride (Murry et al., 2009). The authors conclude that targeting adaptive racial socialization messages in preadolescence was key to establishing the long-term impact of the broader intervention itself (Murry et al., 2007, 2009). *The EMBRace program* (Engaging, Managing, and Bonding through Race) is a five-session manualized intervention that was developed to target racial socialization processes in Black families with early adolescents (Anderson et al., 2018). The intervention provides information about types of RES messages (e.g., cultural socialization, preparation for bias) with a focus on coping and message delivery (e.g., building familial bonds). In a pilot study with 10 families of African American 10- to 14-year-old youth, participants in EMBRace reported that the intervention was useful and taught important skills, and there was evidence for both parents and youth engaging in more coping responses throughout the five sessions.

BPSS is an evidenced-based program that aims to promote cultural, social, and behavioral health among African American families, and consideration of universal and culturally specific strategies warrants attention. BPSS (Coard et al., 2007) is an evidence-based parenting program designed to promote cultural, social, and emotional health and academic success in elementary-age African American children. The 12-session BPSS is a strength- and culturally based intervention that integrates evidenced-based universal parenting strategies with the inherent strengths and processes empirically found in Black families (e.g., RES). This body of work demonstrates that Black/African American families welcome interventions that focus on RES and view them as critical to their child's development. Furthermore, these interventions can lead to effective coping, positive parenting practices, and improvement in youth behavioral outcomes. This body of work demonstrates Black/African American parents benefit from not only increasing their knowledge about key RES processes but understanding its relationship to their parenting goals and child outcome.

## 4.3 Black Parenting Strengths and Strategies (BPSS) Program

BPSS was initially developed in response to the lack of evidence-based interventions that spoke to the lived experiences of families of color, particularly Black/African American families. BPSS was developed with the intent of integrating evidenced-based preventive intervention research and practice with culturally relevant theories and approaches specific to Black child development and Black family strengths. When this program was initially developed, research that considered culturally specific approaches and relevant theories was void in the area of prevention science. The BPSS program has been developed to incorporate universal parental processes (monitoring, positive parenting, discipline) and the most successful strategies used by parenting and child development specialists, while drawing on the strengths, unique parental strategies, and processes inherent in African American families (e.g., racial socialization). BPSS was tested (Coard et al., 2007) via a randomized waitlist-controlled pilot study with 38 families assigned to the BPSS prevention program ($n$ = 16) or to a wait-list control condition. Relative to control caregivers, intervention caregivers used significantly more racial socialization strategies, positive parenting practices, and less harsh discipline. Also, despite caregivers' multiple risk factors (e.g., residing in financially underresourced households and communities), high rates of attendance and satisfaction were achieved. The results of this study support the feasibility, acceptability, and efficacy of this culturally relevant intervention program. BPSS successfully balances the need for integrity, fidelity, and cultural specificity in the adaptation and development of interventions. Coard et al. (2013) describe the challenges, added value, and lessons learned in doing so, and address racial, ethnic, and cultural factors, nuances, and competencies in both content and delivery adaptations.

Interested in how BPSS compares when implemented in the community's real-world realm, it was recently abbreviated by undergoing a dismantling and community-centered approach in response to an expressed need in the community. This dismantling resulted in Black Parenting Strengths and Strategies – Racialized Short (BPSS-RS), a three-week version of the 12-week intervention composed solely of racialized parenting and RES components. The evaluation of BPSS-RS (Coard et al., 2021) sought to determine its effectiveness in a real-world community-based setting void of the constraints of a heavily controlled pilot. The results of this study provide additional support for the feasibility and receptibility of the BPSS program and highlight the effectiveness of culturally relevant intervention programs in improving parenting strategies believed to be most instrumental in helping youth respond to racism and fostering African American parents' use of culturally relevant coping strategies with their children (i.e., racial socialization) to guard against the negative effects of racial discrimination and racism.

## 4.4 Translational Process (Efficacy to Effectiveness)

The dismantling of BPSS in the transition from *efficacy* (lab-centered) to *effectiveness* (a real-world practice application) involved unique considerations and conceptual shifts in (a) intervention design and conceptualization; (b) recruitment, participant selection, and characteristics; (c) intervention facilitators and delivery context; and (d) measurement and methodology, each of which resulted in lessons learned.

## 4.5 Intervention Design and Conceptualization

### 4.5.1 Focus on Community-Based Participatory Research and Organizational Context

This implementation was grounded in a community-based participatory research (CBPR) model (Israel et al., 2005), where the emphasis was on bringing BPSS to Black/African American families in a community in need and in collaboration with community partners. The importance of organizational context to the success of interventions is undeniable. For this study, we implemented the BPSS intervention across three ($N = 3$) nonprofit community center (NCC) settings located in central North Carolina in collaboration with center leadership and staff. The NCC settings all predominately served Black/African American youth and families but varied in context and with unique and historical significance.

The first NCC is a recreation center housed in a community with a unique story of perseverance. The community became a haven for ex-slaves and African American migrants through the turn of the century. Over time, the community has faced hardships of many kinds, the most obvious being racism. Despite the disruption urban renewal caused within the community, the residents of this community continue to exhibit a fierce sense of pride in their community to this day. The second NCC is the oldest and largest multicultural women's organization in the world. The organization is dedicated to eliminating racism, empowering women, and promoting peace, justice, freedom, and dignity for all. The third NCC is housed on the campus of the first state-supported liberal arts college for African American students in North Carolina. This NCC works to enhance the quality of life for individuals and families in a variety of contexts via preschool programs, youth programs, family resource centers, childcare resources and referral agencies, and social services. All three of the NCCs are established in the community with close ties and commitments to the betterment of Black/African American families and communities. As such, it was key that these community partners have a voice in all aspects of the research process. Through multiple discussions via in-person site visits and phone meetings with center directors and program leads, center needs were clearly articulated. Given the sociopolitical climate and racial unrest during this time, NCCs were concerned with its impact on the families, parents, and children they served. Given the direct impact of racism and discrimination on educational outcomes and psychological well-being (Jones & Neblett, 2019; Serchen et al., 2020), public discussions about race and racism had increased in volume and intensity. NCC leadership and staffers felt a heightened sense of responsibility to acknowledge and help address the realities of these lived experiences. NCC staff collectively voiced the importance of implementing a program to support Black/African American parents and families which was intensive (i.e., "short and sweet"). It addressed what they perceived as immediate needs and concerns of African American families participating in their programming (i.e., navigating parenting in the context of racism and discrimination). NCCs also sought a program that would be sustainable within the context of their existing and typically hectic programming schedule. We sought guidance from center leadership and staff on many important decisions, such as effective recruitment strategies and intervention delivery methods that would fit within their respective NCC milieu. Organizational leadership provided the necessary preliminary data on aspects of the organizational context. This included social environment and physical facilities, organizational structure and resources, staffing roles and responsibilities, population(s) served, and NCC participant profiles. The purpose of this intentional pre-assessment was to uncover as many details as possible to set the context for which implementation would take place. Furthermore, we needed to determine the center intervention fit. The data obtained provided insight into the level of difficulty expected in the implementation process and revealed general structural and process factors warranting attention. Detailed meeting logs kept by the intervention director later illuminated the context issues believed to bolster or weaken the intervention's effectiveness.

## 4.6 Core Elements, Length, and Dosage

The efficiency and portability of interventions are key in effectiveness studies. An initial step in our effectiveness study involved determining the optimal dosage of BPSS that could produce the desired outcomes, be of optimal length, and be easy to implement. BPSS required dismantling in order to respond effectively to these expressed needs. The goal was a brief parenting intervention designed for low-income African American families that attend to African American parenting concerns thought to encumber their parenting practices, along with identifying inherent strengths and promoting resilience in African American parents and children. The Black Parenting Strengths and Strategies – Racialized Short (BPSS-RS) program was comprised solely of BPSS RES and racialized parenting components (as opposed to universal and racialized components found in the original version). The racialized parenting components were extracted from each of the 12 sessions and condensed to address 3 broad focal areas: *Parenting in Context: Yourselves as Black Parents* and Black Discipline, *Young Children and Racial-Ethnic Matters: Development and Competence*, and *Black Children and the School and Community Experience: Racial Ethic Learning, Literacy, and Advocacy.* Across the three areas, parents learned content and skills known to be most instrumental in assisting youth to respond to racism, discrimination, and fostering African American parents' use of culturally relevant coping strategies with their children (i.e., RES) to guard against the negative effects of racism and discrimination (cultural pride, preparation for bias). Each session consisted of discussion, handouts, and role-playing exercises. Participants were also given session "homework" to encourage the generalization of content and skills to their home and community settings.

BPSS-RS addressed racial socialization by defining the concept, assisting parents in identifying their own practices, and strengthening and reinforcing their parenting skills with a better understanding of the process and its effects on their children. In this session, parents learned that the racial socialization process promotes racism preparation by emphasizing racial barriers, strategic racial protocol, and adaptive racial orientation, racial pride by emphasizing racial and ethnic pride and commitment to cultural history and heritage, racial equality by emphasizing humanitarianism and multiethnic coexistence, and achievement by emphasizing individual and academic achievement and good work ethic. Additionally, the session emphasized the positive impact racial socialization can have on a child's racial competence, academic achievement, self-efficacy, and self-esteem. Finally, the BPSS-RS model encouraged healthy and productive communications regarding race-related issues between Black parents and their children. For example, the parents are facilitated in an open group discussion of various race-related topics in order to foster collaborative efforts in developing relevant solutions and sharing ideas. Several of the topics of discussion included specific challenges faced by Black boys in society, how to debunk negative stereotypes, how to handle racial incidences, and understanding how race influences behavior.

BPSS-RS incorporated its model of ineffective communication to illustrate how racism, prejudice, and discrimination can cause increased distress for the Black family, in addition to the normal daily life stressors. According to the model, this increase in distress perpetuates ineffective communications that often lead to a breakdown of family relationships. Black families' relationships and individual member success may be extremely vulnerable to racism, prejudice, and discrimination, particularly when they lack racial identity. Racial identity refers to one's acceptance and internalization of the race to which one belongs. This includes embracing the strengths and vulnerabilities of the group. Racism, prejudice, and discrimination can exploit minoritized members' uncertainty and lack of commitment to their race. One of the many ways in which the BPSS model addresses the issue of racial identity with Black families is through the illustration of Black culture and success outside of the immediate family structure. The objective was to provide parents with examples of ways in which Blacks have contributed to America and abroad. For example, in BPSS-RS, the developer exposed parents to a chronological evolution of Black plight from the slave trades of the 1500s to more current events beginning with the Black Lives Movement in 2013. An essential purpose of this session was to equip parents with a knowledge base from which to educate their children on the many struggles and accomplishments of Blacks.

## 4.7 Recruitment, Participant Selection, and Characteristics

Parents/caregivers were recruited on-site at NCCs, as well as through flyers, word of mouth, and local community networks. BPSS-RS was implemented with 28 parents/caregivers who racially-ethnically self-identified as Black/African American. The mean age for this sample of caregivers was 38.4 years ($SD = 8.2$). Their children consisted of 15 girls and 13 boys, with a mean age of 8 years and 4 months ($SD = 2.6$). Among primary caregivers, 26 were biological mothers, one was a biological father, and one was the target child's biological aunt who was identified as the primary caregiver. Fifty percent of the caregivers were single mothers, 82.1% had some college education, and 53.6% of the caregivers had a household gross income of $25,000 or less. While the BPSS efficacy trial was restricted to parents of children ages 5 and 6, the *effectiveness* study warranted flexibility and relaxation of the age requirements given the populations served by the NCCs. Parents of children of all ages were welcome to participate. Furthermore, while assessments were completed on the primary caregiver only, all family members (kin or chosen) were permitted to participate in the intervention. Flexibility in accommodating NCCs and families was key.

The intervention was administered in the respective NCC settings to accommodate participants and to reduce perceptions of unequal power between researchers and participants. Doing so aided in recruitment efforts and in establishing familiarity among participants. The community agencies referred the BPSS-RS to eligible participants and advocated for the program's benefit. Participants tended to be current participants in NCC programming. Others resided in the area and were familiar with the NCC. Implementing BPSS-RS in NCC settings allowed for greater access to/for families by eliminating barriers related to trust, location, and transportation for participants.

## 4.8 Intervention Facilitators and Delivery Context

Across the three sites, BPSS-RS sessions were conducted via group format conducted by two Black/African American facilitators. Facilitators ranged in levels of experience and were trained in the BPSS-RS curriculum by the first author (BPSS and BPSS-RS developer). Paraprofessionals consisted of students and staff, while professionals were doctoral level and clinically trained. Parent groups were held in a room separate from the youth area. Parent groups were conducted by a professional and a paraprofessional. Youth group sessions were facilitated by paraprofessionals only. Parenting groups were consistently led by two facilitators, regardless of the number in attendance (ranging from 5 to 10 parents/caretakers per group across groups), and significant fluctuations in the youth attendance warranted additional staffing ranging from 2 to 4 facilitators per group. At times restrictions in physical space (due to existing programming), distracting noise levels, and privacy challenges resulted in last-minute room shifts and on-the-spot shuffling. While BPSS-RS is manualized, flexibility in the delivery of content was necessary. For example, the initial plan was the use of a BPSS children's curriculum based on the BPSS Child (Coard, 2008). BPSS Child was originally developed for children ages 5 and 6 and as a companion to BPSS. However, due to the variation in ages and developmental levels, structured play activities and homework assistance were provided to youth. Each family was compensated a total of $60 for the completion of pre-group ($20) and post-group ($40) measures and offered dinner at each group. NCCs often sponsored these meals. The partnership and support of community centers not only aided in our appeal in reaching participants, but it showcases the benefits of developing relationships and strengthening ties between academic institutions and community pillars.

BPSS-RS group initially functioned with the assistance of 3–4 staff, including 1–2 parent group facilitators and 2 child group facilitators. Although this was feasible, it was a significant amount of responsibility for the various responsibilities of the intervention to rely on a small group of people. During later rounds of implementation, the assistance of BPSS expanded to 6–7 people. This adjustment allowed for better delegation of tasks that limited the stress and strengthened the flexibility of BPSS staff members. An increase in staff allowed members to rotate during sessions, as well as assist with weekly planning. Planning for weekly sessions included sending caregivers reminders, planning dinner options for families, and preparing session materials.

## 4.9 Measurement and Methodology

The assessment battery was developed to mirror the assessment battery used in evaluating the original version of BPSS (see Coard, 2007). However, it was immediately clear that we needed to streamline in order to accommodate participants' availability and life circumstances (e.g., reports of multiple life stressors at the time of data collection; neighborhood crime concerns). Psychometric properties had already been established with the target population: *The Family Demographic Interview* (Coard et al., 2003)*; The Parent Experiences of Racial Socialization Scale* (*PERS*; Stevenson, 1994); *The Behavioral Assessment System for Children-Parent Report Scale* (BASC-PRS; Reynolds & Kamphaus, 1992, 2002); *The Social Skills Rating Scale-Parent* (*SSRS-P;* Gresham & Elliot, 1990)*; and The Parent Satisfaction Questionnaire*

(Coard, 2003). Finally, a *Program Satisfaction Survey* (adapted from Long & Forehand, 2002) was conducted post-intervention.

This real-world implementation required an allowance for flexibility and accommodation, as needed. While assessments were completed during assessment appointments, at times we had to complete assessments on-site prior to the start of the first session or hand-deliver them to families to complete and be brought at the start of the program.

## 4.10 Overall Lessons Learned

Many lessons have been learned when implementing BPSS-RS as an effectiveness trial. These include the following:

- The need for flexibility and for accommodations at all stages. For example, we learned to tailor material on the spot (context, age, circumstance) and to demonstrate versatility and the ability to pivot and adapt to unexpected circumstances that may arise during implementation.
- Developing realistic expectations including the researcher's attitudes and to expect the unexpected.
- Being prepared to acknowledge and manage the triggering nature of material results and varied responses (engagement and avoidance). This may be in part due to the population likely to utilize the NCCs that we implemented BPSS-RS.
- The importance of rapport building, communication, open discussion, providing clarity, and making the time for face-to-face contact. Black families want to see you. They want to get a feel for your intentions beyond what you state in recruitment materials.
- To make our approach in advertising BPSS-RS, recruiting parents, and implementing the program intentional in not considering participants at risk but at promise.
- For future directions, this program could be held online. However, parents would need a device and reliable internet access.

## 4.11 Recommendations

Based on the lessons learned we share recommendations for practitioners and interventionists.

- Build genuine community relationships – Whether "community" is a group or a geographic location, building genuine community relationships and engaging with that community are paramount to building mutual trust and respect, accurately identifying challenges, and developing more efficient and effective interventions. Leveraging these relationships in order to work together and foster "collective intelligence" will also assist in minimizing conflict given that credibility has been established and there is a chance to "buy into" the process and resulting product (e.g., treatment program, preventive intervention). Building genuine relationships and engaging the community via these relationships are a highly beneficial and fundamental practices.

- Offer face-time when working with Black/African American families – a generally accepted belief among Blacks/African Americans is the notion that "eyes don't lie" or 'laying eyes' is important in order to feel one's energy or get a sense of their motivations, trustworthiness, and authenticity. As such, considering that Black/African Americans may view in-person contact and the ability to be in one's presence (at least initially) may be influential in recruitment, participation, and retention.
- Validation of experiences – unless you validate existing practices (even if maladaptive or less desirable), any openness to new strategies will be limited. Validation of experiences includes understanding the motivations and intent behind their behaviors and practices. What is the goal of the behavior and are there additional skills, perspectives, and practices that one can arm themselves with in order to optimally reach that goal? For example, BPSS does not teach parents not to spank. It does, however, validate its use by examining the sociohistorical context of spanking and the legacy of discipline as protection among Blacks/African Americans in order to encourage parents to consider its use or nonuse contemporarily.
- Consider the use of kinesthetic strategies and skills – Do not just talk about it but do it. Our experience in collaborating with Black/African American communities and implementing BPSS with youth and parents is that strategies that are kinesthetic in nature (i.e., use of modeling, role-plays, and hypothetical scenarios that involve movement and hands-on application) are often preferred and promote engagement with the material. Kinesthetic strategies are consistent with the dimensions of African American culture identified by Boykins (1983) that encompass the essence of African American experiences and interactions (e.g., movement, verve, affect, communalism, expressive individualism, oral tradition).
- Engage frequent check-ins and "temperature" checks – These check-ins communicate to participants that you are interested in them and their experience with the program/intervention and provide an opportunity to identify potential facilitators and/or barriers to their participation. In our experience with BPSS, this strategy was critical to keeping parents attending and engaged. It also communicates to participants that we are approachable and accessible.

- Request feedback from participants – This recommendation is a strategy directly tied to building genuine community relationships discussed earlier. Engaging the community and/or participants before, during, and after the intervention allows for full discovery of the relationships established. That is requesting feedback from participants is central to their ability to have input and to program developers' and interventionists' ability to learn from their participants.
- Utilize a collaborative approach – You have the theoretical/clinical knowledge, but the parent is the expert of their child and family. Valuing their expertise is critical to establishing and maintaining productive collaborative and effective outcomes.
- Facilitators ideally should share the same racial/ethnic background as parents/caregivers – This is particularly important given that the focus of BPSS-RS is fostering racialized parenting in Black parents. The question remains if/how BPSS-RS can be implemented by non-Black facilitators. We contend that teaching racialized parenting content for Black parents to Black parents via a parenting curriculum is distinct from providing therapeutic service to a Black clientele that allows for free expression of racialized experiences without "teaching" the content per se.

## 4.12 Implications for Practitioners

It is imperative that African American children develop a positive sense of self and racial identity in order to foster resilience and strength. Therefore, programs must target documented culturally relevant protective factors (e.g., racial identity, racial socialization) and purposefully and strategically incorporate content and delivery strategies relevant to these constructs. A cultural and ecological perspective of optimal social development interventions provides the opportunity to leverage change in African American children's and adolescents' development. This intervention approach engages stakeholders (e.g., NCC admin) in a co-constructive process that builds broad consensus around program goals, objectives, practices, and evaluation. Empowering youth and their primary socializing agents increases the prospect of authentic and sustainable initiatives.

It is recommended that practitioners:

- develop policy and implement practices ensuring that African American youth are empowered and strengthened through evidence-based, culturally informed strategies,
- implement prevention programs that recognize the legacy of systemic barriers and oppression and that foster active engagement and ownership among community stakeholders,

- train clinicians and other service providers and practitioners in strength-based assessment and therapies,
- support community leaders and partnerships within African American communities,
- advocate for use of evidence-based practices with African American children and youth,
- engage in practice that integrates the cultural competence guidelines and recommendations made by nationally accredited organizations (e.g., Society for Prevention Research),
- promote collaborative decision-making among providers, parents, and youth (as developmentally appropriate), involving a careful risk-benefit analysis and informed treatment decision-making.

## 4.13 Conclusion

The sociopolitical landscape and realities of race in the United States lead to experiences of discrimination, racism, and stress in Black/African American families that cannot be ignored when targeting Black/African Americans in prevention programming and among providers seeking to promote their mental health and wellness. The intervention development process for BPSS and BPSS-RS has involved key actions the consideration of which results in a process that is labor-intensive, systematic, and slow. We view intervention development as a dynamic iterative process, involving targeted youth, parents, families, and community stakeholders, reviewing published research evidence, drawing on existing theories, articulating program theory, undertaking primary data collection, understanding context and culture, paying attention to future implementation in the real world and designing, and refining an intervention using iterative cycles of development with stakeholder input throughout. We need to continue to provide training, resources, and exemplary illustrations of evidence-based prevention programs for students, practitioners, researchers, educators, and policymakers to utilize in developing, adapting, and implementing their prevention initiatives in their communities. BPSS and BPSS-RS are potential resources for students, practitioners, educators, researchers, public health professionals, and communities about what works and what is promising in evidence-based prevention targeting Black/African American families. We recognize that providing tools for practitioners to develop, implement, and evaluate prevention programming and "knowing how" to do culturally and contextually relevant and responsive prevention programming is paramount.

To learn more about BPSS and BPSS-RS the following resources are recommended:

Coard, S. I., Wiley, K. C. & Evans, A. (2021). The Black Parenting Strengths and Strategies Program–Racialized Short (BPSS-RS): "Real-World" Dismantle, Implementation, and Evaluation. *ADV RES SCI 2*, 235–245. doi.org/10.1007/s42844-021-00046-6

Coard, S.I., Herring, M., Watkins, M., McCoy, S., & Foy-Watson, S. (2013). Adapting and implementing a culturally specific preventive intervention program for use with African American families. In C. S. Clauss-Ehlers et al. (Eds)., *Handbook of culturally responsive school mental health: Advancing research, training, practice, and policy* (pp. 77–87). Springer.

Coard, S.I., Foy-Watson, S., Zimmer, C., & Wallace, A. (2007). Considering culturally relevant parenting practices in intervention development and adaptation: A randomized control trial of the Black Parenting Strengths and Strategies (BPSS) Program. *The Counseling Psychologist, 35*(6), 797–820.

Coard, S.I., Wallace, S., Stevenson, H. & Miller Brotman, L. (2004). Towards culturally competent preventive interventions: The consideration of racial socialization in parent training with African American families. *Journal of Child and Family Studies, 13*(3), 277–293.

To learn more about other racial and ethnic socialization-based interventions the following resources are recommended:

## RECAST

Anderson, R. E., & Stevenson, H. C. (2019). RECASTing racial stress and trauma: Theorizing the healing potential of racial socialization in families. *American Psychologist, 74*, 63–75.

## EMBRace

Anderson, R. E., McKenny, M. C., & Stevenson, H. C. (2019). EMBRace: Developing a racial socialization intervention to reduce racial stress and enhance racial coping among black parents and adolescents. *Family Process, 58*(1), 53–67. doi.org/10.1111/famp.12412

## One Talk at a Time

Stein, G. L., Coard, S. I., Gonzalez, L. M. et al. (2021). One talk at a time: Developing an ethnic-racial socialization intervention for Black, Latinx, and Asian American families. *Journal of Social Issues, 77*, 1014–1036. doi.org/10.1111/josi.12482

## Strong African American Families (SAAF)

Murry, V. M., Berkel, C., Brody, G. H., Gerrard, M., & Gibbons, F. X. (2007). The Strong African American Families program: Longitudinal pathways to sexual risk reduction. *The Journal of Adolescent Health: Official Publication of the Society for Adolescent Medicine, 41*(4), 333–342. doi.org/10.1016/j.jadohealth.2007.04.003

### Pathways to African American Success (PAAS)

https://my.vanderbilt.edu/paasresourceid/promgram-overview/#:~:text=Pathways%20for%20African%20American%20Success,their%20potential%20to%20be%20successful

Murry, V. M., Berkel, C., Inniss-Thompson, M. N., & Debreaux, M. L. (2019). Pathways for African American success: Results of three-arm randomized trial to test the effects of technology-based delivery for rural African American families. *Journal of Pediatric Psychology*, *44*(3), 375–387. doi.org/10.1093/jpepsy/jsz001

To learn more about the importance of talking to Black children about race and racism, the following resources are recommended:

### American Psychological Association – RES

www.apa.org/res/about/racial-ethnic-socialization

### EMbraceRace

www.embracerace.org/

National Black Child Development Institute: www.nbcdi.org/

The Conscious Kid: www.theconsciouskid.org/

Talking about race–National Museum of African American History & Culture: https://nmaahc.si.edu/learn/talking-about-race

Center for Racial Justice in Education:

https://centerracialjustice.org/resources/resources-for-talking-about-race-racism-and-racialized-violence-with-kids/

### Successful Black Parenting

https://successfulblackparenting.com/

## References

Anderson, R. E., McKenny, M., Mitchell, A., Koku, L., & Stevenson, H. C. (2018) EMBRacing racial stress and trauma: Preliminary feasibility and coping responses of a racial socialization intervention. *Journal of Black Psychology*, *44*(1), 25–46. doi.org/10.1177/0095798417732930

Boykin, A. W. (1983). The academic performance of Afro-American children. In J. Spence (Ed.), *Achievement and achievement motives* (pp. 321–371). San Francisco: Freeman

Boykin, A. W. (1986). The triple quandary and the schooling of Afro-American children. In U. Neisser (Ed.), *The school achievement of minority children: New perspectives*. Lawrence Erlbaum Associates.

Brody, G. H., Gerrard, M., & Gibbons, F. X. (2004). The strong African American families program: Translating research into prevention programming. *Child Development*, *75*(3), 900–917. doi.org/10.1111/j.1467-8624.2004.00713.x

Brody, G. H., Murry, V. M., Gerrard, M., Gibbons, F. X., McNair, L., Brown, A. C., Wills, T. A., Molgaard, V., Spoth, R., Luo, Z., & Chen, Y. F. (2006a) The strong African American families program: Prevention of youths' high-risk behavior and a test of a model of change. *Journal of Family Psychology*, *20*(1), 1. doi.org/10.1037/0893-3200.20.1.1

Brody, G. H., Murry, V. M., Kogan, S. M., Gerrard, M., Gibbons, F. X., Molgaard, V., Brown, A. C., Anderson, T., Chen, Y.-f., Luo, Z., & Wills, T. A. (2006b). The Strong African American Families Program: A cluster-randomized prevention trial of long-term effects and a mediational model. *Journal of Consulting and Clinical Psychology*, *74*(2), 356–366. doi.org/10.1037/0022-006X.74.2.356

Brown, D. L., & Tylka, T. L. (2011) Racial discrimination and resilience in African American young adults: Examining racial socialization as a moderator. *Journal of Black Psychology*, *37*(3), 259–285. doi.org/10.1177/0095798410390689

Cheeks, B. L., Chavous, T. M. & Sellers, R. M. (2020) A daily examination of African American adolescents' racial discrimination, parental racial socialization, and psychological affect. *Child Development*, *91*(6), 2123–2140. doi.org/10.1111/cdev.13416

Coard, S. I. Black Parenting Strengths and Strategies – Child (BPSS-C) Department of Human Development and Family Studies. University of North Carolina-Greensboro; Greensboro, North Carolina: 2008, 2010, 2012, 2017 Unpublished Curriculum, and Manual.

Coard, S. I., Foy-Watson, S., Zimmer, C. & Wallace, A. (2007). Considering culturally relevant parenting practices in intervention development and adaptation: A randomized controlled trial of the Black Parenting Strengths and Strategies (BPSS) Program. *The Counseling Psychologist*, *35*(6), 797–820. doi.org/10.1177/0011000007304592

Coard, S. I., Herring, M. H., Watkins, M. H., Foy-Watson, S. A., & McCoy, S. Z. (2013). Black Parents Strengths and Strategies (BPSS) program: A cultural adaptation of the strong-willed child program. In *Handbook of culturally responsive school mental health* (pp. 77–87). Springer.

Coard, S. I., Wallace, S. A., Stevenson, H. C., & Brotman, L. M. (2004). Towards culturally relevant preventive interventions: The consideration of racial socialization in parent training with African American families. *Journal of Child and Family Studies*, *13*(3), 277–293. doi.org/10.1023/B:JCFS.0000022035.07171.f8

Coard, S. I., Wiley, K. C., & Evans, A. G. (2021). The Back Parenting Strengths and Strategies Program–Racialized Short (BPSS-RS): "Real-world" dismantle, implementation, and evaluation. *Adversity and Resilience Science: Journal of Research and Practice*, *2*(4), 235–245. doi.org/10.1007/s42844-021-00046-6

Dotterer, A. M., & James, A. (2018). Can parenting microprotections buffer against adolescents' experiences of racial discrimination? *Journal of Youth and Adolescence*, *47*(1), 38–50. doi.org/10.1007/s10964-017-0773-6

Gresham, F. M., & Elliot, S. N. (1990). *Social skills rating system*. Circle Pines, MN: American Guidance Service

Harrell, C. J., Burford, T. I., Cage, B. N., Nelson, T. M., Shearon, S., Thompson, A., & Green, S. (2011). Multiple pathways linking racism to health outcomes. *Du Bois Review: Social Science Research on Race*, *8*(1), 143–157. doi.org/10.1017/S1742058X11000178

Harris-Britt, A., Valrie, C. R., Kurtz-Costes, B., & Rowley, S. J. (2007). Perceived racial discrimination and self-esteem in African American youth: Racial socialization as a protective factor. *Journal of Research on Adolescence*, *17*(4), 669–682. doi.org/10.1111/j.1532-7795.2007.00540.x

Heard-Garris, N. J., Cale, M., Camaj, L., Hamati, M. C., & Dominguez, T. P. (2018). Transmitting trauma: A systematic review of vicarious racism and child health. *Social Science & Medicine*, *199*, 230–230. doi.org/10.1016/j.socscimed.2017.04.018

Hughes, D., Rodriguez, J., Smith, E. P., Johnson, D. J., Stevenson, H. C., & Spicer, P. (2006). Parents' ethnic-racial socialization practices: A review of research and directions for future study. *Developmental Psychology*, *42*(5), 747–770. doi.org/10.1037/0012-1649.42.5.747

Hughes, D. L., Watford, J. A., & Del Toro, J. (2016) A transactional/ecological perspective on ethnic–racial identity, socialization, and discrimination. *Advances in Child Development and Behavior*, *51*, 1–41. doi.org/10.1016/bs.acdb.2016.05.001

Huguley, J. P., Wang, M. T., Vasquez, A. C., & Guo, J. (2019) Parental ethnic–racial socialization practices and the construction of children of color's ethnic–racial identity: A research synthesis and meta-analysis. *Psychological Bulletin*, *145*(5), 437. doi.org/10.1037/bul0000187

Israel, B. A., Parker, E. A., Rowe, Z., Salvatore, A., Minkler, M., López, J., Butz, A., Mosley, A., Coates, L., Lambert, G., Potito, P. A., Brenner, B., Rivera, M., Romero, H., Thompson, B., Coronado, G., & Halstead, S. (2005). Community-based participatory research: Lessons learned from the Centers for Children's Environmental Health and Disease Prevention Research. *Environmental Health Perspectives*, *113*(10), 1463–1471. doi.org/10.1289/ehp.7675

Jones, S. C. T., & Neblett, E. W., Jr. (2019). The impact of racism on the mental health of people of color. In M. T. Williams, D. C. Rosen, & J. W. Kanter (Eds.), *Eliminating race-based mental health disparities: Promoting equity and culturally responsive care across settings* (pp. 79–97). Context Press/New Harbinger Publications.

Lloyd, C. M., Alvira-Hammond, M., Carlson, J., & Logan, D. (2021). Family, economic, and geographic characteristics of Black families with children. In *Racial equity: Child trends*. Eric Institute of Educational Science.

Long, N., & Forehand, R. (2002). *Parenting the strong-willed child: Leader's guide for the six-week parenting class, Version 2.0*. Unpublished manual available from Dr. Nicholas Long, Department of Pediatrics, UAMS/ACH, 800 Marshall St., Little Rock, AR 72202 or at LongNicholas@uams.edu.

Mendoza-Denton, R., Downey, G., Purdie, V. J., Davis, A., & Pietrzak, J. (2002). Sensitivity to status-based rejection: Implications for African American students' college experience. *Journal of Personality and Social Psychology*, *83*(4), 896. doi.org/10.1037/0022-3514.83.4.896

Murry, V. M., Berkel, C., Brody, G. H., Gibbons, M., & Gibbons, F. X. (2007). The Strong African American Families program: Longitudinal pathways to sexual risk reduction. *Journal of Adolescent Health*, *41*(4), 333–342. doi.org/10.1016/j.jadohealth.2007.04.003

Murry, V. M., Berkel, C., Brody, G. H., Miller, S. J., & Chen, Y. F. (2009) Linking parental socialization to interpersonal protective processes, academic self-presentation, and expectations among rural African American youth. *Cultural Diversity and Ethnic Minority Psychology*, *15*(1), 1. doi.org/10.1037/a0013180

Neblett, E. W. Jr. (2019). Racism and health: Challenges and future directions in behavioral and psychological research. *Cultural Diversity and Ethnic Minority Psychology*, *25*(1), 12. doi.org/10.1037/cdp0000253

Neblett Jr., W. E., White, R. L., Ford, K. R., Philip, C. L., Nguyen, H. X., & Sellers, R. M. (2008) Patterns of racial socialization and psychological adjustment: Can parental communications about race reduce the impact of racial discrimination? *Journal of Research on Adolescence*, *18*(3), 477–515. doi.org/10.1111/j.1532-7795.2008.00568.x

Osborne, K. R., Caughy, M. O. B., Oshri, A., Smith, E. P., & Owen, M. T. (2020). Racism and preparation for bias within African American families. *Cultural Diversity and Ethnic Minority Psychology*. doi.org/10.1037/cdp0000339

Pachter, L. M., & Coll, C. G. (2009). Racism and child health: A review of the literature and future directions. *Journal of Developmental and Behavioral Pediatrics*, *30*(3), 255–255. doi.org/10.1097/dbp.0b013e3181a7ed5a

Priest, N., Paradies, Y., Trenerry, B., Truong, M., Karlsen, S., & Kelly, Y. (2013). A systematic review of studies examining the relationship between reported racism and health and wellbeing for children and young people. *Social Science & Medicine*, *95*, 115–115. doi.org/10.1016/j.socscimed.2012.11.031

Priest, N., Walton, J., White, F., Kowal, E., Baker, A. & Paradies, Y. (2014) Understanding the complexities of ethnic-racial socialization processes for both minority and majority groups: A 30-year systematic review. *International Journal of Intercultural Relations*, *43*, 139–155. doi.org/10.1016/j.ijintrel.2014.08.003

Reynolds, C. R., & Kamphaus, R. W. (1992). *Manual for the Behavioral Assessment System for Children (BASC)*. Circle Pines, MN: American Guidance Service.

Reynolds, C. R., & Kamphaus, R. W. (2002). *The clinician's guide to the Behavior Assessment System for Children (BASC)*. New York: Guilford.

Serchen, J., Doherty, R., Atiq, O., Hilden, D., & Health and Public Policy Committee of the American College of Physicians. (2020). Racism and health in the United States: A policy statement from the American College of Physicians. *Annals of Internal Medicine*, *173*(7), 556–557. doi.org/10.7326/M20-4195

Smalls, C. (2009). African American adolescent engagement in the classroom and beyond: The roles of mother's racial socialization and democratic-involved parenting. *Journal of Youth and Adolescence*, *38*(2), 204–213. doi.org/10.1007/s10964-008-9316-5

Smalls, C. (2010). Effects of mothers' racial socialization and relationship quality on African American youth's school engagement: A profile approach. *Cultural Diversity and Ethnic Minority Psychology*, *16*(4), 476. doi.org/10.1037/a0020653

Stevenson, H. (1994). Racial socialization in African American families: The art of balancing intolerance and survival. *The Family Journal*, *2*, 190–198. 10.1177/1066480794023002

Trent, M., Dooley, D. G., Dougé, J. (2019). Section on adolescent health, council on community pediatrics, & committee on adolescence. The Impact of Racism on Child and Adolescent Health. *Pediatrics*, *144*(2), e20191765. doi.org/10.1542/peds.2019-1765

Umaña-Taylor, A. J. & Hill, N. E. (2020). Ethnic–racial socialization in the family: a decade's advance on precursors and outcomes. *Journal of Marriage and Family*, *82*(1), 244–271. doi.org/10.1111/jomf.12622

U.S. Department of Health and Human Services. (2001). *Mental health: Culture, race, and ethnicity – A supplement to mental health: A report of the surgeon general*. U.S. Department of Health and Human Services, Substance Abuse and Mental Health Services Administration, Center for Mental Health Services. www.ncbi.nlm.nih.gov/books/NBK44243/

Wang, M. T., Henry, D.A., Smith, L. V., Huguley, J. P. & Guo, J. (2020a) Parental ethnic-racial socialization practices and children of color's psychosocial and behavioral adjustment: A systematic review and meta-analysis. *American Psychologist*, *75*(1), 1–22. doi.org/10.1037/amp0000464

Wang, M. T., Smith, L.V., Miller-Cotto, D. & Huguley, J. P. (2020b) Parental ethnic-racial socialization and children of color's academic success: A meta-analytic review. *Child Development*, *91*(3), e528–e544. doi.org/10.1111/cdev.13254

# 5 The Right Supports to the Right Students at the Right Time over Time: How Schools and Communities Can Make It Happen

Mary E. Walsh, Quang D. Tran, and Anna N. Hamilton

> The degree to which one can tailor experiences to each child's unique qualities increases the likelihood that the child will grow up physically, intellectually, and emotionally healthy and thus able to meet the expectations of family and society.
>
> —Brazelton and Greenspan (2007)

Children are deeply impacted by the various contexts in which they spend time, across time. Child development is a multifaceted and complex process that is interactive and does not occur in simple linear fashion (Lerner et al., 2022; Masten, 2018). Therefore, it is critically important to view children in a comprehensive manner that incorporates their strengths and needs and that provides them with tailored developmentally appropriate services and opportunities so that they can attain competencies across domains throughout their lives. Comprehensive approaches to supporting children should be grounded in developmental science, specifically, relational developmental systems theory, which accounts for how mutually influential relations between individuals and their contexts impact change across the course of the lifespan (Lerner, 2018).

While the theoretical debate about the nature of prevention and its distinction from intervention continues, there has been a notable shift in making prevention efforts more multidimensional, integrated, and social justice-oriented in order to address the many interacting challenges that each child faces (Kenny & Hage, 2009; Romano, 2015; Romano & Hage, 2000). This multidimensional approach is critical to addressing complex social problems that adversely affect development, such as poverty. Poverty creates complex and unique developmental challenges for individuals, families, and communities. Therefore, a response to poverty requires comprehensive, complex systems of support. Endeavors to address cumulative risks and to prevent deleterious outcomes should aim to be adaptable, systematic, and comprehensive and should engage prevention as well as intervention processes (Masten, 2018; Walsh et al., 2014).

This chapter will begin by distinguishing among *prevention*, *intervention*, and *promotion efforts*, giving particular attention to how these processes operate in the context of schools. One example of a school-based, evidence-based practice – City Connects – will illustrate how prevention, promotion, and intervention can be operationalized in the contexts of schools and their local communities. This clinical/public health model is responsive to the unique strengths and needs of each child, as well as every child in the school. The chapter will conclude with a summary of challenges and possibilities involved in implementing high-quality prevention and promotion approaches, as well as several resources for readers to gain a deeper understanding of how the example might operate in practice.

## 5.1 Current Status and Challenges of Prevention

The concept of prevention is hotly debated among researchers, practitioners, and policymakers. Within human or health services, prevention is often defined as "the arresting of adverse developmental, psychological, educational, health and other life outcomes" (Reese & Vera, 2007, p. 764). A "preventive intervention" typically targets a specific deficit or risk factor (e.g., substance abuse, teen pregnancy, academic difficulties) within a multidimensional and complex system (Hage et al., 2007; National Research Council and Institute of Medicine [NRCIM], 2009). "Primary prevention" is often conceptualized in terms of halting the onset of future problems (Reese & Vera, 2007). Differentiating between related and overlapping constructs, such as treatment (*secondary prevention*), rehabilitation (*tertiary prevention*), capitalizing on strengths rather than focusing on deficits (*promotion*), and avoiding negative outcomes given present risks (*protection*), continues to be a challenge in theory and practice, as it has been for many decades (Caplan, 1964; Hage et al., 2016; NRCIM, 2009; Romano, 2015; Romano & Hage, 2000).

Beyond semantic precision, it is especially difficult to move theories of prevention into practice in the fields of human behavior and psychosocial development due to the complex interplay of environmental and personal factors that impact an individual's developmental outcomes over the lifespan (Lerner, 2018; NRCIM, 2009; Sameroff, 2009). For example, within the context of schools, well-designed and effective prevention and intervention efforts should take into account ecological and individual (e.g., temperament, family, and medical history) data, population demographics, cultural diversity, multiple developmental domains (e.g., social, emotional, and behavioral), and contextual circumstances across time (Kenny & Hage, 2009; Lerner, 1991; Walsh et al., 2002, 2014). Further, the operationalization and measurement of relevant constructs are not as straightforward in the social sciences as, for instance, in epidemiological studies (NRCIM, 2009). The prevention power of vaccines against viral infections is more easily tested than a middle school online bullying intervention. While it is typically clear whether or not someone had a certain disease based on their lab results, bullying can be difficult to define objectively and to get an accurate assessment of how frequently it occurs as well as its social-emotional impact. Thus, quantifying the outcomes of preventative programs that target the whole person (e.g., psychosocial, emotional, behavioral development) and the contexts within which they exist is a complex process that lacks universally agreed-upon best practices (Kenny & Hage, 2009; NRCIM, 2009).

Debates in the literature on prevention have elucidated the need for practices that are comprehensive, flexible, and integrated in order to meet the needs of the heterogeneous, diverse populations they serve (Hage et al., 2007; Kenny & Hage, 2009; Romano, 2015; Romano & Hage, 2000). This recognition has led to a critical shift. Historically, psychosocial and developmental needs have been conceptualized as discrete problems located within the individual at one point in time and have been treated as such in prevention and intervention efforts (Hage & Kenny, 2009; Kenny & Hage, 2009). A social justice approach to prevention and contemporary theories in developmental science have moved in the direction of more integrated care of the whole person that takes their context into account (Kenny & Hage, 2009; Lerner, 2018; National Center for Complementary and Integrative Health [NCCIH], 2021; Romano, 2015; Walsh et al., 2009). Efforts to provide "wrap-around" services have been notably rising in the past three decades through school-based programs/interventions and community health centers in collaboration with multiple institutions (e.g., universities, community agencies) (Brabeck et al., 2003; Walsh et al., 2019; Weiss & Reville, 2019).

Guided by social justice values and strong evidence of the social determinants of health, researchers in youth development, and counseling psychologists in particular, have encouraged viewing individuals and communities in terms of assets to be promoted instead of problems to be treated or "fixed" (Hage et al., 2007; Lerner, 2001; Reese & Vera, 2007; Walsh et al., 2009). Rather than having deficits and risks be the primary loci of prevention and intervention models, researchers and practitioners have begun to capitalize on youths' strengths and skills in order to promote their potential to thrive (Kirschman et al., 2009; Lerner et al., 2022; Masten, 2018). Providing children with a caring and protective environment, for example, has been shown to reduce risks related to adverse experiences (e.g., poverty, racism), but above all, growing up in such an environment makes it more likely for children to develop cognitive and psychosocial skills that have benefits beyond prevention of negative outcomes (Jessor, 1992; Masten, 2018; Masten & Labella, 2016). When "promotion is promoted" from an early age, individuals are able to develop the resources they need to better cope with life's unpredictable obstacles and adversities, such as the COVID-19 pandemic (Kirschman et al., 2009; Lerner, 2001; Lerner et al., 2022).

Instead of associating problems or deficiencies with particular individuals or groups, promotive efforts with preventative and protective potential are emphasized. This also means intervening at the systems level to influence structural and cultural changes that are conducive to healthy development (Hage & Kenny, 2009; Kenny & Hage, 2009). Community collaboration, advocacy, and policy reforms can increase a child's access to cognitively and socially stimulating environments, as well as supportive resources and structures (e.g., enrichment activities matched with children's interests, nutritious meals, safe play space) in the early, critical stages of development (Dearing, 2008; Masten & Labella, 2016; McEwen, 2016; Walsh et al., 2019). Targeting these crucial enrichments at a period of peak neuroplasticity facilitates an individual's development of competencies and overall capacity for future success. "Targeting" resources is facilitated by identifying and utilizing a family's and its community's cultural and social opportunities that are often untapped or underappreciated (Masten, 2014; Theron et al., 2022).

Developing and maintaining malleable, adaptive systems that tailor support to children's and families' diverse strengths and needs, promote resilience, and foster healthy development in spite of adversity and life's vicissitudes is a daunting and complex operation (Ghate, 2016; Masten & Labella, 2016). Attempts through the years to develop and implement sustainable adaptive systems in schools, though well meaning, have resulted in fragmented or disconnected services, and evidence of positive outcomes that is scant and inconclusive (Walsh et al., 2019). Having resources is generally better than not having resources, but without a systematic, organized approach guided by the integration of theory, research, and practice, the costs are likely to outweigh the benefits (Bowden et al., 2015; Fisher, 2018).

The remainder of this chapter will describe the challenges associated with designing, implementing, and measuring the outcomes of a complex and adaptive system that promotes lasting and quantifiable ecological changes. The focus will be on how one particular evidence-based approach – City Connects – has successfully created a school-based system that promotes children's thriving. After outlining the practice, theoretical foundations and outcome research will be described.

## 5.2 Prevention and Promotion in Schools

Schools represent a key context in children's lives that can provide a nurturing, predictable environment in which their strengths are recognized and drawn upon and where their challenges are understood and addressed. However, traditional school systems, and specifically the structures of student support within these school systems, are not often set up in a way that can respond flexibly and efficiently to students' developmental strengths and needs (Walsh et al., 2014). Student support structures greatly vary school-to-school and between districts, with nonacademic services often being provided in a decentralized, fragmented way by school nurses, counselors, psychologists, and/or social workers (Walsh et al., 2014, 2019). These siloed systems of student support that operate at the periphery of the school community are ill-equipped to manage the complex contextual factors that many students present, especially in underserved communities (Adelman & Taylor, 2012).

Policymakers and educators have been increasingly calling for a comprehensive, coordinated approach to student support (Adelman & Taylor, 2002; Walsh et al., 2014). This type of approach would empower teachers and administrators to focus on their core roles and responsibilities rather than constantly putting out "fires" and managing crises outside of their expertise. As a result, schools are better positioned to meet their full potential as a key environment to facilitate children's growth and healthy development.

In order to address the barriers to student achievement and thriving, school systems need to understand and to be equipped to address the role of out-of-school challenges with comprehensive and multifaceted methods (Adelman & Taylor, 2002; Reardon, 2011). Schools must (a) understand their students' cultures, contexts, and backgrounds, (b) have a network of school-based and community-based supports and services, and (c) have systems and structures that measure accountability and outcomes to effectively provide all students with opportunities for promotion, prevention, and early intervention (Reardon, 2011; Walsh et al., 2014). Few models of student support have effectively implemented this type of approach as it requires cooperation and coordination from the entire school and surrounding community.

### 5.2.1 Integrated Student Support

One promising strategy for providing networks of support for students is referred to as integrated student support (ISS) (Moore & Emig, 2014). ISS has been defined as "a school-based approach to promoting students' academic success by developing or securing and coordinating supports that target academic and non-academic barriers to achievement" (Moore & Emig, 2014, p. 1). ISS approaches utilize a wide range of student supports, ranging from more traditional school-based interventions, such as tutoring, to broader supports that impact students' contexts outside of school, such as assistance with finding housing, food, and clothing (Wasser Gish, 2019). Many of these approaches work in partnerships, which are external to the school. They involve collaboration with school leaders and sometimes a small number of teachers to support children experiencing difficulties or to provide more universal school-wide programming. In addition to securing a wide range of supports for students that promote their healthy development across domains (e.g., social, emotional, physical, cognitive), ISS approaches are most effective when they are embedded in the day-to-day school environment and when they tailor supports to meet students' unique needs.

ISS approaches should be grounded in research and theory on child and youth development. ISS implementation is most effective when it situates the child within their larger context and considers how the child's success in school is impacted by the various environments they interact with, both inside and outside of school (Moore & Emig, 2014; Reardon, 2011). Some ISS approaches are implemented by family or community workers, while the in-school models are typically led by school-based student support staff (e.g., school counselor, school social worker) (Moore & Emig, 2014). The latter's clinical expertise and training in systems of equity and social justice make them ideal ISS practitioners and coordinators (Pollack et al., 2021).

The next sections of this chapter will describe City Connects, a school-based ISS model that simultaneously prevents, promotes, and intervenes, not just in the area of academics, but also across social-emotional-behavioral, health, and family domains. This model offers an intervention that aims to prevent negative outcomes downstream by promoting positive development and intervening both early and intensively, as well as addressing challenges that are already occurring.

## 5.3 Description of City Connects

### 5.3.1 Brief Background

City Connects was developed in 1999 to address the out-of-school needs impacting the ability for students to thrive, particularly for youth attending high-poverty schools (Walsh & Brabeck, 2006). The City Connects model recognized the critical importance of addressing challenges faced by children outside of school, which account for up to two-thirds of the variance in student achievement (Leigh et al., 2022; Rothstein, 2010). It is an evidence-based approach to supporting students across developmental domains (i.e., academic, social, emotional, physical) by connecting them with a tailored set of school- and community-based supports and services (City Connects, 2022). The model was developed around best practice recommendations for integrated systems of holistic school-based support (Walsh et al., 2014). Aligned with these best practices, schools implementing City Connects have prioritized moving effective student support from a peripheral to a central role in their educational mission and day-to-day work (City Connects, 2022). Strong relationships with a wide variety of community agencies facilitate each school's ability to support student thriving (City Connects, 2022).

Started initially as a partnership between Boston College and Boston Public Schools, City Connects has significantly expanded over the past two decades, and in that time has been implemented in urban centers in the states of New York, Minnesota, Connecticut, Massachusetts, Indiana, Tennessee, as well as in Dublin, Ireland. City Connects continues to primarily operate in underserved elementary and middle schools serving predominantly students from marginalized backgrounds in terms of race and socioeconomic status. City Connects has also been implemented in early childhood centers, a small number of high schools, and experimentally in a community college setting (City Connects, 2022).

### 5.3.2 The City Connects Model

The core tenet that undergirds the City Connects model is equity. The City Connects model does not just serve the students with the most significant behavioral issues or those who are the furthest below grade level. It does not only prepare students who are planning to go to college. The City Connects model is for and seeks to serve every single student who attends a City Connects school: Straight A students, shy students, chronically absent students, popular students, and special education students are all included in the City Connects practice.

The City Connects coordinator, a master's-level social worker or school counselor, implements the City Connects model in schools. Early on in the school year, they review each student in the school with that student's classroom teacher. The coordinator supports the teacher in identifying each student's unique strengths and needs across four developmental domains (family, health, social-emotional, and academic). The structured Whole Class Review (WCR) discussion also involves matching students and their families with identified services based on students' strengths and needs. Based on the information discussed during the WCR, the teacher and coordinator assign the strength/risk level of each student to one of four tiers: Tier 1 (strengths and minimal risk), Tier 2A (strengths and mild risks), Tier 2B (strengths and moderate risks), and Tier 3 (strengths and severe/intensive risks) (City Connects, 2020). Students' strength/risk level are assigned to a tier relative to the other students in their classroom.

A subset of students identified as having intensive, complex needs at any point in the school year (typically 10–15% of the student population) are referred to an Individual Student Review (ISR) (City Connects, 2022). During the ISR, a larger team of professionals (i.e., counselors, teachers, nurses, principals, community agency representatives) are gathered together for an in-depth discussion about the identified student and to develop measurable goals and strategies for the student.

Coordinators' work is guided by a local program manager. Program managers are typically assigned to one district and are responsible for overseeing the City Connects practice in that district's schools. The duties of the program manager include recruiting coordinators, delivering professional development to coordinators, and coaching, as well as, if appropriate, supervising coordinators (City Connects, 2022). The partnership with Boston College is leveraged as program managers participate in regular professional development offered by City Connects staff at the university to best support coordinators in implementing the practice.

City Connects utilizes a proprietary web-based student support information system called MyConnects to ensure secure collection of data around the WCR, ISR, and service referral processes. Examples of the types of data that are tracked and stored in MyConnects include individual support plans for each student in a school, service referrals, community agencies, and implementation of core practices (Leigh et al., 2022). These dynamic and "real-time" data on students, schools, and their surrounding communities help streamline the work of the coordinator and facilitate their ability to effectively implement student support plans, track progress and follow-up on plans, see patterns related to service referrals and community partnerships, and provide tailored implementation support and coaching to schools and districts (Leigh et al., 2022). The utilization of this system aids the coordinator in managing and keeping track of a caseload of approximately 400 students (City Connects, 2020).

One of the key components of City Connects is its close work with agencies in the community. The City Connects coordinator builds and maintains partnerships with a number of community agencies that provide a variety of services across intensity levels. The coordinator also gathers information from students about their interests and works with agencies to help them shape programming to fill the gaps between what is currently available in the community and what students in their schools could benefit from. Students are matched with tailored in-school and out-of-school services and supports that align with their strengths, needs, and interests. Students' service referrals and providers (in-school and out-of-school) are then collected and tracked in MyConnects. During the 2018–2019 school year, over 261,000 services were delivered to students in City Connects schools by over 1,200 community agencies (City Connects, 2020). Services are classified into three overarching categories: prevention and enrichment (e.g., before- and after-school programming, health and wellness classes, sports, summer programs), early intervention (e.g., adult mentoring, academic support, social skills interventions, family assistance, tutoring), and intensive/crisis intervention (e.g., mental health counseling, health services, screening or diagnostic testing, violence intervention, family counseling) (Walsh et al., 2014).

### 5.3.3 Theoretical Underpinnings and Practice-Informed Research

Children's needs, within the context of their continuously changing internal and external environments, require supportive systems that have well-articulated, organizing principles based on sound theory and empirical research that is also informed by practice. During the past two decades of working with schools, community partners, and other stakeholders, City Connects has not only turned to developmental science and research to guide best practices, but also allowed the rich lessons and experiences of real-world application to inform theory and research. This section presents the theoretical/philosophical road map and the real-world experiences that have informed City Connects' guiding principles and best practices.

The core components of City Connects ensure that the program meets the requirements of a practice grounded in developmental science; that is, it is comprehensive, customized, coordinated, and continuous (City Connects, 2022; Moore & Emig, 2014). Consistent with the scientific understanding that children develop as whole people, City Connects is comprehensive in that it focuses simultaneously on multiple developmental domains (i.e., academic, social/emotional/behavioral, health, and family) within multiple contexts. Understanding that a child's development incorporates both strengths and needs, City Connects is customized; that is, it tailors individualized plans of services and supports for each individual child. Relying on the knowledge of developmental science that multiple contexts impact development, City Connects is coordinated; it serves as a bridge between families, school personnel, and community partners, including universities, to optimize cohesive and collaborative efforts to support students. Recognizing the ever-evolving nature of developmental progress, City Connects ensures that its efforts are continuous by using a rigorous and data-driven system for monitoring progress, facilitating self-evaluation in order to promote accountability, responding to evolving needs, and improving delivery of services.

Addressing the developmental needs of the "whole child" based on these components involves attentiveness to many details and moving parts and requires multiple perspectives and expertise. For this reason, through the years, City Connects' staff, including graduate research assistants, have become increasingly multidisciplinary. The diverse skill sets among the staff are systematically directed toward optimizing student support from different angles and at different levels of child development in context. City Connects attempts to actualize the phrase "It takes a village" by building a system across schools, communities, and families (Hayward, 2022).

Given that child development occurs within multilevel contexts and systems, City Connects follows a clinical/public health model to guide intervention efforts. It addresses and provides a unique support plan for each student that is clearly not "one size fits all." Simultaneously, the intervention delivers the assessment and tailored plan to all students in a school – and to the larger population in all City Connects schools. In short, City Connects holds in tension a customized treatment for each student while using the same practice for all students. City Connects collaborates with multiple stakeholders to identify and respond to as many risks as possible in order to avoid the "snowball effect" or negative cascades when risk factors accumulate and lead to more detrimental and less modifiable outcomes (Masten & Cicchetti, 2010). At the same time, City Connects also identifies and supports as many strengths as possible at a given moment in time in order to promote positive cascades at the individual and systems levels.

In addition to identifying the challenges and strengths of each child, City Connects is able to aggregate the strengths and needs across populations – at the level of classroom, school, and/or district. That is to say, in addition to being a "whole child" support system, City Connects is also a "whole school" and "whole community" support system. While City Connects, in collaboration with numerous community partners, has developed and implemented this comprehensive and holistic approach for over two decades, the Association for Supervision and Curriculum Development (ASCD) formally proposed a similar approach – the Whole School, Whole Community, Whole Child (WSCC) model – in 2014 with the support of the Centers for Disease Control and Prevention (CDC) (ASCD, 2014). This approach to intervention comes out of the efforts in the past decades to integrate personalized/clinical care and public health interventions (ASCD, 2014; Unger et al., 2020). Bringing together an understanding of the needs of specific individuals and the cumulative risks that specific populations face optimizes risk reduction and facilitates the use of resources in an equitable and just manner (Unger et al., 2020).

While this WSCC model is widely promoted today, few approaches have successfully actualized it (Moore & Emig, 2014). City Connects embodies the WSCC vision of designing sustainable interventions that integrate education, health, and wellness rather than targeting specific problems in a fragmented and compartmentalized manner. While City Connects places heavy emphasis on the care of each student and all students, the intervention also tailors school- and community-based services and supports according to the strengths and needs of the child's context (Bowden et al., 2015; City Connects, 2018; Pollack et al., 2021). Schools are embedded in communities, and community demographics vary from one school district to another. Besides considering the risks that these communities face, seeking out and forming relationships with community partners/agencies, recognizing strengths, identifying resources, and systematically allocating those resources to students, families, and schools generate a mutually transformative network and culture of support at both the individual and group population levels.

Besides the tension that arises from strategically planning to intervene at both the individual and group levels, there is also the tension of targeting deficits *and* fostering strengths. Drawing from the risk and resilience literature from the past decades, City Connects uses a strengths-based approach that also aims to remediate specific deficits (Masten, 2011; Masten & Cicchetti, 2016; Masten & Labella, 2016). For example, a large number of the services that City Connects provides for the majority of the students via multiple agencies offer enrichment/prevention (e.g., sports, summer enrichment programs, arts and music programs). At the same time, at a specific school in a specific district, most students might also receive an intervention to address a specific prevalent problem (e.g., bullying, homelessness, substance abuse). In other words, caring for the whole child and building on their talents also involve identifying and tackling notable challenges. Promoting strengths and human development is inseparable from addressing adversity and risks, since the latter, if left unaddressed, could undermine the efforts to achieve the former.

In developing preventive interventions that might address the complex needs of students and their families, the North Star for City Connects holds the empirically based conviction of developmental science that children and their developmental pathways can be modified (Cicchetti & Rogosch, 1996). Their fate is not predetermined by a single or even several risk factors and adverse experiences. Developmental research confirms that children with similar backgrounds and who face similar risk factors do not necessarily follow the same developmental trajectory or have the same outcomes (Beauchaine et al., 2009; Cantor et al., 2019). Further, providing the right supports at the right time can change the course of a maladaptive pathway, particularly for younger children when developmental plasticity is highly impressionable and can be altered in a positive direction (Belsky & Pluess, 2013; Cicchetti & Crick, 2009).

While many interventions aim primarily to change students' developmental pathways, City Connects also pays attention to how students, along with their schools, families, and communities, shape City Connects' own approach to intervention. Masten and Labella (2016) argued that "malleable" systems are critical in helping children address risks and build resilience. Individuals and systems/environments change each other in a transactional relationship (Sameroff, 2009). Thus, City Connects regularly evaluates how efforts to maintain high fidelity in implementation and practice affect its capacity to be strategically flexible to respond to the unpredictability of life's circumstances. Quantitative measures of "fidelity of implementation" were developed by researchers as soon as the positive effects of the intervention became apparent (Foley et al., 2015).

## 5.4 City Connects Evaluation Processes

### 5.4.1 Process Evaluation

Annually, City Connects publishes detailed, empirical reports that include both outcome evaluation and process evaluation (e.g., City Connects, 2020, 2022). The process evaluation involves receiving feedback from school personnel as a way to gauge how well City Connects supports teachers and principals in meeting the specific needs of individual students and the general needs of the schools. One way that City Connects does this is by gathering anonymized feedback from teachers, principals, coordinators, and community partners who work with or in City Connects schools through surveys. Using several types of questions (e.g., Likert scale, open-ended), the surveys are designed to assess participants' levels of satisfaction with City Connects, identify areas of strength, and detect opportunities for improvement (City Connects, 2022). The spring 2021 surveys showed that the majority of principals, teachers, community partners, and coordinators were satisfied with the practice (City Connects, 2022).

### 5.4.2 Implementing with Fidelity

One key aspect of City Connects that has been paramount to its successful expansion over the years is a rigorous evaluation process for quality assurance and improvement to ensure consistent delivery of the practice across all sites (City Connects, 2022). Various aspects of implementation are operationalized and measured in order to inform the work of coordinators and highlight areas of strength and potential improvement (City Connects, 2022). Information gathered during the course of typical day-to-day work is entered into MyConnects and utilized to assess fidelity across the core components of the practice (i.e., WCR, ISR, community partnerships) (City Connects, 2022). This information is utilized to aid the program manager in targeting their support for the coordinators in their district.

### 5.4.3 City Connects Outcomes

City Connects outcome evaluation involves the tracking of student outcomes across a number of domains in the short term and long term (e.g., academics, attendance, dropout rates, postsecondary achievement) to ensure that the model is continuously promoting positive outcomes for all students. Continuous evaluation of City Connects indicates that the model promotes a number of positive outcomes for students across multiple stages of development (i.e., elementary school, middle school, high school, and postsecondary). The strong evidence that City Connects promotes positive outcomes for students remains consistent across a number of methods, samples, and geographic areas (City Connects, 2022).

At the elementary school level, students who attend City Connects schools have better academic outcomes than their peers who never attended City Connects schools (City Connects, 2010, 2014; Khanani, Raczek, & Walsh, 2021). Specifically, findings indicate that students who attended City Connects in elementary school have:

- stronger academic effort (Khanani, O'Dwyer, Walsh, & Raczek, 2021);
- higher report card scores in reading, writing, and math (Walsh et al., 2014);
- higher performance on standardized tests in English and mathematics (An, 2015; Walsh et al., 2014); and
- fewer days absent from school (City Connects, 2014)

These findings were consistent across various types of schools and student groups. For example, the higher performance on statewide tests persisted for students attending "turnaround" and "transformation" (consistently low-performing) schools. Within the first few years of implementation of City Connects, gaps in performance between turnaround and transformation schools narrowed to insignificant levels for test scores on statewide English and math assessments. English language learner (ELL) immigrant students who received City Connects performed better on reading and math achievement assessments, compared to immigrant students who never got the City Connects model (Dearing et al., 2016).

At the middle school and high school level, studies continue to show that students who received City Connects in elementary school have better outcomes on several key indicators of educational achievement and overall success. Specifically, findings indicate that at the middle school/high school level, students who received City Connects in elementary school are:

- less likely to repeat a grade in middle school compared to similar students who never received City Connects (City Connects, 2010);
- more likely to have lower rates of chronic absenteeism in middle school and high school (defined as missing at least 10% of the school year) (City Connects, 2014); and
- less likely to drop out of high school (Lee-St. John et al., 2018).

These findings provide evidence that receiving the City Connects intervention early on in development (i.e., elementary school) prevents the likelihood of negative outcomes later on in development.

### 5.4.4 Evaluation Challenges and Opportunities

The complexity of the contextual and individual challenges that City Connects seeks to address mandates evaluation approaches that are equally complex. Not all City Connects work can be easily quantified or measured but is no less critical for constructive feedback and intervention enhancement. For example, providing students with dance classes might not have a clear and direct effect on academic outcomes, but one immediate consequence is that these students have learned a new skill they might not have learned before. Similarly, providing children with thick coats for the winter might not have a direct impact on the children's socioemotional skills, but the immediate consequence is that these children have something to wear in the cold. Because there is no straightforward, simple way to quantify the impact of providing dance classes and coats for evaluation purposes, City Connects' team members brainstorm creative ways to provide enriching and essential services that have benefits beyond certain traditional measures of achievement and success. As noted in the previous sections, City Connects navigates these challenges by continuously evaluating the practice and outcomes of students across methods, samples, and sites.

There are challenges to evaluating a preventative K-12 intervention in high-poverty schools. Families, caregivers, and students are among the most important stakeholders, and their voices are critical in evaluating an intervention. However, there are several prohibitive barriers that make it difficult for researchers to accurately and fully capture student and family voices in evaluations. Acquiring consent for incorporating students' voices through surveys or interviews is complex. Additionally, one of the most critical barriers is a family's ability to access a survey due to a myriad of factors, such as language barriers, other commitments and stressors taking priority over survey participation, and lack of access to reliable internet. When survey translation is not available in each of the languages spoken by families in a school community, only a subset of voices are heard. It is critical for researchers to compare the demographic makeup of school communities to their respondents to identify groups who might not have been able to easily access the evaluation and whose feedback is missing. Researchers can further address some of these evaluation challenges by developing strong, trusting relationships with school communities, having open lines of communication with school staff and families to be able to hear and respond to concerns as they arise, and continuously increasing the accessibility of survey administration processes.

## 5.5 Ideas for Practical Development, Adaptation, and Implementation

### 5.5.1 Leveraging the Power of Student Voice and Community Agency Relationships to Build Competence

While it has long intuitively made sense to school staff that building on students' strengths is just as important as addressing their needs, this has not always been one of the primary focuses of school-based interventions. To solely focus on remediating deficits ignores critical research on child development. Recognizing students' strengths and setting them up with opportunities for success in areas of interest can increase their feelings of competence, which in turn leads to positive patterns of adaptation in the face of adverse situations (i.e., resilience) (Masten & Obradovic, 2006). One unique aspect of the City Connects model is its collection and use of information on student interests and activities. At the beginning of the school year, each family is given a student activities and interests survey to complete on behalf of their elementary school-age student(s). This survey collects information from the perspective of the student and/or family about each student's unique skills, areas of interest, activities in which they would like to participate, and activities or services in which they are already participating.

This information is used in conjunction with academic data, observation data, and health data from the nurse to guide the discussion of every student's strengths and needs across developmental domains during the WCR. The information on students' strengths and interests is used to connect them with services that can help them build areas of competence. The coordinator utilizes their connections with and knowledge of community agencies to get students access to tailored services and resources. Further, the coordinator considers each student's family situation to ensure that referrals are accessible and works to obtain transportation and/or scholarships to increase accessibility. Many of the interests and skills that these referrals help foster are outside of academics (e.g., music, sports, electronics).

The data collected on student interest forms can also facilitate the creation of new services in a community. Through a simple analysis of the data collected on interest surveys, the coordinator is able to notice where the majority of students' interests lie. For example, say the coordinator in school A sees that 50% of the students in his school are interested in Legos and 30% are interested in taking dance lessons. The coordinator is then able to investigate what community agencies exist that currently provide those services and if they are a match for the students who are interested in them. If the majority of students interested in Legos are in 3rd–4th grade, but all of the Lego clubs in the community only serve middle school students, that is an important service gap. With this knowledge, coordinators can liaise with community agencies and schools to make them aware of these service gaps so that they can be filled.

Data-driven practices are possible, due to the coordinator's access to rich data on student interests and community agency offerings. Coordinators are not making assumptions about what students want and need; rather, they are utilizing parents' and students' voices to drive the practice. Systematic processes for matching students with services that are a good fit enable school staff to shift from firefighting mode to prevention mode. They do not have to scramble to get supports for a student when they are in crisis. Instead, all students' strengths and needs are regularly considered at set intervals throughout the school year, and tailored services/supports are put in place to promote and prevent, rather than to "fix" something that is already wrong. This also means that some of the higher tiered services that have lower levels of availability, such as individual therapy, are less in demand. Students have spaces to grow their interests and feel competent through lower intensity-level services that have higher capacity, such as sports teams or after-school music classes.

While identifying gaps in services based on students' interests is one part of the puzzle, getting buy-in from caregivers is another critical piece. Schools, and specifically coordinators, need to have open, honest lines of communication with their students' families in order to work together to get students involved in services. In order to do this, positive and supportive relationships with each family need to be established. When these types of relationships exist, parents and coordinators can work together as a team to get students involved in activities that match their interests and skills.

These practices illustrate how school–community–family partnerships can work together to (a) identify students' strengths (rather than focusing solely on deficits); (b) match students to appropriate services, supports, and extracurricular activities that build their competence; (c) identify any service gaps in the community based on the interests and needs of the students they serve; and (d) utilize their relationships with community agencies to fill those gaps. These practices not only promote positive student development, but also support community agencies' ability to serve students who have the most interest and potential to benefit from their services.

## 5.6 Conclusion

Prevention must be about promoting equity and a just society. These aims have been central to the design and implementation of City Connects. By focusing on all students across the entire school, City Connects is able to avoid an exclusive preoccupation with either the subset of students who are in severe crisis or those who are highest performing and most likely college bound. Support provided to every student is comprehensive, taking into consideration their development across domains (e.g., social/emotional, health, family) and contexts (e.g., culture, school, neighborhood).

Prevention-in-action requires working across polarities, such as intervening at both the individual and the group levels, targeting challenges while fostering strengths and interests, and promoting healthy development while simultaneously intervening in existing difficulties. City Connects has relied on a public health/clinical model to intervene at individual and group levels in a school setting in which each student receives a support plan tailored to their unique strengths and needs. Additionally, whole classrooms, whole schools, and/or whole districts benefit from the universal strategy that City Connects provides. In City Connects, as in other prevention/intervention programs, fostering strengths/interests and targeting areas of challenge are inextricably tied:

To overlook, one would make it impossible for the efforts of the other to fully come to fruition. When working with the complex challenges that poverty presents to children and families, prevention efforts necessitate a simultaneous focus on intervention. Complex social problems require solutions that match their complexity in order to make a measurable impact. In City Connects, the continuum of supports, ranging from prevention through early intervention to intensive intervention, is essential in supporting all children in an individualized way. With both prevention and intervention, one size does not fit all.

Prevention and intervention efforts, such as City Connects, can be actualized through the rich theoretical framework of developmental science, which provides very clear guidance on the design of intervention and prevention strategies. In developing City Connects, a theory of change based on developmental science was specified at the outset. Importantly, the theory of change included measurable outcomes, that is, indicators that the intervention led to prevention and other life changes.

## Recommended Resources

America's Promise (2019). Building systems of integrated student support: https://americaspromise.org/resources/building-systems-integrated-student-support/

City Connects (2016). Principles of effective practice in integrated student support. www.bc.edu/content/dam/bc1/schools/lsoe/centers/city-connects/coss/Principles%20of%20Effective%20Practice%20policy%20brief.pdf

City Connects 2022, 2020, and 2018 Progress Reports. www.bc.edu/content/bc-web/schools/lynch-school/sites/city-connects/results.html

Mary E Walsh Center for Thriving Children (2019). The whole child: Building systems of integrated student support during and after COVID-19: An action guide. www.bc.edu/content/dam/bc1/schools/lsoe/centers/city-connects/coss/pdfs-for-ctc/CTC%20Action%20Guide.pdf

Project Evident (2022). An actionable data system approach at City Connects. https://projectevident.org/case-study/an-actionable-data-system-approach-at-city-connects%EF%BF%BC/

## References

Adelman, H. S., & Taylor, L. (2002). Building comprehensive, multifaceted, and integrated approaches to address barriers to student learning. *Childhood Education*, *78*(5), 261–268. doi.org/10.1080/00094056.2002.10522738

Adelman, H. S., & Taylor, L. (2012). Mental health in schools: Moving in new directions. *Contemporary School Psychology*, *16*(1), 9–18.

An, C. (2015). *Estimating the effectiveness of City Connects on middle school outcomes* (Publication No. 3716216) [Doctoral Dissertation, Boston College] ProQuest Dissertations Publishing.

ASCD. (2014). *Whole school, whole community, whole child: A collaborative approach to learning and health*. Center for Disease Control and Prevention. www.cdc.gov/healthyschools/wscc/wsccmodel_update_508tagged.pdf

Beauchaine, T. P., Klein, D. N., Crowell, S. E., Derbidge, C., & Gatzke-Kopp, L. (2009). Multifinality in the development of personality disorders: A biology x sex x environment interaction model of antisocial and borderline traits. *Development and Psychopathology*, *21*(3), 735–770. doi.org/10.1017/S0954579409000418

Belsky, J., & Pluess, M. (2013). Beyond risk, resilience, and dysregulation: Phenotypic plasticity and human development. *Development and Psychopathology*, *25*, 1243–1261. doi.org/10.1017/S095457941300059X

Bowden, A. B., Shand, R., Belfield, C. R., Wang, A., & Levin, H. M. (2017). Evaluating educational interventions that induce service receipt: A case study application of City Connects. *American Journal of Evaluation*, *38*(3), 405–419. doi .org/10.1177/1098214016664983

Bowden, B., Belfield, C. R., Levin, H. M., Shand, R., Wang, A., & Morales, M. (2015). *A benefit-cost analysis of City Connects*. https://repository.upenn.edu/cbcse/6

Brabeck, M. M., Walsh, M. E., & Latta, R. E. (Eds.) & National Society for the Study of Education. (2003). *Meeting at the hyphen: Schools-universities-communities-professions in collaboration for student achievement and well-being*. (The 102nd yearbook of the National Society for the Study of Education; Vol. pt. 2).

Brazelton, T. B., & Greenspan, S. I. (2007). Why children need experiences tailored to their uniqueness. *Early Childhood Today*, 21(4), 10–11.

Cantor, P., Osher, D., Berg, J., Steyer, L., & Rose, T. (2019). Malleability, plasticity, and individuality: How children learn and develop in context. *Applied Developmental Science*, *23*(4), 307–337. doi.org/10.1080/10888691.2017.1398649

Caplan, G. (1964). *Principles of preventive psychiatry*. Basic Books.

Cicchetti, D., & Crick, N. R. (2009). Precursors and diverse pathways to personality disorder in children and adolescents. *Development and Psychopathology*, *21*(3), 683–685. doi.org/10.1017/S0954579409000388

Cicchetti, D., & Rogosch, F. A. (1996). Equifinality and multifinality in developmental psychopathology. *Development and Psychopathology*, *8*(4), 597–600. doi.org/10.1017/S0954579400007318

City Connects (2010). *The impact of City Connects: Annual report 2010*. Boston College Center for Optimized Student Support. www.bc.edu/content/dam/city-connects/Publications/CityConnects_AnnualReport_2010.pdf

City Connects (2014). *The impact of City Connect: Progress report 2014*. Center for Optimized Student Support. www.bc.edu/content/dam/city-connects/Publications/CityConnects_ProgressReport_2014.pdf

City Connects (2016). *The impact of City Connects: Student outcomes*. Center for Optimized Student Support. www.bc.edu/content/dam/files/schools/lsoe/cityconnects/pdf/City%20Connects%20Progress%20Report%202016.pdf

City Connects (2018). *City Connects: Intervention and impact*. Center for Optimized Student Support. www.bc.edu/content/dam/bc1/schools/lsoe/sites/coss/pdfs-for-ctc/CityConnectsProgressReport2018%20updated%20Feb.%202022.pdf

City Connects (2020). *City Connects: Intervention and impact*. Center for Optimized Student Support. www.bc.edu/content/dam/city-connects/Publications/City%20Connects%20Intervetion%20%20Impact%20Progress%20Report%202020.pdf

City Connects (2022). *City Connects: Intervention and impact*. Center for Optimized Student Support. www.bc.edu/content/dam/city-connects/Publications/The%20Impact%20of%20City%20Connects-Progress%20Report%202022.pdf

Dearing, E. (2008). Psychological costs of growing up poor. *Annals of the New York Academy of Sciences*, *1136*(1), 324–332. doi.org/10.1196/annals.1425.006

Dearing, E., Walsh, M. E., Sibley, E., Lee-St. John, T., Foley, C., & Raczek, A. E. (2016). Can community and school-based supports improve the achievement of first-generation immigrant children attending high-poverty schools? *Child Development*, *87*(3), 883–897.

Fisher, J. F. (2018). *Who you know: Unlocking innovations that expand students' networks*. John Wiley & Sons.

Foley, C., Theodorakakis, M., Walsh, M. E., DiNatale, P., & Raczek, A. (2015). Building a sustainable intervention to address the out-of-school factors affecting achievement: A primer and case study. *Center for Optimized Student Support*. www.bc.edu/content/dam/city-connects/Publications/Policy%20Brief%20-%20Building%20Sustainable%20Interventions%20Final%20WEBSITE.pdf

Ghate, D. (2016). From programs to systems: Deploying implementation science and practice for sustained real world effectiveness in services for children and families. *Journal of Clinical Child and Adolescent Psychology*, *45*(6), 812–826. doi.org/10.1080/15374416.2015.1077449

Hage, S. M., & Kenny, M. E. (2009). Promoting a social justice approach to prevention: Future directions for training, practice, and research. *The Journal of Primary Prevention*, *30*(1), 75–87. doi.org/10.1007/s10935-008-0165-5

Hage, S. M., & Romano, J. L. (2010). History of prevention and prevention groups. *Group Dynamics*, *14*(3), 199–210. doi.org/10.1037/a0020736

Hage, S. M., Romano, J. L., Conyne, R. K., Kenny, M., Matthews, C., Schwartz, J. P., & Waldo, M. (2007). Best practice guidelines on prevention practice, research, training, and social advocacy for psychologists. *The Counseling Psychologist*, *35*(4), 493–566. doi.org/10.1177/0011000006291411

Hage, S. M., Schwartz, J., & DeMartino, S. (2016). International issues in the ethics of prevention. In M. Israellashvili & J. L. Romano (Eds.), *Cambridge handbook of international prevention science* (pp. 63–80). Cambridge University Press. doi.org/10.1017/9781316104453

Hayward, E. (2022, February). *Lynch school prof's work in support of children recognized by $10M gift: BC's Center for Optimized Student Support will be renamed the Mary E. Walsh Center for Thriving Children*. BC News. www.bc.edu/bc-web/bcnews/nation-world-society/education/major-gift-honors-kearns-professor-mary-walsh.html

Jessor, R. (1992). Risk behavior in adolescence: A psychosocial framework for understanding and action. *Developmental Review*, *12*(4), 374–390. doi.org/10.1016/0273-2297(92)90014-S

Kenny, M. E., & Hage, S. M. (2009). The next frontier: Prevention as an instrument of social justice. *The Journal of Primary Prevention*, *30*(1), 1–10. doi.org/10.1007/s10935-008-0163-7

Khanani, N., O'Dwyer, L., Raczek, A., & Walsh, M. E. (2021, October 1). *The impact of integrated student support on non-cognitive outcomes* [Paper presentation]. Society for Research on Educational Effectiveness, Virtual.

Khanani, N., Raczek, A., & Walsh, M. E. (2021, October 1). *Integrated student support and academic achievement* [Paper presentation]. Society for Research on Educational Effectiveness, Virtual.

Kirschman, K. J. B., Johnson, R. J., Bender, J. A., & Roberts, M. C. (2009). Positive psychology for children and adolescents: Development, prevention, and promotion. In C. R. Snyder & S. J. Lopez (Eds.), *Oxford handbook of positive psychology* (2nd ed., pp. 133–148). Oxford University Press.

Lee-St. John, T. J., Walsh, M. E., Raczek, A. E., Vuilleumier, C. E., Foley, C., Heberle, A., Sibley, E., & Dearing, E. (2018). The long-term impact of systemic student support in elementary school: Reducing high school dropout. *AERA Open*, *4*(4), 1–16. doi.org/10.1177/2332858418799085

Leigh, Y., Foley, C., & Walsh, M. E. (2022). *Actionable evidence initiative case study: An actionable data system approach.* Project Evident. www.projectevident.org/updates/2022/1/5/an-actionable-data-system-approach

Lerner, R. M. (1991). Changing organism-context relations as the basic process of development: A developmental contextual perspective. *Developmental Psychology*, *27*(1), 27–32.

Lerner, R. M. (2001). Promoting promotion in the development of prevention science. *Applied Developmental Science*, *5*(4), 254–257. doi.org/10.1037/0012-1649.27.1.27

Lerner, R. M. (2018). *Concepts and theories of human development* (4th ed.). Routledge. doi.org/10.4324/9780203581629

Lerner, R. M., Bornstein, M. H., & Jervis, P. (2022). The development of positive attributes of character: On the embodiment of specificity, holism, and self-system processes. *Human Development*, *66*(1), 34–47. doi.org/10.1159/000521583

Manekin, S. (2016). City Connects: Redesigning student support for academic success. *The Abell Report*, *29*(3), 1–16. https://files.eric.ed.gov/fulltext/ED570922.pdf

Masten, A. S. (2011). Resilience in children threatened by extreme adversity: Frameworks for research, practice, and translational synergy. *Development and Psychopathology*, 23(2), 493–506. doi.org/10.1017/S0954579411000198

Masten, A. S. (2014). *Ordinary magic: Resilience in development.* Guilford Publications.

Masten, A. S. (2018). Resilience theory and research on children and families: Past, present, and promise. *Journal of Family Theory & Review*, *10*(1), 12–31. doi.org/10.1111/jftr.12255

Masten, A. S., & Cicchetti, D. (2010). Developmental cascades. *Development and Psychopathology*, *22*(3), 491–495. doi.org/10.1017/S0954579410000222

Masten, A. S., & Cicchetti, D. (2016). Resilience in development: Progress and transformation. In D. Cicchetti & D. J. Cohen (Eds.), *Developmental psychopathology: Risk, resilience, and intervention* (3rd ed., pp. 271–333, Volume 4). John Wiley & Sons, Inc.

Masten, A. S., & Labella, M. H. (2016). Risk and resilience in child development. In L. Balter & C. S. Tamis-LeMonda (Eds.), *Child psychology: A handbook of contemporary issues* (pp. 423–450). New York, NY: Taylor & Francis.

Masten, A. S., & Obradović, J. (2006). Competence and resilience in development. *Annals of the New York Academy of Sciences*, *1094*(1), 13–27. doi.org/10.1196/annals.1376.003

McEwen, B. (2016). In pursuit of resilience: Stress, epigenetics, and brain plasticity. *Annals of the New York Academy of Sciences*, *1373*(1), 56–64. doi.org/10.1111/nyas.13020

Moore, K., & Emig, C. (2014). *Integrated student supports: A summary of the evidence for policymakers. Child Trends.* www.childtrends.org/wp-content/uploads/2014/02/2014-05ISSWhitePaper3.pdf

National Center for Complementary and Integrative Health. (2021). *NCCIH strategic plan FY 2021–2025: Mapping a pathway to research on whole person health.* www.nccih.nih.gov/about/nccih-strategic-plan-2021-2025

National Research Council and Institute of Medicine. (2009). Defining the scope of prevention. In M. E. O'Connell, T. Boat, & K. E. Warner (Eds.), *Preventing mental, emotional, and behavioral disorders among young people: Progress and possibilities* (pp. 59–70). The National Academies Press. doi.org/10.17226/12480

Pittman, K. (1996). Community, youth, development: Three goals in search of connection. *New Designs for Youth Development, 12*(1), 4–8.

Pollack, C., Theodorakakis, M., & Walsh, M. E. (2021). Leveraging integrated student support to identify and address COVID-19-related needs for students, families, and teachers. *AERA Open, 7*(1), 1–18. doi.org/10.1177%2F23328584211058473

Reardon, S. F. (2011). The widening academic achievement gap between the rich and the poor: New evidence and possible explanations. In G. J. Duncan & R. J. Murnane, *Whither opportunity: Rising inequality, schools, and children's life chances* (pp. 91–115). Russell Sage Foundation.

Reese, L. R. E., & Vera, E. M. (2007). Culturally relevant prevention: The scientific and practical considerations of community-based programs. *The Counseling Psychologist, 35*(6), 763–778. doi.org/10.1177/0011000007304588

Romano, J. L. (2015). *Prevention psychology: Enhancing personal and social well-being.* American Psychological Association. doi.org/10.1037/14442-001

Romano, J. L., & Hage, S. M. (2000). Prevention and counseling psychology: Revitalizing commitments for the twenty-first century. *The Counseling Psychologist, 28*(6), 733–763. doi.org/10.1177%2F0011000000286001

Rothstein, R. (2010). How to fix our schools. *Economic Policy Institute, 286*, 1–6. www.epi.org/publication/ib286/

Sameroff, A. (2009). The transactional model. In A. Sameroff (Ed.), *The transactional model of development: How children and contexts shape each other* (pp. 3–21). American Psychological Association. doi.org/10.1037/11877-001

Theron, L., Rothmann, S., Höltge, J., & Ungar, M. (2022). Differential adaptation to adversity: A latent profile analysis of youth engagement with resilience-enabling cultural resources and mental health outcomes in a stressed Canadian and South African community. *Journal of Cross-Cultural Psychology, 53*(3–4), 403–425. doi.org/10.1177%2F00220221221077353

Unger, J., Morales, I., De Paepe, P., & Roland, M. (2020). Integrating clinical and public health knowledge in support of joint medical practice. *BMC Health Services Research, 20*(Suppl 2), 1073–1073. doi.org/10.1186/s12913-020-05886-z

Walsh, M., & Brabeck, M. (2006). Resilience and risk in learning: Complex interactions and comprehensive interventions. In R. J. Sternberg & R. F. Subotnik (Eds.), *Optimizing student success in school with the other three Rs: Reasoning, resilience, and responsibility* (pp. 113–142). Information Age.

Walsh, M., DePaul, J., & Park-Taylor, J. (2009). Prevention as a mechanism for promoting positive development in the context of risk: Principles of best practice. In M. E. Kenny, M. Horne, P. Orpinas, & L. E. Reese (Eds.), *Realizing social justice: The challenge of preventive interventions* (pp. 57–78). American Psychological Association. doi.org/10.1037/11870-000

Walsh, M. E. (2021). *The whole child: Building systems of integrated student support during and after COVID-19: An action guide.* Boston College Center for Optimized Student Support. www.bc.edu/content/dam/bc1/schools/lsoe/sites/coss/COVID%20Action%20Guide_V7.pdf

Walsh, M. E., Galassi, J. P., Murphy, J. A., & Park-Taylor, J. (2002). A conceptual framework for counseling psychologists in schools. *The Counseling Psychologist, 30*(5), 682–704. doi.org/10.1177/0011000002305002

Walsh, M. E., Hamilton, A., & Tran, Q. (2019). Role of the university in building schools for the whole child. In R. F. Kronick (Ed.), *Emerging perspectives on community schools and the engaged university* (pp. 40–61). IGI Global. doi.org/10.4018/978-1-7998-0280-8

Walsh, M. E., Madaus, G. F., Raczek, A. E., Dearing, E., Foley, C., An, C., Lee-St. John, T. J., & Beaton, A. (2014). A new model for student support in high-poverty urban elementary schools: Effects on elementary and middle school academic outcomes. *American Educational Research Journal*, *51*(4), 704–737. doi.org/10.3102%2F0002831214541669

Wasser Gish, J. (2019). Building systems of integrated student support: A policy brief for local and state leaders. *Center for Promise*. www.bc.edu/content/dam/bc1/schools/lsoe/sites/coss/FederalPolicyBrief_v4.pdf

Weiss, E., & Reville, P. S. (2019). *Broader, bolder, better: How schools and communities help students overcome the disadvantages of poverty*. Harvard Education Press.

# 6 Systemic Interventions to Promote Well-Being in Black, Indigenous, and People of Color Students Attending K-12 Schools

Elizabeth Vera, Claire Furtado, and Chelsea Yanuaria

> Educators need to know what happens in the world of the children with whom they work. They need to know the universe of their dreams, the language with which they skillfully defend themselves from the aggressiveness of their world, what they know independently of the school, and how they know it.
>
> —Paulo Freire (Freire, 1988, p. 72)

> Our wonderful ability to reason must be combined in education with a warm heart and a sense of responsibility, in order to bring about a peaceful, happy world.
>
> —Dalai Lama (Dalai Lama, 2022, p. 8)

Recent sociopolitical events in the United States have reminded us of the ongoing social injustices impacting Black, Indigenous, and People of Color (BIPOC) communities, as evidenced in acts of racially motivated, discriminatory legislation, and a worsening of ethnic–racial health and economic disparities. At the onset of the COVID-19 pandemic, the murders of unarmed Black Americans at the hands of law enforcement sparked public outrage, activism, countless protests, and the Black Lives Matter movement to refocus our nation's attention to the systemic racism and discrimination that people of color are continually forced to endure in contemporary US society. This context has important implications for promoting the healthy development and well-being of BIPOC students attending US schools.

While one might assume that our history of racial injustices would be a necessary focus of educational experiences of all students, an increasing number of states have passed legislation banning discussions and teachings that critique race relations in K-12 schools, thereby limiting dialogues that educate youth about racism and bias in and out of school contexts. These policies are not only overtly discriminatory and antithetical to freedom of speech, but also stifle critical perspectives about the historical and systemic oppression of BIPOC communities in the United States. Further, they send a clear message to BIPOC youth that the comfort of White students is more important than acknowledging their lived experiences of discrimination and challenging systems of oppression and social injustice.

The COVID-19 pandemic has also had adverse health consequences for BIPOC communities, creating even more challenges to the positive development of youth. Although BIPOC groups have long faced significant health and mental health disparities in the United States, the pandemic exacerbated these disparities. Prior to COVID-19, although racial and ethnic minority groups experienced mental health disorders at rates similar to the general US population, they were substantially less likely to receive mental health treatment (SAMHSA, 2020). A wide range of social and economic factors have contributed to these inequities in access to mental health care, such as racial disparities in health insurance and access to affordable healthcare, as well as overrepresentation of BIPOC families in low-wage jobs, leading to food and housing insecurity and related financial concerns (Artiga et al., 2020). For BIPOC youth, virtual learning and social distancing mandates limited their access to social support (e.g., friends at school) and consistent, safe environments (e.g., schools, after-school programs, community centers), all of which are important to well-being.

Beyond the stressors associated with the pandemic, BIPOC youth, unlike their White peers, must still contend with ongoing experiences of discrimination across contexts, which has clear implications for their well-being. Benner et al. (2018) conducted a meta-analysis to investigate the relationship between BIPOC adolescents' experiences of racial/ethnic discrimination and various well-being outcomes, which yielded a number of significant findings. Experiences of racial/ethnic discrimination were associated with increased socio-emotional distress (i.e., depression, internalizing symptoms, and lower self-esteem and well-being), as well as lower academic achievement, motivation and engagement, and increased engagement in risky health behaviors (i.e., externalizing behaviors, risky sexual behaviors, substance use).

Another noteworthy challenge specific to BIPOC adolescents which has adverse consequences for their mental health is racial trauma that refers to instances in which an individual directly experiences or witnesses dangerous race-based events or discrimination (Comas-Diaz et al., 2019). Because communities of color repeatedly live amid these stressful experiences, racial trauma results in ongoing injuries to BIPOC individuals and their communities (Saleem et al., 2020). Such experiences were pervasive during the summer of 2020, as countless BIPOC youth witnessed physical assaults against people of color who were protesting play out in the media. As a key context in which BIPOC youth operate, school systems are particularly influential in shaping youths' experiences of racial trauma, as they may serve as environments in which youth both experience racial trauma and, alternatively, have access to supporting services that help them combat these experiences and help mitigate the consequences of such experiences (Saleem et al., 2020).

The role of contexts and larger systems in youth development cannot be understated, as BIPOC youth not only are forced to confront racism and discrimination in public policies and their local communities but may also contend with these experiences in school settings. Research has indicated that BIPOC youth report experiences of discrimination from peers as well as from educators and administrators in school settings (Montoro et al., 2021). Of note, when adolescents experienced discrimination from peers, they reported poorer mental health outcomes, whereas when confronted with discrimination from school personnel, they exhibited worse academic performance and lower sense of belonging at school (Benner & Graham, 2013). Collectively, this information underscores the need for professionals to go beyond universal individual-level interventions to promote the well-being of BIPOC youth and to develop culturally relevant interventions that not only account for the aforementioned challenges facing BIPOC students, but also target school systems (e.g., teachers, administrators, school policies).

To date, the vast majority of empirically supported social and emotional learning (SEL) interventions for K-12 students have been developed and tested with predominantly White samples and implemented universally. As a result, the voices and needs of BIPOC students are markedly underrepresented in intervention development and evaluation processes, which limits the generalizability and relevance of said interventions for BIPOC students. In order to elucidate the need for culturally relevant, comprehensive systems-level interventions to support the well-being of BIPOC youth, this chapter will first review some of the shortcomings with existing universal SEL interventions.

## 6.1 Critique of Existing Prevention Programs

As indicated earlier, BIPOC youth face a variety of unique challenges that can impair their well-being, underscoring the need for culturally relevant interventions that explicitly address their social and emotional needs. Although past research has supported the positive effects of universal SEL interventions for K-12 students (Durlak et al., 2011), compelling reasons exist to examine this claim with skepticism. In a review of over 100 studies, Rowe and Trickett (2018) found that only one-third of the studies included any analyses to test for diverse program effects, leading them to assert that researchers must exercise considerable caution in drawing conclusions about the generalizability of universal SEL intervention effectiveness for diverse groups of students. Likewise, other SEL scholars have criticized the overreliance on individual, decontextualized approaches that fail to acknowledge or address the unique needs of BIPOC students, given their minoritized identities (Jagers et al., 2019).

Apart from neglecting the distinct mental health needs of BIPOC students, universal SEL interventions also have the potential to reinforce existing inequities. School systems exist within the larger context of US society and, as such, inherently reflect and reproduce the central ideologies, values, norms, and systemic inequities of dominant US culture. Consequently, because US systems have historically served to reinforce the oppression of racial and ethnic minority groups, while privileging the rights, values, and norms of the White majority, school systems may, by default, center Whiteness and prioritize the success and well-being of mainstream students (Jagers et al., 2019).

To illustrate this point, the work of Voight and colleagues (2015) on school climate examined subjective perceptions of safety, support, and connectedness among middle school students and found that *within the same school environments,* Black and Latinx students reported poorer perceptions of school climate than did White students. These racial school climate gaps were also associated with racial disparities in academic achievement. Furthermore, the results of the study revealed that when schools carried out universal efforts to improve school climate and reduce racial achievement gaps, White students benefited significantly more than BIPOC students. Certainly, these findings highlight the need for schools to go beyond universal interventions to promote the well-being of BIPOC youth, as even well-intended interventions that address issues relevant to these students may be limited in effectiveness at best and may reproduce ethnic/racial inequities at worst.

In a similar vein, scholars have argued that universal SEL interventions may inherently reflect the dominant US culture's emphasis on individualism, normative views of appropriate expressions of emotion, and perceptions of power, and individual choice and control (Hoffman, 2009). This perspective suggests that simply making surface-level modifications to universal SEL interventions (e.g., using culturally diverse illustrations, translating into multiple languages) is not enough to ensure that interventions are culturally appropriate, as such efforts do not address implicit biases that are embedded in the underlying assumptions and content of universal SEL programs. Relatedly, research has supported an association between universal SEL, increased teacher classroom management, and control of student behavioral issues (Lewkowicz, 2006; Hoffman, 2009). These findings raise the question of whether universal SEL programs are intended to cultivate social and emotional skills that are in the best interest of *all* students, or if they are actually serving to condition students to function more optimally within systems that represent dominant Western culture that was designed to reinforce systems of power, privilege, and oppression. Collectively, the considerations presented earlier highlight the limitations and potential consequences of relying on universal SEL interventions to foster equitable outcomes and promote the well-being of BIPOC students. Therefore, we argue that there is a clear need for the implementation of systems-level interventions explicitly designed to address the unique mental health needs of BIPOC students.

In addition to concerns about the lack of attention to culture and diversity in universal school-based SEL interventions, the vast majority of these interventions are also significantly limited in scope. More specifically, interventions that solely target individual students fail to address other important members of the school community (e.g., teachers, administrators, students' families), as well as key characteristics of the school environment which have a profound impact on students' experiences at school (e.g., policies, norms, school climate) (Mahoney et al., 2021). Moreover, individual-level interventions do not take advantage of students' family systems or members of the broader community, all of whom could be leveraged to increase the support for BIPOC students at multiple levels and across critical developmental contexts. Further, because these interventions do not address many of the actors and issues within school systems that contribute to the inequitable and harmful experiences that BIPOC students face, they place a tremendous burden on the individual students to manage the stress and extensive negative impacts of navigating oppressive systems.

Given the embeddedness of racism, discrimination, and social inequalities throughout US systems, policies, and the dominant culture at large, interventions that target only students' social and emotional competencies simply are not equipped to confront the root causes of these systems-level problems. Indeed, a paramount advantage of adopting a comprehensive systems-level focus in school-based interventions lies in the potential they have to transform entire school systems and, in turn, promote change that is more enduring. In the upcoming segments of this chapter, we will provide an in-depth review of the role of systemic interventions in the promotion of well-being for BIPOC youth, but first we will briefly present an argument for centering culture in the development and implementation of systems-level interventions for BIPOC.

## 6.2 Culture and Prevention Programs

Given the overall dearth of existing culturally relevant prevention programs for BIPOC youth, in conjunction with the potential for increased intervention effectiveness that may result from a more robust consideration of the cultural background of the target community, a clear rationale exists for prevention efforts to strive for cultural relevance. To ensure conceptual clarity, cultural relevance of an intervention refers to the degree to which it aligns with the values, beliefs, and needs of a specific community (Reese & Vera, 2007).

In the development of culturally relevant interventions, it is essential for researchers to first establish a foundational understanding of the cultural worldview (i.e., norms, values, lived experience, understanding of the world) of members of the community that the intervention plans to target. This involves contextualizing the problems in a way that is consistent with the community members' lived experiences and understanding of the given problems (Reese & Vera, 2007). If executed effectively, not only does this help ensure that the voices and needs of the community members of interest serve as the basis upon which the intervention will be developed, but it may also help prevent researchers from imposing their personal values and worldviews on the intervention design and characteristics.

Also critical to the development of culturally relevant interventions is the cultivation of personal relationships between researchers and members of the community (Reese & Vera, 2007). By interacting with community members and getting involved in community events, researchers can build enduring partnerships with members of the community they hope to serve and, importantly, demonstrate their investment in the community. Beyond establishing these relationships, inviting community members to serve as partners in all phases of program development and evaluation is an important way to give voice to the community and to ensure that interventions meaningfully address their needs; such involvement can also serve as a source of empowerment and provide opportunities for skill development (Trickett et al., 2011). Additionally, the utilization of community-based participatory research and transformative research methodologies can help guide these efforts. While the recommendations presented herein are by no means exhaustive, they serve as a starting point. We next outline the ways in which systems influence the well-being of BIPOC youth in school settings.

## 6.3 Systems' Influences on BIPOC Well-Being

Given that important contexts such as school, family, and the larger community influence well-being of BIPOC students, relying on prevention programs and SEL frameworks that overemphasize self-awareness, self-management, social awareness, decision-making, and relational skills is inadequate. BIPOC students are directly impacted by not only school experiences but also the larger contexts in which they live shape expectations of and needs that can be met in schools. We next discuss how specific components of school systems, namely, teachers, school climate issues, and parent involvement, play a role in mitigating the well-being of BIPOC students.

### 6.3.1 Teachers

Teachers are integral to creating and sustaining environments where all students can thrive. However, research indicates that teachers are not always sufficiently trained to understand student diversity issues (Shim, 2019; Liang et al., 2020); furthermore, the majority of teachers are still not as racially diverse as the students they serve (Gay, 2018). This is not solely a US reality.

In most Western countries, teachers tend to be English-speaking, middle-class females of European descent (Sleeter, 2001). This often leads to a mismatch in the worldviews of teachers and BIPOC students.

Further, research indicates that racial microaggressions from teachers occur frequently and creates a threatening environment that negatively impacts not only BIPOC students' social and emotional well-being but also their ability to learn (Vera et al., 2018, 2021). In a recent study, the need for teachers to interrogate their own assumptions and biases and better understand the nuances of their sociocultural experiences was highlighted by students' desire for teachers to better understand their lived experiences and get to know their families and circumstances outside of school (Heineke & Vera, 2022). Student participants wanted teachers to develop a more personalized understanding of their lives and how their unique struggles influence their social and emotional well-being, a finding echoed in previous literature (Vera et al., 2021). Notably, students further indicated a need for teachers to understand the impact of adverse in-school experiences (e.g., microaggressions from peers and educators) on their well-being and wanted to intervene on their behalf. Vera et al. (2021) found that teachers often minimize the impact their words and actions have on students and underestimate the degree to which teachers were modeling to other students that insensitive and microaggressive behavior is acceptable. Cultural insensitivities and unintended racism serve as barriers to positive relationships that teachers must have with BIPOC students; thus, the cultural competencies of teachers must be a focus of systems-level interventions.

### **6.3.2** School Climate

Schools serve as a microcosm of a broader society that treats differences as deficits, and unfortunately, school climate is often not as supportive for BIPOC students as their White counterparts (Voight et al., 2015). Indeed, educators frequently hold deficit views of immigrant and BIPOC families, treating their languages and cultures as problems to be fixed. For example, Valenzuela (1999) highlights the historical bias of English as a Second Language Programs that often convey the message that languages such as Spanish are second rate, regarding youth as "limited English proficient" instead of "Spanish dominant" or bilingual. Such educational practices are regarded as "subtractive," as they signal a goal to "disinfect" students of their language and culture, crippling both their educational success and positive ethnic identity development (Menken & Kleyn, 2010). In addition, research shows that students are negatively impacted when schools fail to take a stand on social problems relevant to their lives. In Vera et al.'s (2021) study, many students were sensitive to the fact that their schools failed to take a position on the growing anti-immigrant sentiments in the United States, negatively impacting their social and emotional well-being.

Within a school climate that devalues diverse languages, cultures, and experiences, it is not surprising that BIPOC students are more likely to experience bullying than those from the cultural majority. According to Polanin and Vera (2013), it is imperative that educators recognize school bullying as a social justice issue as it threatens access to a safe and equitable learning environment. Educators must also recognize the influence they hold through promoting and modeling acceptance for students of all cultures. Unfortunately, students' regular experiences of microaggressions and bullying from peers are not typically reported to school personnel (Vera et al., 2018). Indeed, if children feel teachers will not assist in such situations, they are not only less likely to report these experiences, but they are also less likely to stand up for targeted peers (Vera et al., 2019). It is unreasonable to expect a behavioral change in the majority student population without teachers, staff, and school leadership first addressing their own biases and harmful interactions with BIPOC students and modeling respect and appreciation for cultural diversity.

However, a strong need also exists for majority students to be challenged about their own values, attitudes, and biases, which show up not only in negative events such as bullying, but also in patterns of friendships between BIPOC and White students (Byrd, 2019; Vera et al., 2021). Furthermore, school curricula often insufficiently reflect the cultures of students (Gay, 2018), which suggests that school administrators must be monitoring to what extent their BIPOC students' sense of belonging is impacted by school climate issues. However, there is often a dearth of knowledge and opportunities available for them to do so (Heineke & Vera, 2022), This is due to several factors, one being that examining the impact of racism in education has been "stymied by a lack of coherence in the many conceptualizations and operationalizations in the educational and psychological literatures" (Byrd, 2019, p. 137). In addition, there are few valid measures available that can be used to monitor BIPOC perceptions of school racial climates (Bustamante, 2006; Byrd, 2019).

### 6.3.3 Parent Involvement

Research shows that parents represent a too often untapped resource for teachers which, if engaged as equals, could transform the culture of schools and communities (Warren, 2005; Warren et al., 2009; Hong, 2011). If engaged, BIPOC parents could serve as a gateway for teachers to better understand students' lives outside of the classroom, and while parent educational involvement has been demonstrated to be an important contributor to children's educational success, traditional forms of parent involvement cater to White middle-class families, making school engagement less accessible to many BIPOC families (Hong, 2011). Traditional forms of parent involvement tend to be school-centric and activity-based, focusing on ways individual parents can assist with school operations. Involving parents in this way fails to give parents any measure of power over school processes, which is problematic given that BIPOC parents may have different ideas and values for their children's education (Warren et al., 2009).

BIPOC parents may also be reluctant to seek involvement due to longstanding legacies of racism and mistrust between parents and educators, and they may lack the social and cultural capital necessary to have their voices heard (Fine, 1993; Warren et al., 2009; Vera et al., 2016). As previously indicated, educators frequently hold deficit views of immigrant and BIPOC families, treating parents as "less than" school professionals (Fine, 1993). Given these challenges, it is not surprising that parents and teachers often become adversaries instead of collaborative partners in the education of children (Fine, 1993; Hong, 2011). Thus, to engage BIPOC parents as partners, active efforts need to undo potential harm and biases that have led BIPOC parents to assume that they are not valued as assets.

## 6.4 Systemic Interventions

Prevention best practice literature identifies cultural relevance and the inclusion of systemic influences as key ingredients of successful intervention design (Hage et al., 2007), despite the reality that too many prevention programs continue to over-rely on universal, individually focused strategies. However, in a recent article, Mahoney et al. (2021) discuss systemic SEL as a new framework that includes systemic-centered interventions, such as those that strengthen adults' competencies, cultivate family, and community partnerships, and examine school-wide practices and policies, identifying each of these three factors as being a critical ingredient of successful SEL. We argue that by adopting a systemic lens, SEL and other prevention frameworks used with BIPOC students are significantly strengthened (Jagers et al., 2019; Mahoney et al., 2021). We next highlight several systems-level intervention frameworks that have been successfully used in school-based prevention with BIPOC students: parent-centered interventions, teacher-centered interventions, and examinations of school-wide practices that impact climate.

## 6.5 Parent-Centered Interventions

Collaborations between schools and community-based organizations have emerged as a means of bridging the cultural gap between schools and families (Warren, 2005; Warren et al., 2009). These collaborations highlight that engaging BIPOC parents in schools requires attending to and transforming underlying processes of power and recognizing their cultures and experiences as assets in the education of children (Hong, 2011). Community-based organizations act as cultural brokers between families and schools, affording educators an opportunity to better meet the needs of the families they serve and parents an avenue to greater influence in schools and communities (Hong, 2011; Ishimaru et al., 2016). Beyond this, family, community, and school partnerships give parents an opportunity to build relational networks, develop as leaders, and engage in community activism. These collaborations demonstrate how intimately linked community and school life are and the necessity of understanding the needs of the neighborhoods and influences of the larger social systems in which schools are embedded (Warren, 2005; Warren et al., 2009; Hong, 2011). We next briefly discuss three community–school collaboration models as proposed by Warren et al. (2009), paying special attention to the work the Logan Square Neighborhood Association is doing in Chicago (Hong, 2011). We then highlight Hong's (2011) ecology of parent engagement model and Warren et al.'s (2009) community-based relational model of parent engagement.

### 6.5.1 The Community Service Approach

The community service model is predicated on the assumption that schools cannot serve children without attending to their basic needs (Warren et al., 2009). Through partnerships with service delivery organizations, this model mandates that public schools provide access to a range of health and social services as well as after-school programs, such as adult education and ESL courses for community residents. Through the provision of services, families are brought into the life of the school and teachers develop a more holistic understanding of how to support children (Warren, 2005). As an example, Warren et al. (2009) discuss the partnership between the Quitman School and the Community Agencies Corporation of New Jersey (CACNJ). Through the creation of a community school, Quitman became a safe place for families struggling to survive day-to-day. Beyond receiving services, parents were given the opportunity to become group leaders providing supervision to children in after-school programs and becoming bridges between teachers and the larger parent population. Quitman School demonstrates the importance of meeting the basic needs of families as a necessary first step to parent engagement. A critique of this model is that it tends to emphasize family needs over family assets and fails to address the extent to which parents exercise any power within the school community (Warren et al., 2009).

### 6.5.2 The Community Development Approach

The community development model involves the creation of a new school, usually a charter school that is explicitly committed to community engagement and change. United by a shared pedagogy and values, sponsored schools make efforts to engage families through the hiring of staff that families can relate to and by engaging them in community development efforts to strengthen ownership of their neighborhoods (Warren, 2005). Warren et al. (2009) discuss the Camino Nuevo Charter Academy in Los Angeles, which was established by the Pueblo Nuevo Development (PND) Corporation, to revitalize the MacArthur Park neighborhood and to better serve the Latinx families who live there. To make the school a place families felt welcomed, 50% of the teachers, administrators, and paraprofessionals spoke Spanish. Through required participation, parents became an important presence in the school with some becoming paraprofessionals via participation in leadership workshops. Like with the Quitman School, these parents served as a bridge between the school and the larger community. The school also sponsored neighborhood cleanups, environmental campaigns, and health fairs. A critique of this model is it does not foster parent leadership in the school and community (Warren et al., 2009).

### 6.5.3 The Community Organizing Approach

The community organizing approach is the most political of all models discussed focusing on schools becoming vehicles for social and political change. This model highlights the importance of developing parents as leaders not just within schools, but also in the greater community (Warren, 2005; Warren et al., 2009; Hong, 2011). Hong (2011) discusses the work of Chicago's Logan Square Neighborhood Association (LSNA) which, through their Parent Mentor Program, leadership training, and the cultivation of strong relational networks, develops parents into school–community leaders and activists. Through the Parent Mentorship Program, parents are paired with teachers and work alongside them as equals throughout the course of the school year, affording parents insight into the inner workings of schools and teachers' much-needed support in the classroom. Working together builds the mentality that parents and teachers are on the same team when culture and language differences previously served as a real or perceived barrier. Parents reach out to other parents not yet involved and build a supportive parent community that sustains their continued involvement. Parents also set their own goals for the year, such as getting their GED or learning English and participating in leadership training where they can cultivate a critical consciousness and better understand how power operates in their encounters with schools and other institutions. Many parents also participate in the Grow Your Own Teachers Program, taking tuition-free college courses leading to certification as bilingual teachers. Through these experiences, parents develop as school leaders and community activists. What this model of parent engagement teaches us is that parents possess a multitude of too often untapped resources that can benefit not only schools but the fabric of the communities in which they live.

Through studying the work of the LSNA, Hong (2011) developed the ecology of parent engagement model that consists of three stages. The first phase, induction, begins when parents begin to develop an understanding of schools through initial participation and educators begin to understand the culture and assets that parents bring to the classroom. The second phase, integration, occurs when parents develop an identity as part of the school community and are working collaboratively with teachers on the education of children. The third phase, investment, occurs when parent leaders emerge, and their interests are not just for their own children but for all children and the needs of the greater community. Hong (2011) highlights that the success of parent engagement is shaped by three driving processes, including mutual engagement, relationship building, and the sharing of leadership and power.

Warren et al. (2009) also offer a framework for parent engagement via community and school partnerships that they describe as the community-based relational approach. While the previously discussed models offer different means of parent engagement, their success is driven by three core elements including relationship building among parents and between parents and educators, developing parents as leaders, and bridging the power and culture gap between families and educators. Opportunities for such partnerships are dependent on teachers and school leadership being open to change. As Hong (2011) highlights, the culture of schools is critical and whether or not parents are welcomed and viewed as assets will influence their engagement. In one of our own studies on parent leadership (Vera et al., 2016), we found that teacher attitudes toward parents and the encouragement of their involvement impacted parents' leadership interests. We next discuss teacher-centered interventions that focus on building teacher capacities for working with diverse communities.

## 6.6 Teacher-Centered Interventions

Given that self-awareness impacts the capacity of prevention interventionists to deliver culturally relevant interventions, teachers' self-awareness and cultural competence are important aspects of successful school-based prevention efforts and transformational SEL (Jagers et al., 2019). This is not only because teachers often serve as interventionists for SEL and other prevention efforts, but also because teachers' expectations and relationships with students are so critically tied to students' successes and feelings of acceptance (Shapiro & MacDonald, 2017; Shi, 2018). Thus, improving the well-being of BIPOC students must involve strengthening the cultural competence of teachers.

It is important to state that teachers and other school professionals are educated in the same higher education institutions as most other professionals. Thus, teachers are not *less* well trained to understand cultural diversity than are other professionals. In fact, Starck et al. (2020) found that teachers as a profession are no more biased than nonteachers, but implicit biases that exist in educators can result in misattributions about student behaviors, differential academic expectations for BIPOC students, and inequities in the way students are graded (Chin et al., 2020). Furthermore, biases in academic teaching and advising can have significant implications for students' postsecondary paths (Oseguera, 2013), often through inequitable access to advanced coursework for BIPOC students (Chajewski et al., 2011). Thus, strengthening teachers' cultural competencies, expectations for BIPOC students, and self-awareness of diversity issues can take on a variety of forms.

### 6.6.1 Interrogating Beliefs and Biases

Self-awareness is the cornerstone of cultural competence (Sue et al., 2019), and a plethora of education scholars have argued that the first step in strengthening cultural competence of teachers is helping them gain greater awareness of their beliefs and biases, both those that are explicit and those that are implicit (Samuels, 2014). Historically, teachers were not trained to explicitly attend to the cultures of their students, in favor of a colorblind approach that encourages a view where "all students are the same." However, without understanding the importance of larger societal contexts of racism and educational disparities, teachers can adopt deficit mindsets (Gay, 2018) that lower expectations of individual students who are not part of the so-called mainstream.

It may be that the biases teachers are unaware of can do the most damage. For example, a 2010 study that examined teachers' implicit and explicit ethnic biases found that their implicit – not explicit – biases were responsible for different expectations of achievement for students from different ethnic backgrounds (van den Bergh et al., 2010). Fortunately, mechanisms for identifying and reducing implicit biases have been developed over the last decades, and in the context of education, Whitford and Emerson (2019) found that implicit bias can be reduced through psychoeducational programs with preservice teachers.

### 6.6.2 Microaggressions

A second area that is critical for teachers to build awareness of is the topic of microaggressions. Microaggressions can appear as unintentional racism, such as when teachers mispronounce ethnic names (Thorpe, 2017), hold erroneous beliefs about bilingualism (Reeves, 2006), or discourage BIPOC students from taking academically challenging classes in an effort to "protect" them (Oseguera, 2013). While not intentionally mean-spirited, teachers' microaggressions can have unintended consequences of reducing BIPOC students' feelings of belonging, validation, and self-confidence (Vera et al., 2021).

However, it is not merely the prevention of teachers' own microaggressive beliefs or behaviors that should be included in professional development. Teachers are also often the primary adults who witness microaggressions that happen between students, and their ability to respond appropriately can also affect students' sense of safety and well-being in school settings. Eisenberg et al. (2021) studied racial and other culturally targeted microaggressions in students and found that teachers' responses, when they were in the position to interrupt or intervene, were virtually nonexistent. Inaction can be a sign of complicity at worst, but even when it is not meant as such, passivity models a lack of accountability and signals to BIPOC students that they are on their own to handle racism in its many forms.

### 6.6.3 Expanding Knowledge of Diverse Cultures

Given the changing demographics of most communities in the United States, teachers' students are likely to be of different cultural backgrounds than teachers themselves (Gay, 2018). Therefore, there is a need for teachers to engage in cross-cultural learning (Milner, 2003; Killoran et al., 2004; Brown & Howard, 2005; Garmon, 2005). This may be particularly true for newer immigrants and refugees, but also for groups of students from cultures that are a part of the history of the United States such as African American, Asian American, and Latinx ethnic groups.

Professional development can focus on building knowledge about the histories, customs, and values of specific cultural groups and can feature parents of students who can serve as teachers about their cultures. Professional learning communities can identify books, speakers, and cultural immersion opportunities to learn about unfamiliar cultures. Ideally, this expansion of knowledge would occur while teachers are still preservice. Studies have shown that teacher preparation courses and activities can successfully enhance teacher candidates' level of intercultural sensitivity (Mahoney & Schamber, 2004; Sobel & Taylor, 2005). Nonetheless, teachers acknowledge that professional development focused on cultural knowledge building enhances their ability to teach BIPOC, immigrant, and refugee students (Heineke & Vera, 2022).

## 6.7 Examining School-Wide Practices and Policies

Many activities encompass a holistic examination of school-wide practices and policies important to promoting a positive climate for BIPOC students. The end goal of these examinations, however, is capacity building, such that schools can monitor their own strengths and growth edges in a sustainable way. Meyers et al. (2012) noted that schools function best when they diagnose their own strengths and weaknesses. There are several helpful models that assist schools in this examination. Bustamante's (2006) "cultural audit" is a framework and set of questions that schools can ask themselves which allow for the development of action plans that can be implemented locally. Examples of areas where schools can self-assess include examining the existence (or lack thereof) of diversity-affirming mission statements and strengthening the use of culturally inclusive curricula. Importantly, the audit also calls for assessing the representation of students in advanced placement, special education, and honors programs. This type of data monitoring is key to identifying educational disparities. Also, the audit helps schools in creating mechanisms that monitor the functioning of student voice feedback loops such as student advisory boards.

Additionally, the audit focuses on helping schools identify and design areas for ongoing professional development of teachers and staff in areas that are specific to their schools' populations (e.g., BIPOC, immigrant groups). The audit also provides guidance on how schools can set up processes for tracking the success of differentiated instructional strategies, examining success in community outreach efforts, and monitoring inclusivity in parent involvement. Once schools can identify areas in which they are successful as well as growth edges, plans can be developed for areas of need.

Similarly, Byrd (2019) developed a survey that allows school professionals to capture the experiences of BIPOC students with respect to their perceptions of inclusivity, representation, and to ascertain how successful schools have been in fostering opportunities for intercultural relationships and friendships. This kind of a tool not only helps schools identify areas for growth, but also whether specific groups of students feel better represented than other groups. For example, if one particular group of students felt that their cultures were not well represented in student activity opportunities, schools could invest resources in new clubs or organizations and monitor changes in students' attitudes and feelings. These types of surveys also help school professionals identify areas where students perceive bias and discrimination in curricular efforts as well as in peer relations. Thus, schools can greatly enhance opportunities for promoting well-being in BIPOC students by investing in systems that allow for monitoring of school climate.

## 6.8 Illustrations of Systems-Centered Interventions

As prevention practitioners and scholars, we have been involved in partnerships between our home institution, Loyola University Chicago, and local Chicagoland school districts for the past several decades. Our long-term goals have been to help schools build their capacities for identifying and responding to the needs of culturally and linguistically diverse students (e.g., see Israel et al., 2017). The core activities of our collaborations have been to help schools engage in self-assessments, review their districts' policies and practices as they relate to the well-being of BIPOC students, facilitate ongoing teacher professional development sessions, and consult with parent organizations to help them increase their representation and inclusivity. While we have had opportunities to work directly with BIPOC students, we have been cautious of overemphasizing these efforts, to avoid overfocusing on the empowerment of these students to advocate for their own needs. We have preferred to view ourselves as student-centered advocates (Oyen et al., 2019) by giving power to their voices as informants and collaborators. At the same time, our collaborations have also allowed us to identify gaps in community resources and larger societal systems that will require political advocacy for policy change at state and federal levels.

Each collaboration has led to an individualized set of recommendations and interventions based on needs assessments and constituent focus groups. With administrators, we have generally focused our interventions on improving school climate and educational resources. With teachers, we have designed and implemented professional development to help them better understand the needs of their students and to adjust their instructional methods to be more inclusive. Additionally, in the parent sphere, we have helped schools strengthen the representation and participation of parents of BIPOC students within school environmental structures such as School Boards, Parent-Teacher Associations (PTAs), and Local School Councils. This work has included raising the awareness of parent and community leaders to better understand the nuances of engaging their BIPOC parents in such structures and helping them to create better recruitment policies that result in inclusivity and representative of the diversity of the student base (Vera et al., 2017).

Another focal point of our work has focused on empowering the constituency of parents of BIPOC, immigrant, and refugee children, so that they are prepared to serve as advocates within the school system for their children (Vera et al., 2016). This has included participating in Parent Mentoring programs and doing outreach and education of parents that represent BIPOC as well as White parents. By working with parent communities, teachers, and administrators, we aim to enhance communication among school stakeholders and actors and also to empower leaders within the school to be active advocates for the needs of all students.

There have been opportunities for us to monitor short-term outcomes of our work such as the extent to which interventions resulted in greater insight about the challenges that face BIPOC students and their families (see Vera et al., 2022). We have also attended meetings of parent organizations to ascertain changes in attitudes (e.g., a shift in beliefs away from “they are not interested in coming to our meetings” to a focus on how parent organizations can be more welcoming). Furthermore, we have helped schools track the success of adopting practices that will improve outreach efforts (e.g., allocating resources to have interpreters on hand for School Board, PTA, and LCS meetings). Another example of evaluating outcomes was monitoring changes in the degree to which BIPOC parents express greater interests in advocacy and leadership positions within school districts, and whether or not representation in school-sponsored activities (e.g., Literacy Nights) became more inclusive.

What is most encouraging has been watching the capacity of our partner schools to commit to and engage in this work independently, after our involvement. For example, we have observed that schools continue to monitor the success of new structures aimed at enhancing a sense of school belonging for BIPOC students, such as ambassador programs for newly arriving immigrant students and after-school culture clubs that allow immigrant parents to serve as cultural liaisons and help teach students about the diverse cultures represented in the schools. Additionally, many of our partners have instituted professional learning communities that allow school leaders, teachers, and parents to work collectively at learning best practices with respect to school climate and program evaluation. Thus, we feel confident that schools are more than capable of engaging in successful systems-level interventions that benefit the well-being of BIPOC students and communities, given the will and capacity to make such commitments.

## 6.9 Conclusion

Given the legacy of racism and social inequalities in schools and other contexts, SEL and prevention interventions that target only students' social and emotional competencies are not sufficiently equipped to confront the system-level, root causes of challenges to BIPOC students' well-being. We have adopted Mahoney et al.'s (2021) Systemic SEL framework in arguing for the inclusion of systemic-centered interventions (e.g., strengthening adults' competencies, cultivating family and community partnerships, and examining school-wide practices and policies) in programs designed to enhance the well-being and success of BIPOC students. We argue that SEL and other prevention frameworks used with BIPOC students are significantly strengthened by adopting a systemic lens and have seen success in such efforts.

## Resources

Bustamante, R. M. (2006). The culture audit: A leadership tool for assessment and strategic planning in diverse schools and colleges. *International Journal of Educational Leadership Preparation*, *1*(2), n2. https://files.eric.ed.gov/fulltext/EJ1066685.pdf

This article describes a tool that facilitates a cultural audit of schools' DEI practices (e.g., mission statements, inclusive curricula, representation of students in advanced placement, honors programs, feedback loops, professional development of teachers and staff; differentiated instructional strategies, community outreach, parent involvement).

Byrd, C. M. (2019). A measure of school racial socialization and quality of intergroup interactions. *Cultural Diversity and Ethnic Minority Psychology*, *25*(2), 137–147.

This article describes a survey tool that can be used with students to assess perceptions of inclusion and intercultural group relations.

Hong, S. (2011). *A cord of three strands: A new approach to parent engagement in schools.* Harvard Education Press.

This book discusses the Logan Square Neighborhood Association and their approach to parent engagement. The author describes the ecology of parent engagement which includes three elements – induction, integration, and investment – as well as three essential processes including mutual engagement, building relationships, and sharing leadership and power.

Jagers, R. J., Rivas-Drake, D. & Williams, B. (2019). Transformative Social and Emotional Learning (SEL): Toward SEL in service of educational equity and excellence. *Educational Psychologist*, *54(3)*, 162–184. doi.org/10.1080/00461520.2019.1623032

This article describes a framework for SEL that emphasizes DEI goals integrated with traditional student outcomes.

Mahoney, J. L., Weissberg, R. P., Greenberg, M. T., Dusenbury, L., Jagers, R. J., Niemi, K., Schlinger, M., Schlund, J., Shriver, T. P., VanAusdal, K., & Yoder, N. (2020). Systemic social and emotional learning: Promoting educational success for all preschool to high school students. *American Psychologist*, *76(7),* 1128–1142.

This article describes a systemic model of SEL that emphasizes the importance of strengthening adult SEL competencies and capacity, building family and community partnerships, and monitoring school-wide practices and policies in the design and implementation of SEL.

Samuels, D. R. (2014). *The culturally inclusive educator: Preparing for a multicultural world.* Teachers College Press.

This book describes opportunities to expand the cultural capacities of teachers through professional development in education and college campus settings.

Warren, M. R., Hong, S., Rubin, C. L., & Sychitkokhong, P. U. (2009). Beyond the bake sale: A community-based relational approach to parent engagement in schools. *Teachers College Record*, *111*(9), 2209–2254. doi.org/10.1177/016146810911100901

This article describes examples of three types of school–community collaborations – community service, community development, and community organizing – and the community-based relational approach at the heart of these partnerships, emphasizing the importance of relationship building, leadership development, and bridging the gap in culture and power between families and schools.

## References


Artiga, S., Garfield, R., & Orgera, K. (2020). *Communities of color at higher risk for health and economic challenges due to COVID-19*. Kaiser Family Foundation. www.kff.org/coronavirus-covid-19/issue-brief/communities-of-color-at-higherrisk-for-health-and-economic-challenges-due-to-covid-19/?utm_campaign=KFF-2020Uninsured&utm_source=hs_email&utm_medium=email&utm_content=2&_hsenc=p2ANqtz-_UqLIoowVMibewUsBF8kGfwwkh4ndUc-Ng7RZ8if–KZNFdsVsWt8UG2un7FH2DxliVe3nEefuXSQR1155GRcIUWd7mg&_hsmi=2

Benner, A. D., & Graham, S. (2013). The antecedents and consequences of racial/ethnic discrimination during adolescence: Does the source of discrimination matter? *Developmental Psychology*, *49*(8), 1602. doi.org/10.1037/a0030557

Benner, A. D., Wang, Y., Shen, Y., Boyle, A. E., Polk, R., & Cheng, Y. P. (2018). Racial/ethnic discrimination and well-being during adolescence: A meta-analytic review. *American Psychologist*, *73*(7), 855. dx.doi.org/10.1037/amp0000204

Brown, E., & Howard, B. (2005). Becoming culturally responsive teachers through service learning. *Multicultural Education*, *12*(4), 2–8. https://files.eric.ed.gov/fulltext/EJ727793.pdf

Byrd, C. M. (2019). A measure of school racial socialization and quality of intergroup interactions. *Cultural Diversity and Ethnic Minority Psychology*, *25*(2), 137–147. doi.org/10.1037/cdp0000202

Chajewski, M., Mattern, K. D., & Shaw, E. J. (2011). Examining the role of Advanced Placement® exam participation in 4-year college enrollment. *Educational Measurement: Issues and Practice*, *30*(4), 16–27. doi.org/10.1111/j.1745-3992.2011.00219.x

Chin, M. J., Quinn, D. M., Dhaliwal, T. K., & Lovison, V. (2020). Bias in the air: A nationwide exploration of teachers' implicit racial attitudes, aggregate bias, and student outcomes. *Educational Researcher*, *49*(8), 566–578. doi.org/10.3102/0013189X20937240

Comas-Díaz, L., Hall, G. N., & Neville, H. A. (2019). Racial trauma: Theory, research, and healing: Introduction to the special issue. *American Psychologist*, *74*(1), 1–5. doi.org/10.1037/amp0000442

Dalai Lama (Gyatso, T.D.L.T.) (2022). His Holiness the Dalai Lama: Education of the heart for a happy life. In R.S. Webster, T. Airaksinen, P. Batra, & M. Kozhevnikova (Eds.), *Humanizing education in the 3rd millennium*. SpringerBriefs in Education. Springer. doi.org/10.1007/978-981-19-1205-4_1

Durlak, J. A., Weissberg, R. P., Dymnicki, A. B., Taylor, R. D., & Schellinger, K. B. (2011). The impact of enhancing students' social and emotional learning: A meta-analysis of school-based universal interventions. *Child Development*, *82*(1), 405–432. doi.org/10.1111/j.1467-8624.2010.01564.x

Eisenberg, M. E., Gower, A. L., Brown, C., Nam, Y. S., Rider, G., & Ramirez, M. (2021). "It was never really bullying, but …": Reflections of adolescents and parents on experiences of microaggressions in school. *International Journal of Bullying Prevention*, 1–12. doi.org/10.1007/s42380-021-00103-9

Fine, M. (1993). [Ap]parent involvement: Reflections on parents, power, and urban public schools. *Teachers College Record*, *94*(4), 682–710. www.tcrecord.org/books/Content.asp?ContentID=147

Freire, P. (1998). *Teachers as cultural workers: Letters to those who dare teach*. Boulder: Westview.

Garmon, M. A. (2005). Six key factors for changing preservice teachers' attitudes/beliefs about diversity. *Educational Studies*, *38*, 275–286. doi.org/10.1207/s15326993es3803_7

Gay, G. (2018). *Culturally responsive teaching: Theory, research, and practice* (3rd ed.). Teachers College Press.

Hage, S. M., Romano, J. L., Conyne, R. K., Kenny, M., Matthews, C., Schwartz, J. P., & Waldo, M. (2007). Best practice guidelines on prevention practice, research, training, and social advocacy for psychologists. *The Counseling Psychologist*, *35*(4), 493–566. doi.org/10.1177/0011000006291411

Heineke, A. J., & Vera, E. M. (2022). Beyond language and academics: Investigating teachers' preparation to promote the social-emotional well-being of emergent bilingual learners. *Journal of Education*, *73*(2), 145–158. doi.org/10.1177/00224871211027573

Hoffman, D. M. (2009). Reflecting on social emotional learning: A critical perspective on trends in the United States. *Review of Educational Research*, *79*(2), 533–556. doi.org/10.3102/0034654308325184

Hong, S. (2011). *A cord of three strands: A new approach to parent engagement in schools*. Harvard Education Press.

Ishimaru, A. M., Torres, K. E., Salvador, J. E., Lott, J., Williams, D. M. C., & Tran, C. (2016). Reinforcing deficit, journeying toward equity: Cultural brokering in family engagement initiatives. *American Educational Research Journal*, *53*(4), 850–882. doi.org/10.3102/0002831216657178

Israel, M., Vera, E., Heineke, A., Goldberger, N. (2017). An unlikely destination: Meeting the educational needs of immigrant, migrant and refugee children in the suburbs of Chicago, IL. *International Journal of Educational Management*, *31*(5), 580–597. doi.org/10.1108/IJEM-09-2016-0190/full/html

Jagers, R. J., Rivas-Drake, D., & Williams, B. (2019). Transformative social and emotional learning (SEL): Toward SEL in service of educational equity and excellence. *Educational Psychologist*, *54*(3), 162–184. doi.org/10.1080/00461520.2019.1623032

Killoran, I., Panaroni, M., Rivers, S., Razack, Y., Vetter, D., & Tymon, D. (2004). Rethink, revise, react: Using an anti-bias curriculum to move beyond the usual. *Childhood Education*, *80*(3), 149–156. doi.org/10.1080/00094056.2004.10522794

Lewkowicz, A. B. (Ed.). (2006). *Teaching emotional intelligence: Strategies and activities for helping students make effective choices*. Corwin Press.

Liang, C. T., Rocchino, G. H., Gutekunst, M. H., Paulvin, C., Melo Li, K., & Elam-Snowden, T. (2020). Perspectives of respect, teacher–student relationships, and school climate among boys of color: A multifocus group study. *Psychology of Men & Masculinities*, *21*(3), 345. doi.org/10.1037/men0000239

Mahoney, J. L., Weissberg, R. P., Greenberg, M. T., Dusenbury, L., Jagers, R. J., Niemi, K., Schlinger, M., Schlund, J., Shriver, T. P., VanAusdal, K., & Yoder, N. (2021). Systemic social and emotional learning: Promoting educational success for all preschool to high school students. *American Psychologist*, 76(7), 1128–1142.

Mahoney, S., & Schamber, J. (2004). Exploring the application of a developmental model of intercultural sensitivity to a general education curriculum diversity. *The Journal of General Education*, *53*(3), 311–334. www.jstor.org/stable/27797998

Menken, K., & Kleyn, T. (2010). The long-term impact of subtractive schooling in the educational experiences of secondary English language learners. *International Journal of Bilingual Education and Bilingualism*, *13*(4), 399–417. doi.org/10.1080/13670050903370143

Meyers, A. B., Meyers, J., Graybill, E. C., Proctor, S. L., & Huddleston, L. (2012). Ecological approaches to organizational consultation and systems change in educational settings, *Journal of Educational and Psychological Consultation*, *22*(1–2), 106–124. doi.org/10.1080/10474412.2011.649649

Milner, H. R. (2003). Teacher reflection and race in cultural contexts: History, meanings, and methods in teaching. *Theory into Practice*, *42*(3), 173–180. doi.org/10.1207/s15430421tip4203_2

Montoro, J. P., Kilday, J. E., Rivas-Drake, D., Ryan, A. M., & Umaña-Taylor, A. J. (2021). Coping with discrimination from peers and adults: Implications for adolescents' school belonging. *Journal of Youth and Adolescence*, *50*(1), 126–143. doi .org/10.1007/s10964-020-01360-5

Oseguera, L. (2013). Importance of high school conditions for college access. *Research Brief*, *7*(7), 1–18. https://pathways.gseis.ucla.edu/publications/publications/201307_HSConditionsRB.pdf

Oyen, K. A., Eklund, K., & von der Embse, N. (2019). The landscape of advocacy in public schools: The role of school psychologists. *Psychological Services*, *17*(1), 81–85. doi.org/10.1037/ser0000373

Polanin, M., & Vera, E., (2013). Bullying prevention and social justice. *Theory into Practice*, *52*(4), 303–310. doi.org/10.1080/00405841.2013.829736

Reese, L. R. E., & Vera, E. M. (2007). Culturally relevant prevention: The scientific and practical considerations of community-based programs. *The Counseling Psychologist*, *35*(6), 763–778. doi.org/10.1177/0011000007304588

Reeves, J. R., (2006). Secondary teacher attitudes toward including English-language learners in mainstream classrooms. *The Journal of Educational Research*, *99*, 131–143. doi.org/10.3200/JOER.99.3.131-143

Rowe, H. L., & Trickett, E. J. (2018). Student diversity representation and reporting in universal school-based social and emotional learning programs: Implications for generalizability. *Educational Psychology Review*, *30*(2), 559–583. doi.org/10.1007/s10648-017-9425-3

Saleem, F. T., Anderson, R. E., & Williams, M. (2020). Addressing the "myth" of racial trauma: Developmental and ecological considerations for youth of color. *Clinical Child and Family Psychology Review*, *23*(1), 1–14. doi.org/10.1007/s10567-019-00304-1

Shapiro, S., & MacDonald, M. T. (2017). From deficit to asset: Locating discursive resistance in a refugee-background student's writing and oral narrative. *Journal of Language, Identity, and Education*, *16*(2), 80–93. doi.org/10.1080/15348458.2016.1277725

Shi, H. (2018). Self-efficacy beliefs and effective instructional strategies: US university English learners' perspective. *International Journal of Teaching and Learning in Higher Education*, *30*(3), 477–496. https://files.eric.ed.gov/fulltext/EJ1199328.pdf

Shim, J. M. (2019). Toward a more nuanced understanding of White teachers of English learners: Increasing capacity and capabilities. *Journal of Language Teaching & Research*, 10(1), 1–10. dx.doi.org/10.17507/jltr.1001.01

Sleeter, C. (2001). Preparing teachers for culturally diverse schools: Research and the overwhelming presence of Whiteness. *Journal of Teacher Education*, *52*(2), 94–106. doi.org/10.1177/0022487101052002002

Sobel, M., & Taylor, S. (2005). Diversity preparedness in teacher education. *Kappa Delta Pi Record*, *41*, 83–86. doi.org/10.1080/00228958.2005.10532050

Starck, J. G., Riddle, T., Sinclair, S., & Warikoo, N. (2020). Teachers are people too: Examining the racial bias of teachers compared to other American adults. *Educational Researcher, 49*(4), 273–284. doi.org/10.3102/0013189X20912758

Substance Abuse and Mental Health Services Administration. (2020). *Double jeopardy: COVID-19 and behavioral health disparities for Black and Latino communities in the U.S.* www.samhsa.gov/sites/default/files/covid19-behavioral-healthdisparities-blacklatino-communities.pdf

Sue, D. W., Sue, D., Neville, H. A., & Smith, L. (2019). *Counseling the culturally diverse: Theory and practice.* John Wiley & Sons.

Thorpe, H. (2017). *The newcomers: Finding refuge, friendship, and hope in an American classroom.* Scribner.

Trickett, E. J., Beehler, S., Deutsch, C., Green, L., Hawe, P., McLeroy, K., Miller, R. L., Rapkin, B. D., Schensul, J. J., Schulz, A. J., & Trimble, J. E. (2011). Advancing the science of community-level interventions. *American Journal of Public Health, 101*(8), 1410–1419. https://ajph.aphapublications.org/doi/full/10.2105/AJPH.2010.300113

Valenzuela, A. (1999). *Subtractive schooling: U.S.-Mexican youth and the politics of caring.* State University of New York Press.

van den Bergh, L., Denessen, E., Hornstra, L., Voeten, M., & Holland, R. (2010). The implicit prejudiced attitudes of teachers: Relations to teacher expectations and the ethnic achievement gap. *American Educational Research Journal, 47*(2), 497–527. doi .org/10.3102/0002831209353594

Vera, E. M., Heineke, A., Camacho, D., Israel, M. S., Goldberger, N., Clawson, A., Hill, M., & Carr, A. (2016). Predicting school leadership interests in parents of English learners: An exploratory study. *TESOL Journal, 7*(3), 645–666. doi .org/10.1002/tesj.236

Vera, E. M., Heineke, A., Carr, A., Camacho, D., Israel, M., Goldberger, N., Clawson, A., & Hill, M. (2017). Latino parents of English Learners in Catholic schools: Home vs. school based educational involvement. *Journal of Catholic Education, 20*, 1–29.

Vera, E. M., Heineke, A., Daskalova, P., Schultes, A. K., Pantoja-Patiño, J., Duncan, B., Yanuaria, C., Furtado, C. (2021). Emergent bilingual high school students' social and emotional experiences. *Psychology in the Schools, 58*(10), 1932–1961. doi .org/10.1002/pits.22559

Vera, E. M., Heineke, A., Israel, M., Goldberger, N., & Hill, M. (2022). Learning about English learners: Teachers' and leaders' perceptions of effective professional development. *International Multilingual Research Journal, 16*(2), 93–112. doi.org/10.1080/19313152.2021.1971474

Vera, E. M., Hill, L., Daskalova, P., Chander, N., Galvin, S., Boots, T., & Polanin, M. (2019). Promoting upstanding behavior in youth: A proposed model. *Journal of Early Adolescence, 39*(7), 1020–1049. doi.org/10.1177/0272431618798514

Vera, E. M., Hook, K., Daskalova, P., Hill, L., Galvin, S., Fritsche, S., Catellier, J., Haywood, S., Raziuddin, A., Anderson, B., Roche, M., Floro, M., Mutuyemariya, C., Thomas, K., Heerwagen, K., Camacho, D., Boots, T., & Gruber, E. O. (2018). Understanding the socioemotional worlds of English learners: A retrospective study. *Journal of Educational and Psychological Consultation, 28*(2), 137–163. doi.org/10.1080/10474412.2017.1305279

Voight, A., Hanson, T., O'Malley, M., & Adekanye, L. (2015). The racial school climate gap: Within-school disparities in students' experiences of safety, support, and connectedness. *American Journal of Community Psychology, 56*(3), 252–267. doi .org/10.1007/s10464-015-9751-x

Warren, M. R. (2005). Communities and schools: A new view of urban education reform. *Harvard Educational Review*, *75*(2), 133–173. doi.org/10.17763/haer.75.2.m718151032167438

Warren, M. R., Hong, S., Rubin, C. L., & Sychitkokhong, P. U. (2009). Beyond the bake sale: A community-based relational approach to parent engagement in schools. *Teachers College Record*, *111*(9), 2209–2254. doi.org/10.1177/016146810911100901

Whitford, D. K., & Emerson, A. (2019). Empathy intervention to reduce implicit bias in pre-service teachers. *Psychological Reports*, *122*(2), 670–688. doi.org/10.1177/0033294118767435

# 7 Building Race-Centered, Trauma-Responsive Schools: One Path toward Justice in Education

**Christopher T. H. Liang, Brooke Kohler, Keya Williams, Teresa Rosenberger, Jessica M. Safi, and Malaïka Gutekunst**

> The practice of love is the most powerful antidote to the politics of domination.
>
> —bell hooks, *Toward a Worldwide Culture of Love*

Mental health problems, as well as internalizing and externalizing symptoms among youth, have been trending upward even before the onset of the COVID-19 pandemic (Center for Disease Control, n.d.). The ongoing COVID-19 pandemic has likely resulted in an increase in the prevalence of childhood trauma, mental health problems (Centers for Disease Control and Prevention, 2022), and internalized and externalized behavioral health problems. Such problems include social withdrawal and acts of physical and verbal aggression among adolescents and children (Hanno et al., 2022). These behaviors present many challenges for teachers and school administrators, leading schools to find ways to support students, while also enforcing consequences. Although data regarding office discipline referrals (ODRs) (i.e., students referred by teachers to the principal or dean of students for disciplining) during the pandemic are not readily available, research published prior to 2020 suggests that children of the global majority (CGM; i.e., Black, Indigenous, Asian, Latinx, the Global South), particularly those who are Black or Brown, are punished more frequently and severely when compared to their peers (Losen & Martinez, 2020; Skiba et al., 2011).

Data regarding school punishment for externalizing behaviors have led scholars and activists to consider the powerful role of schools in the *school-to-prison pipeline* (i.e., the causal relationship between racially disproportionate ODRs, academic disengagement and/or dropout, and engagement with the justice system including incarceration). When Black or Brown children and adolescents are not referred for discipline, they may be directed for special education services instead of mental health support (Annamma et al., 2013).

Disparities in referrals for special education services for Black and Brown children can also lead to negative academic outcomes, including school drop-out (Newman et al., 2011). The majority of those in the school-to-prison pipeline, as well as those who are referred for special education services, may be students who live in poverty and who experience family-based and community-based trauma (Mallet, 2014).

Given the mental health problems found in schools, as well as the high levels of trauma and disproportionate numbers of Black and Brown students referred for discipline or special education services, a shift in focus away from ameliorative change efforts to those that are transformative is necessary. Although broad and overarching social change is necessary, localized efforts for transformation are also needed. Specifically, transformations within schools are one way to remove some conditions for suffering and re-traumatization. Potential change efforts include a school's reevaluation of how they understand and respond to symptoms of trauma and mental health problems, particularly from a race-centered lens. A race-centered, trauma-responsive school approach is a framework we developed to help educators understand student experience in a way that is sensitive to educator racial bias and responsive to family-based and community-based trauma. This approach fits within a social justice framework because it shifts attention away from a sole focus on individual-level (e.g., teaching mindfulness skills) and punishment-based (e.g., suspension) interventions, and instead understands the problem and solutions within their greater context. This chapter provides an overview of adverse childhood experience (ACE: Felitti et al., 1998) and the psychosocial impacts of disparities in the prevalence of ACEs, reviews the trauma-responsive school framework, and discusses how race-centered, trauma-responsive schools can be used as a preventive strategy to reduce negative outcomes for CGM.

## 7.1 Understanding ACEs and Its Impacts

In their landmark study, Felitti and colleagues (1998) coined the term ACEs, to encapsulate a person's exposure to multiple, chronic, prolonged, and developmentally adverse traumatic events. These adversities are often interpersonal in nature and occur prior to age 18. While various research teams have conceptualized ACEs differently, they are typically understood as including events such as (a) sexual and physical abuse, (b) community violence, (c) separation of biological parents, (d) emotional or physical neglect, (e) consistent lack of food, (f) loss of a parent to death or abandonment, (g) parental incarceration, and (h) living with a parent struggling with mental health or substance abuse issues. According to the Children's Defense Fund's 2021 report on The State of America's Children, 45% of children in the United States have experienced at least one ACE. Further, research has consistently demonstrated a dose–response relationship such that adults with more ACEs are at greater risk of contending with mental health and substance abuse issues, obtaining poor educational and occupational achievement, and suffering from chronic physical conditions such as cardiovascular disease and cancer (Felitti et al., 1998).

Some of the psychological impacts of trauma may be understood as arising from the impact of ACEs on physiology. Exposure to traumatic events stimulates the sympathetic nervous system and creates elevated levels of stress hormones including cortisol (Bick & Nelson, 2016; De Bellis & Zisk, 2014). Cortisol release leads to increased activity in the amygdala, the part of the brain responsible for the fear and survival response, and decreased activity in the parts of the brain responsible for executive functioning such as memory, attention, and impulse control (Pechtel & Pizzagalli, 2011). As young people's brains are in the process of developing, they experience neuroplasticity, or the ability to respond and react to new information or experiences much more than adults. The effects of prolonged or chronic stress and resultant cortisol levels may cause permanent changes in the structure and function of these brain areas (Bick & Nelson, 2016), thus negatively impacting optimal psychological, cognitive, and socioemotional development.

Given these developmental impacts, combined with possible continued and chronic exposure to family-based and community-based adversities, students exposed to ACEs are at risk for ongoing academic, cognitive, and psychosocial challenges in school (Perfect et al., 2016). Students' academic performance may suffer as a result of deficits in memory and attention, in addition to the presence of other learning difficulties such as cognitive delays (Bick & Nelson, 2016). Webster (2022) points out that ACEs are significant predictors of grades and school achievement and note that students with four or more ACES are 30 times more likely to have challenges with learning and behavior than their peers with no experience with ACEs. For example, students exposed to adversity demonstrated lower competency in math and reading and are more likely to repeat a grade than peers with lower ACE exposure (Chafouleas et al., 2019).

ACEs may also disrupt a child's affective functioning, leading to deficiencies in social processing, emotional cue response, and stress regulation, which may additionally contribute to difficulty in school (Bick & Nelson, 2016). In their meta-analysis, Mui and colleagues (2022) identified consistent evidence that childhood adversity increased the likelihood of emotional regulation difficulties. An inability to regulate emotions can increase a student's risk of engaging in challenging behaviors in school, such as hyperactivity, impulsivity, defiance, bullying, and physical and verbal aggression (Chafouleas et al., 2019). Additionally, these authors point out that trauma-exposed children may withdraw from peers, decreasing their ability to develop friendships and creating a susceptibility to teasing and bullying in the school environment.

From a trauma-informed perspective, behaviors such as hyperactivity and defiance are conceptualized as symptoms of trauma and represent a child's attempt to secure their safety. However, traditional systems of school discipline dictate that such behaviors be punished, often harshly, with conventional approaches such as classroom removal, suspensions, and expulsions (Garret, 2015). Indeed, research indicates that students with more ACEs are more likely to receive school suspension or expulsion (Pierce et al., 2022), which can lead to decreased school engagement and teacher referrals to special education services (Porche et al., 2016).

## 7.2 ACEs and Racial and Socioeconomic Disparities

According to the US Census Bureau, 11.6 million children lived in poverty in 2020, with CGM representing approximately 71% of that number (Children's Defense Fund, 2021). Poverty and racial bias are argued to influence the ways in which ACEs are experienced by youth, as well as how teachers understand and respond to symptoms of trauma (Liang & Rivera, 2017). A student's socioeconomic status has significant effects on several aspects of their lives, including influencing their exposure to adversities, determining which schools they attend, and affecting how they are treated in school by peers, teachers, and staff (Hughes & Tucker, 2018; Owens, 2018). Poverty is highly comorbid with a child's exposure to adversity, and children living in poverty are at greater risk of exposure to frequent and intense adversities than their higher socioeconomic peers (Hughes & Tucker, 2018). Further, because a significant portion of school funding is from local revenues, including school district property taxes, low-income students tend to attend schools with less funding capacity (Owens, 2018). This suggests that students with the highest economic need and the greatest likelihood of ACEs exposure are often in schools with the fewest resources and lowest capacity to serve them.

Racial bias also has undeniable impacts on the ways in which educators respond to students' expressions of trauma. Strategies such as exclusionary disciplinary practices and referrals for special education services are often used by educators to manage disruptive behaviors that may be indicative of trauma exposure; however, they have clear negative short- and long-term impacts that disproportionately impact CGM. For example, African American students are more likely than their White peers to experience punitive forms of discipline such as suspensions (Noltemeyer et al., 2015). In addition to short-term impacts of harsh school discipline on academic achievement, regular exclusionary discipline is also associated with an increased risk of dropout, grade retention, and involvement in the criminal justice system throughout the lifespan (Marchbanks III et al., 2015).

Referrals to special education, which often result in students' removal from the general education classroom, are another behavioral management method that is informed by racial bias and that may lead to unintended negative outcomes. A review of the literature indicates that race is a strong predictor for identifying students for special education (Cruz & Rodl, 2018) and that Black students were overrepresented in the disability categories of emotional disturbance (ED) and intellectual disability (ID). Additionally, Oswald and colleagues (1999) reported that Black students were more likely than White peers to be labeled with ID. Importantly, referrals for ED – which can be conceptualized as symptoms of trauma – have historically relied on practitioner judgment and represent high levels of racial disparity (Bal et al., 2014).

Although some children do need and can benefit from special education services, placement in special education, particularly with an ED label, can have long-term negative academic and life outcomes for students of color, including a disturbingly low (51%) high school graduation rate for African American and Native American students with this identification (Bal et al., 2019). The psychosocial impacts of being labeled with a learning disability or branded with low intelligence when placed in special education classrooms on CGM must also be taken into account. These studies point to the importance of addressing racial bias among teachers in schools, particularly those located within low-income communities.

*White cultural logic* that is a term we developed and defined as the unconscious use of White norms to understand behaviors, actions, and feelings of people of the global majority plays a pivotal role in teachers referring Black and Brown students for behavioral discipline and special education. In practice, when CGM do not meet the cultural expectation ascribed by the institution, their behavior is labeled as unacceptable and inappropriate, which may lead teachers and staff to make generalized assumptions about their behavior (Annamma et al., 2013). These generalized assumptions play a critical role in the disproportionality of discipline and special education referrals. For instance, Bal et al. (2019) point out that African American, Latinx, and Native American students are disproportionately removed from the classroom for subjective reasons such as disrespect, excessive noise, and insubordination. Such subjective ideals of student behavior may align with White cultural norms of politeness, quietness, and submissiveness, but be otherwise antithetical to the norms of those from the global majority. Thus, while unconscious, teachers may hold beliefs about what characteristics constitute a "good" or "well-behaved" student; these characteristics are informed by White cultural ideals and codified in the institutional rules of the school system (Annamma et al., 2013).

Such exclusion practices are exacerbated as Black and Brown youth are more likely than White students to receive their special education services in self-contained classrooms (Bal et al., 2019), even though research suggests that students receiving special education services have improved educational outcomes when they remain in general education settings for at least 80% of the time (Cole et al., 2021). As noted earlier, these self-contained settings may create a learning environment that is less academically rigorous, with lower expectations for prosocial behaviors, which may lead to further impediments in academic achievement and socio-emotional development over time. Such educational stratification was brought to light in legal cases such as Larry P. vs. Riles (1972), a case that led to the decision to prohibit standard intellectual tests on African American students for placement in special education and may act as an additional layer that perpetuates cycles of undereducation, poverty, and criminality in communities of color.

## 7.3 Systems-Level Change: Trauma-Informed and Trauma-Responsive Schools

Research indicates that ACEs influence how a student engages in school (Bick & Nelson, 2016). Although a systems-level sociopolitical intervention is needed to address the prevalence of trauma, school districts, when engaged in trauma-responsive approaches to discipline, are uniquely positioned to mitigate the impact of a student's exposure to adversities. Given how ACEs disrupt strong attachments, result in dysregulated states, and compromise a student's ability to succeed academically, the National Child Traumatic Stress Network's (NCTSN) attachment, regulation, and competency (ARC) framework provides a simple reminder of the importance of creating conditions within schools to build (a) nurturing environments that strengthen attachments, (b) opportunities for students to develop self-regulation skills that can help facilitate higher order cognitive functioning, and (c) competence among youth (Kinniburgh & Blaustein et al., 2005). In adopting this framework, adults within the school are charged with the responsibility of helping students develop awareness of their own emotional, mental, and physical states, while also fostering increased tolerance, management, and skill-building of emotional and physiological experiences. Central to this work is the development of strong affective–based teacher-student relationships (Souers & Hall, 2018). For example, research suggests that simply having a trusted adult in a child's life can buffer the negative impacts of ACEs (Webster, 2022). School teachers, coaches, and support staff can often fill that role when they prioritize relationship-building with students ahead of punitive discipline.

Schools are a primary system of support for children and have the ability to address the impact of ACEs and their negative academic, behavioral, and psychological consequences. Schools represent an ideal setting for expanding mental health services and for reaching at-risk populations, as the majority of youth experiencing trauma or other mental health concerns lack access to treatment (Weist & Evans, 2005). Leaders in education have begun to adopt a trauma-informed school model as a way to develop systems that promote resilience for all students regardless of their trauma history. In considering the disproportionate experience of trauma for racial or ethnic minorities, the implementation of trauma-responsive care in schools is not only a universal benefit, but a pursuit of social justice.

A trauma-informed school is typified by knowledge and recognition, among all stakeholders, of the multifaceted symptoms associated with exposure to childhood trauma (National Child Traumatic Stress Network, n.d.). Initial findings suggest trauma-informed schools can reduce behavioral issues, improve student–teacher relationships, and improve student mental health (Mendelson et al., 2015; Walkley & Cox, 2013). Importantly, the focus of work within trauma-informed schools begins with developing educators' knowledge and awareness of how trauma affects school children and educators' skills in managing these effects, as well as teacher mindset toward students' trauma responses and an examination of school-level practice and policy (e.g., discipline policy, identification of students in need).

A trauma-responsive approach, like a trauma-informed approach, requires the knowledge of trauma but additionally anticipates the potential existence of trauma, addresses prevention, and supports at all levels of an organization. Thus, a trauma-responsive school should promote (a) feelings of physical, social, and emotional safety in students; (b) a shared understanding among staff about the impact of trauma and adversity on students; (c) positive and culturally responsive discipline policies and practices; (d) access to comprehensive school mental and behavioral health services; and (e) effective community collaboration (National Association of School Psychologists, 2016). In short, a trauma-responsive school is designed to cultivate a positive school climate and encourages integrating mental health learning into the curriculum, such as the development of social–emotional learning (SEL) skills to help students self-regulate and focus on learning (Crosby, 2015).

## 7.4 Race-Centered Trauma-Responsive Schools and Multitiered Systems of Support

A systems-level approach requires that all aspects of the educational environment be grounded in the knowledge of trauma and its impact. The pursuit of trauma-responsive practice also requires a change in mindset where the attitudes and knowledge of trauma-informed care are necessary for sustainable practice. Changes can be implemented in school practice and policies, but what is most important is a change in the culture of the school to uphold these values and practices. The sustainability and effectiveness of school-based mental health intervention implemented by teachers requires administrative support; thus, teachers must be involved in prevention and intervention approaches and receive adequate training related to trauma-informed practices (Reinbergs & Fefer, 2018).

Although a trauma-responsive school approach addresses racial dynamics, including racism, a race-centered, trauma-responsive school explicitly names the role of race and racism. Specifically, a race-centered, trauma-responsive school involves a shift in practices, policies, and procedures across different levels and functional units within a school. It takes into account the role of racial bias and White cultural logic that are embedded within systems. Addressing White cultural logic reduces the likelihood that youth of the global majority, including those with intersectional identities, are viewed from a deficit-oriented perspective – as a problem to be corrected.

Implementation of a race-centered, trauma-responsive school approach is multifaceted and can be framed through the use of multitiered systems of support (MTSS; Fondren et al., 2020). MTSS relies on a philosophy that preventing problems is more effective than treating them after they have been identified. By following this philosophy, MTSS provides schools with a structure to organize, implement, and communicate a systematic approach to supporting all students, with increasing intensity of intervention, as needed (Sugai & Horner, 2009). There are three tiers of support within an MTSS. At the first tier (Tier 1), universal strategies are applied with the goal of affecting all students within a school. These strategies may include in-service for all staff, implementation of social-emotional learning programs, a focus on strengthening teacher–student relationships, teaching youth about the brain and trauma responses, or a shift away from punitive discipline to restorative practice. For instance, in an in-service, educators may learn about how they develop the attributions they make regarding the behavior of students. They may also learn about dispositional and situational attributions, as well as the common errors they may make when judging the behaviors or emotions of others, particularly when it comes to events involving CGM. This is one way educators learn how biases are typical and how to disrupt them.

It is estimated that about 80% of students will respond positively to Tier 1 strategies. However, about 15% of students within a school will require additional support. At the second tier (Tier 2), targeted interventions are developed for those students who may be at risk for more serious concerns. Supports at Tier 2 may include the use of *peace rooms* (a designated room in the school which provides interventions to help facilitate students' development and/or use of self-regulation skills) or structured mindfulness groups aimed at helping strengthen students' skills for self-regulation. Some students will require supports that exceed those offered in the first two tiers. The third tier (Tier 3) is reserved for intensive and individualized supports for students with the most serious problems (<5% of students). In addition to support at each of the tiers, MTSS requires active attention to processes of identification of students in need, as well as the development and tracking of action plans for students identified for Tier 2 and Tier 3 supports.

## 7.5 Case Example: Building Trauma-Responsive Schools in the Lehigh Valley

Over the past seven years, the first author established relationships with local school district leaders and community partners through his work on equity, diversity, and inclusion in schools. This work had been rooted in a desire to transform schools as one way to address inequities in education and subsequent life outcomes. The belief was that school, because of its centrality and importance in life outcomes, was a critical space to engage in the work of prevention. To frame the detrimental impacts of racism on students' well-being and academic outcomes, the first author provided an overview of trauma and its influence on the brain to educators during an in-service for teachers and building leaders. Although unintended, this sparked intense interest among district leaders to learn more about trauma and its influence on learning outcomes. One longtime principal shared that "this was the first time all the dots between racism, poverty, and behavior were connected." Another principal commented that they "realized through this work on trauma that they had not been sensitive enough to trauma."

Several additional in-service training sessions were delivered at the request of leaders from several school districts, all located in a small urban area in the Lehigh Valley of Pennsylvania. These presentations provided additional information on the brain and trauma, while still addressing disproportionate referrals for discipline experienced by Black and Brown youth. Specifically, the presentations linked trauma-related symptomatology (e.g., externalizing and internalizing behaviors) with ODRs vis-a-vis the unconscious race-based attributions of those behaviors (e.g., "bad kids"). While these presentations were impactful, they are only the beginning of a sustainable trauma-responsive approach. Individual, one-time trauma-informed care professional development opportunities for educators can be effective in changing attitudes (Liang et al., 2021) and inspiring educators for individual-level change; however, more is needed to transform and sustain systems-level change.

Desiring sustained change efforts, these presentations led to a collaboration between the first author, leaders from the two local school districts, and the United Way of the Greater Lehigh Valley that provided funding. The partners agreed that the effort of the first author and his team should focus on developing sustainable practices within schools, while also providing some in-service sessions on trauma and equity, diversity, and inclusion, when needed. The first author and his team focused their efforts on working with school leaders to build *trauma leadership teams* within each of the three schools they were assigned during the first year, as well as four additional schools over the next three years.

This team of authors led the meetings during the inaugural year of each school's team. A conscious decision was made to model trauma-responsive practices and to communicate the importance of a growth mindset. Goals were individualized to each school and cocreated with the trauma leadership teams. The first author and his team also modeled trauma-responsive strategies at each meeting, including using different strategies for check-ins, offering grounding exercises, modeling race talk, and fundamentally adopting a relationally oriented and strengths-based approach. Using existing peer-reviewed scholarship, books, and articles from websites popular with educators (see resources later in this chapter), these teams deepened their knowledge, developed synergy and cohesion within the staff, and (when needed) established new policies and norms for practice within their schools. The teams were challenged to think critically about their referral processes and mindsets, particularly as they concerned punishment and discipline.

## 7.6 Forming and Function of the Trauma Leadership Team

Within a trauma leadership team model, a race-centered, trauma-responsive approach incorporates a diverse range of school staff, including teachers, counselors, nurses, teaching aids, and any additional formal and informal school leaders (Liang et al., 2023a). Including diverse voices in trauma, leadership teams are designed with the intention of building a systems-level approach that is informed by the integration of rich experiences. Working with the administration, trauma leadership teams were created by identifying school staff who may be "champions" of trauma-informed care. Some team members may also be "fence-sitters" who are learning or in the process of incorporating a trauma-responsive approach into their work.

The trauma leadership teams we have worked with so far have been comprised of 10–15 members per team. Elementary schools have had one trauma leadership team for the entire school. Larger secondary schools ($N = 1{,}800$ students), such as the middle schools we have worked with, have created trauma leadership teams per individual grade level (e.g., sixth-grade team, seventh-grade team, eighth-grade team) to address the needs (and size) of the student body. In our work, we have seen a few different approaches in the assembly of school trauma leadership teams. In one approach, leadership is centralized; this means that the effort for change emanates from the principal, who periodically checks in with team members. A second approach is typified by the distribution of leadership, where the principal facilitates conditions for teachers and staff on the team to create priorities and assign tasks to one another.

The use of trauma leadership teams in schools is an intentional move away from teaching educators a supplementary trauma-responsive curriculum. Rather than school staff learning "another program," which educators view as problematic and unsustainable, trauma leadership teams learn how this approach is centered on intentional organization of existing interventions, and shifting mindsets, practices, and policies to reflect how ACEs and biases shape student interactions and behavior in the classroom.

In the first year of implementation, our team adopts a leadership role to help orient new team members, to educate and share resources around trauma and trauma-responsive approaches, and to support team members in identifying their school's unique strengths and areas of growth they would like to focus on as a team. Throughout this process, we provide experiential learning by modeling a trauma-informed approach: checking in with each other at the beginning of each meeting (e.g., "What is your weather report today?"), sharing out successes we see throughout the school or with our students, allowing for flexibility in "meeting the team where it's at," and offering space for team members to share different perspectives. The sharing of successes, strengths, and appreciations is an additional important component of trauma leadership team meetings. This practice supports team members in connecting with each other and offers insight into moments where educators can see change as a result of their efforts.

A school-centered approach is used to determine how hands-on our team may need to be to support trauma leadership team goals. Our approach often looked like a hands-on approach during the first year of application, a semi-hands-on approach in the second year, and support-as-needed within the third year. Throughout this time, teams started off with monthly meetings, typically 45–60 minutes long. Team members were incentivized with professional development credits they were required to earn. Over time, as team members developed their knowledge, awareness, and ownership within the leadership team, they began to create subgroups, who may focus on specific needs within their school.

Trauma leadership teams incorporate a modified version of the ARC model (Kinniburgh et al., 2005) for school-wide treatment intervention, incorporating the intentional application of *self-care* ("S" or "SARC") as suggested by our team. In the SARC variation, educator self-care is seen as an intentional shift and imperative first step that provides educators with tools to self-regulate and coping strategies to take care of themselves to sustain their race-centered, trauma-responsive work in the classroom. Teachers experience work-related burnout for a multitude of reasons, including decreased feelings of self-efficacy, self-regulation, and social support (Ghanizadeh & Jahadizadeh, 2015).

Regarding the COVID-19 pandemic, heightened feelings of anxiety around COVID-19, teaching, communication with parents, and administrative support have all been identified as predictors for teacher burnout and stress in recent years (Pressley, 2021). Moreover, teacher burnout has been associated with worsened student academic achievement and motivation (Madigan & Kim, 2020). By prioritizing self-care within the SARC model, self-regulated and well teachers are more likely to engage in better decision-making and less likely to retraumatize students. Better self-care practices may also support teachers' emotional well-being, which may help sustain their work overtime.

At first, teams may start in different places in their trauma-responsive knowledge and intended goals. Some schools may have already started incorporating restorative practices (Archibold, 2014), zones of regulation (Kuypers, 2011), and/or begun implementing positive behavioral interventions and supports (PBIS; Center on PBIS, 2022). However, they may not have considered how to monitor the fidelity of intervention implementation. Some may have viewed these programs in isolation, rather than an integrated set of programs that could support student development from a trauma-responsive lens. Other schools may have little or no idea where to begin with race-centered, trauma-responsive work. Our team looks to work with schools whose leadership and staff show some initial interest in becoming trauma-responsive. Some buy-in is warranted, as suggested by Sporleder and Forbes (2016), who recommend that all school administration ought to be committed to a trauma-responsive approach, as well as roughly 75–80% of school staff. Not all staff members need to be "experts," but instead they need to be committed and willing to try out a "new mindset shift" in trauma-informed care. If school administrators or a higher percentage of school staff are not committed to trying out a trauma-responsive approach, making school-wide shifts at the individual and institutional levels may be more challenging and less sustainable over time (Nadeem & Ringle, 2016).

Another common experience we have seen in trauma leadership team implementation is that schools may have lots of enthusiasm and ideas they desire to apply. We recognize this as a strength and also offer educators a caution of moving too quickly to solutions. An emphasis on taking time to build a strong foundation is emphasized so that team members can create the time to identify, plan for, and achieve their goals. As school leaders and team members see the challenges their staff and students experience, there is sometimes a sense of urgency to "fix everything" all at once. Slowing down provides leadership teams time to intentionally think, process, and react or respond to the specific challenges or issues they may encounter. As a result, trauma leadership teams are typically offered more intensive support the first year with increasing levels of responsibility transferred to the teams.

Trauma leadership team subgroups are identified by the teams and what they see as unique to their students and school communities (e.g., Brain group, Classroom Skills, Cultural Diversity and Inclusion, and Teacher Self-Care). Some examples of their deepening work are listed in the following sections.

## 7.7 Teacher Wellness Rooms

Teacher "wellness rooms" are rooms specifically created and designed to promote teacher wellness, relaxation, and self-regulation. Wellness rooms might include resources or materials that promote teacher relaxation, including calming music and visual imagery, ambient lighting, comfortable seating, and resources to support self-regulation, such as guided meditation or mindfulness prompts. Trauma leadership teams have helped create wellness rooms, including the processes for using the rooms. For instance, if a teacher notices that they are beginning to feel dysregulated, they may be able to implement a "tap out" process, in which the teacher "taps out" of their classroom for a few minutes to visit the wellness room, while another staff member "taps in" to oversee the classroom. In the wellness room, some schools have implemented a "no work" rule, in which teachers are prohibited from doing any school-related tasks or work. Within such wellness rooms, teachers have been able to support their own individual self-regulation and relaxation, as well as their relationships with fellow teachers. Outcomes upon implementation of teacher wellness rooms have so far included a reduction in ODRs, as well as a decrease in absenteeism among teachers. A reduction in ODRs is very desirable. However, a reduction in chronic absenteeism among teachers results in more stable environments where strong teacher-student relationships can form, which are important for children with trauma histories (Craig, 2008), and are also predictive of academic wellbeing (Miller et al., 2008).

## 7.8 Strengthening Relationships

Trauma leadership team members are encouraged to develop and strengthen relationships within their school system and school community. Relationships of particular focus include relationships among school staff and administration, between teachers and their students, educator relationships with their colleagues, parents, or caregivers, and relationships among trauma leadership team members. This focus on relationship-building is cited as a key component of success in trauma-responsive literature (Brown et al., 2017; Wolpow et al., 2016). Within trauma leadership team meetings, team members practice and model relationship-building with one another through group check-ins and check-outs. Team members might also incorporate intentional activities into meeting times to foster connection and self-reflection as a person with social identities, such as writing and sharing an "I Am From" poem – a poetry-based activity inspired by writer and teacher, George Ella Lyon, in which writers describe the different components of their lives that make them who they are. Teachers experience how they, their peers, and their students are more than what is presented – that there is more to the book than its cover. Through the activity, they experience perspective-taking, empathize, and connect with their students and colleagues. A deeper understanding of others may support teachers in asking the question "What is going on for them?" rather than "What is wrong with them?," which may instill further judgment or disconnection amongst individuals (Sporleder & Forbes, 2016).

Moreover, trauma leadership team members attempt to foster relationships by "meeting each other where they are at" and acknowledge the strengths as well as challenges throughout the school year. For instance, as schools began to return back to in-person learning after the COVID-19 pandemic, many schools felt pressure to "reverse the loss" and make sure students did not stray from their academic schedules. Although attendance to academic achievement is warranted, students may find it more challenging to learn in an environment that they have not been in for several months, with students and teachers they have not seen in person for the same amount of time. As such, a focus on relationship-building, reconnecting students with their peers and teachers, as well as the school environment itself may support students in feeling more safe and secure and therefore open to learning.

## 7.9 Integration of Existing Socioemotional Learning Programs

It is important to emphasize that the trauma-responsive approach is not "just another program" for teachers to adopt. Framed as a multitiered system of support interventions, a trauma-responsive approach can help integrate existing socioemotional learning (SEL) programs. For example, schools that our team has worked with have utilized the Second Step SEL curriculum and Zones of Regulation (Kuypers, 2011). Both programs include components of trauma-responsive care and can be easily understood within a trauma-responsive framework. Second Step emphasizes skills such as processing emotions, building empathy, and resolving conflicts (Wenz-Gross et al., 2018). These skills can be contextualized within the SARC framework as important for developing healthy and securely attached relationships. Meanwhile, the Zones of Regulation program provides common language and a framework for students and teachers alike to identify emotional states and practice emotional self-regulation.

Our team has helped trauma leadership teams integrate these programs by identifying them generally as Tier 1 supports and discussing how they can be used to help students develop necessary relational and self-regulation skills. In the context of a race-centered, trauma-responsive approach, it is also necessary to discuss how White cultural logic influences educator beliefs about appropriate emotional expression – and how expectations for students may differ based on their sociocultural identities. School leaders and our teamwork with parents and community members identify the behaviors and interactions that are desired and reinforced within their own communities. One outcome of this approach is that schools move away from imposing one set of propositions of appropriate behaviors that are unconsciously rooted in White cultural logic to include other frames, whenever appropriate. Doing so not only allows for greater consistency across school, family, and community settings but also may result in more positive behaviors being recognized by educators.

## 7.10 Self-care and Self-regulation Opportunities

As previously mentioned, the trauma leadership team model incorporates teacher self-care as an essential component of trauma-informed care. One way teacher self-care has been incorporated into school settings is through monthly professional development training in mindfulness strategies. Mindfulness training was intentionally offered as professional development so that teachers could receive continuing education credits for their time, and so they were not asked to perform additional "self-care" practices on top of their already busy and demanding schedules.

During this training, teachers learned mindfulness practices and strategies they could use for themselves to promote teacher self-care and well-being. Teachers were led through and taught a variety of different formal mindfulness practices, including mindful breathing, progressive muscle relaxation, guided imagery, gratitude and loving-kindness, self-compassion, and mindful movement. Teachers also discussed ways to bring mindful awareness into their school days, such as noticing feelings of stress or dysregulation, and using mindfulness to self-regulate. As teachers learned about and developed their own mindfulness practices and strategies, they began to apply these practices in the classroom to support students' self-regulation skills.

## 7.11 Peace Spaces for Students

Alternatives to referrals for discipline needed to be developed for educators to use in response to dysregulated students in the classroom. Similar to the elementary level, trauma leadership teams in secondary schools have identified teacher self-care as an essential component of trauma-informed care. In addition to wellness rooms for teachers, trauma leadership teams have identified "Peace Spaces," or specific areas or rooms for students to deregulate, as important (Liang et al., 2023b). Within Peace Spaces, students have the opportunity to go to either a designated area of a classroom or a separate room altogether when feeling overwhelmed or dysregulated. Within the Peace Spaces, students may find activities to practice on their own (e.g., journal prompt, coloring, breathing exercises) or be led by a specific Peace Space staff member to support self-regulation. Once a student begins to feel more regulated, they return to their classroom or desk if already in the classroom area. The application of

Peace Spaces allows students to practice their own self-regulation awareness and skills and also offers an alternative space for students to go rather than being directly referred for discipline. If Peace Spaces are being used within the classroom (e.g., one example of a classroom Peace Space is the Peace Corner), teachers are able to keep students in the classroom, rather than sending them to guidance or for discipline.

## 7.12 Focus on Diversity, Equity, and Inclusion

Schools incorporate a direct focus on diversity, equity, and inclusion work within their trauma leadership team goals and subgroups. As schools reviewed the demographics of their students receiving discipline referrals, some schools noticed a higher number of male CGM students being referred to than others. Other leaders recognized that male CGM students may not be recognized in the same way as female students as needing mental health support if they are internalizing their symptoms. As a result of these findings, trauma leadership team members (including school administration) intentionally incorporated professional development trainings, working groups, and school-wide goals focused on anti-racist efforts and initiatives.

## 7.13 De-escalating and Preventing Conflict

Teachers across all schools identified a need to strengthen their ability to de-escalate conflicts. Our observation was that some teachers' desire to control the situation and show students who was in charge was grounded in good intentions but counterproductive to creating a safe environment. Indeed, some strategies used to control the classroom resulted in escalating conflict, were more disruptive to learning, and were retraumatizing to the student. Our approach was to focus on prevention of conflict, particularly the importance of developing strong teacher–student relationships. However, because classroom conflict will arise, we provided teams and whole schools our SAFE Model© that consists of (a) scanning for triggers, racial biases, and value violations within oneself; (b) assessing the situation and attending to feelings verbally and nonverbally; (c) providing facts (e.g., reminders of school or classroom processes for de-escalation); and (d) empowering students to make decisions.

## 7.14 Peer-Led Professional Development

At the secondary level, middle school trauma leadership teams have focused on sharing resources with fellow teachers that they can apply with their students throughout the school day, including the use of restorative practices and mindfulness strategies. Trauma leadership team members have conducted book clubs with school staff, in which team members assign readings and guided discussions around restorative practices. As teachers attend such discussions, they then apply restorative practices within their respective classrooms.

## 7.15 Recommendations

Transforming a school's culture to embrace a race-centered, trauma-responsive school approach is one way to address racial disparities in schools. Providing training to educators on the influence of physiological, psychological, familial, and social factors on a student's functioning has facilitated our ability to deepen knowledge and awareness of the experiences of the youth with whom they work. Our ongoing work to transform schools has resulted in educators developing greater empathy for others, awareness of self, perspective-taking, and a deepening of their system-wide and individual efforts to support students from a race-centered, trauma-responsive lens. Several key recommendations emerged from our self-reflection of our efforts to transform schools.

1. Some educators may want to shift the focus of the work onto parents and families. This is understandable, yet training parents does not address systems-level problems that are occurring within the school. Instead, it focuses blame and responsibility solely on parenting. Taking a stepwise approach, where the focus is first placed on school-based practices, is needed. Further, when shifting to parents and caregivers, it is important to engage them not as consumers but as partners. This entails providing information on trauma and listening for their strengths. Incorporating their knowledge and ways of being not only is culturally responsive but also has the potential to strengthen school-based efforts.
2. Some educators are oriented toward finding quick solutions. Thus, it is important to set clear expectations with school leaders and educators that this process takes multiple years of sustained effort. It is also important to remind teams that change is not linear – that there will be setbacks with individual students and educators, as well as in the process of transforming the system.
3. Although it is important to communicate to leaders that the entire process is ongoing and may take multiple years, it is also important to share that they should begin to see some evidence of change within the first year.
4. Noticing incremental changes should be taught and modeled. Some educators may desire to see huge shifts in behavioral disruptions quickly. Although it is reasonable for them to desire this change sooner than later, it is an unrealistic expectation. Thus, it is important to communicate the value of recognizing and celebrating small successes (e.g., teachers building relationships with students by using morning circles). Noticing these successes not only sustains effort and communicates movement forward

but also models for teachers the importance of celebrating strengths over a sole focus on deficits.

5. Because schools are complex systems with many staff, it is important to recognize that there will be divergent viewpoints. Diversity of opinion is a strength. However, members of teams will need to develop effective ways to respond to peers who are ambivalent. Further, it is helpful to remind team members that they need not focus on the small number of their peers who cannot be convinced.
6. One main area of disagreement among teachers is that some deeply hold onto the belief that punishment is needed for students to grow. Some educators have difficulty reconciling their core belief that harsh punishment is needed with our message of accountability through relationships. It is important to communicate the need for both safety and accountability as well as to emphasize that research demonstrates that strong teacher–student relationships increase motivation and reduce the likelihood of behavioral problems among students.
7. It is important to communicate the many small ways that relationships with students can be built. For instance, we have communicated the importance of engaging youth and adolescents in "small talk" or morning check-ins.
8. Promoting a policy and culture of self-care is more important than encouraging teachers to engage in self-care activities. Self-care that ostensibly leads to a stronger ability to employ self-regulation skills is important for all educators and health-care providers. Teachers able to self-regulate are more likely to employ trauma-responsive strategies and acknowledge and disrupt their use of White cultural logic when interacting with students exhibiting symptoms of trauma. However, having a culture and policy where self-care is supported during work hours is critical. Educators who feel supported by their building administrator to engage in self-care are more likely to report better mental health and less burnout (Liu & Liang, under review). Our experience also suggests that it is helpful when building and district-level leaders assure teachers that it is appropriate to spend time developing relationships with students through classroom activities.

## 7.16 Conclusion

Even with the recent mass school shootings, most American parents send their children to school each day with the basic assumption that their child will be safe, well educated, and respected. Many parents feel secure in the idea that their children will be able to engage in social activities with peers, find a sense of belonging, and be given the space and freedom to mature, both academically and personally. While many students do indeed experience school as validating, safe, and communal, many ethnic minority students have quite a different experience of the school environment. Racial disparities in engagement with school discipline systems, referrals for special education, and experiences of discrimination are challenges that communities of color face when they enter schools. The race-centered, trauma-responsive school approach presented in this chapter is one way to transform systems to engage in the work of prevention.

## Resources

### Books

*Fostering resilient learners: Strategies for creating a trauma-sensitive classroom*, by Kristin Souers and Pete Hall

*Relationship, responsibility and regulation: Trauma-invested practices for fostering resilient learners*, by Kristen Van Marter Souers and Pete Hall

*Trauma-sensitive schools for the adolescent years: Promoting resiliency and healing, Grades 6–12*, by Susan E. Craig

*Trauma-sensitive schools: Learning communities, transforming children's lives K-5*, by Susan E. Craig

*Reading with Patrick: A Teacher, a student, and a life-changing friendship*, by Michelle Kuo

*The trauma-informed school, by* J. Sporleder, T. H. Forbes, and N. A. Colflesh. (2016).

*Reaching and teaching children who hurt: Strategies for your classroom* by Susan E. Craig

*Help for Billy: A beyond consequences approach to helping and challenging children in the classroom*, by Heather T. Forbes

### Websites

The National Child Traumatic Stress Network; www.nctsn.org

UCSF HEARTS: Healthy Environments and Response to Trauma in Schools; https://hearts.ucsf.edu

United Way of the Greater Lehigh Valley; www.unitedwayglv.org

Trauma-Responsive MTSS Toolkit; https://sites.google.com/lehigh.edu/mtsstoolkit/about

## References

Annamma, S. A., Connor, D. & Ferri, B. (2013). Dis/ability critical race studies (DisCrit): Theorizing at the intersections of race and dis/ability. *Race Ethnicity and Education*, *16*(1), 1–31. doi.org/10.1080/13613324.2012.730511

Archibold, E. (2014). Restorative approach in schools: Systemic approaches to building positive school climates. *Journal of Pedagogy, Pluralism, and Practice*, *6*(1). https://digitalcommons.lesley.edu/jppp/vol6/iss1/6

Bal, A., Betters-Bubon, J., & Fish, R. E. (2019). A multilevel analysis of statewide disproportionality in exclusionary discipline and the identification of emotional disturbance. *Education and Urban Society*, *51*(2), 247–268. doi.org/10.1177/0013124517716260

Bal, A., Sullivan, A., L., & Harper, J. (2014). A situated analysis of special education disproportionality for systemic transformation in an urban school district. *Remedial and Special Education, 35* (1), 3–14. doi.org/10.1177/0741932513507754

Bick, J., & Nelson, C. A. (2016). Early adverse experiences and the developing brain. *Neuropsychopharmacology, 41*(1), 177–196. doi.org/10.1038/npp.2015.252

Brown, J. D., King, M. A., & Wissow, L. S. (2017). The central role of relationships with trauma-informed integrated care for children and youth. *Academic Pediatrics, 17*(7), S94–S101. doi.org/10.1016/j.acap.2017.01.013

Center for Disease Control. (n.d.). *Mental health among adolescents.* [Fact sheet]. www.cdc.gov/nchhstp/newsroom/docs/factsheets/dash-mental-health.pdf

Center for Disease Control. (2022, March 31). *New CDC data illuminate youth mental health threats during the COVID-19 pandemic.* www.cdc.gov/media/releases/2022/p0331-youth-mental-health-covid-19.html

Center on PBIS. (2022). *Positive behavioral interventions & supports.* www.pbis.org.

Chafouleas, S. M., Koriakin, T. A., Roundfield, K. D., & Overstreet, S. (2019). Addressing childhood trauma in school settings: A framework for evidence-based practice. *School Mental Health, 11*(1), 40–53. doi.org/10.1007/s12310-018-9256-5

Children's Defense Fund. (2021). *The state of America's children 2021.* www.childrensdefense.org/state-of-americas-children/

Cole, S. M., Murphy, H. R., Frisby, M. B., Grossi, T. A., & Bolte, H. R. (2021). The relationship of special education placement and student academic outcomes. *The Journal of Special Education, 54*(4), 217–227. doi.org/10.1177/0022466920925033

Craig, S. E. (2008). *Reaching and teaching children who hurt: Strategies for your classroom.* Brookes Publishing.

Crosby, S. D. (2015). An ecological perspective on emerging trauma-informed teaching practices. *Children & Schools, 37*(4), 223–230.

Cruz, R. A., & Rodl, J. E. (2018). An integrative synthesis of literature on disproportionality in special education. *The Journal of Special Education, 52*(1), 50–63. doi.org/10.1177/0022466918758707

De Bellis, M. D., & Zisk, A. (2014). The biological effects of childhood trauma. *Child and Adolescent Psychiatric Clinics, 23*(2), 185–222. doi.org/10.1016/j.chc.2014.01.002

Felitti, V. J., Anda, R. F., Nordenberg, D., Williamson, D. F., Spitz, A. M., Edwards, V., & Marks, J. S. (1998). Relationship of childhood abuse and household dysfunction to many of the leading causes of death in adults: The Adverse Childhood Experiences (ACE) Study. *American Journal of Preventive Medicine, 14*(4), 245–258. doi.org/10.1016/S0749-3797(98)00017-8

Fondren, K., Lawson, M., Speidel, R., McDonnell, C. G., & Valentino, K. (2020). Buffering the effects of childhood trauma within the school setting: A systematic review of trauma-informed and trauma-responsive interventions among trauma-affected youth. *Children and Youth Services Review, 109*, 104691. doi.org/10.1016/j.childyouth.2019.104691

Ghanizadeh, A., & Jahedizadeh, S. (2015). Teacher burnout: A review of sources and ramifications. *British Journal of Education, Society & Behavioural Science, 6*(1), 24–39. doi.org/10.9734/BJESBS/2015/15162

Hanno, E. C., Cuartas, J., Miratrix, L. W., Jones, S. M., & Lesaux, N. K. (2022) Changes in children's behavioral health and family well-being during the COVID-19 pandemic. *Journal of Developmental & Behavioral Pediatrics, 43*(3), 168–175. doi.org/10.1097/DBP.0000000000001010

Hughes, M., & Tucker, W. (2018). Poverty as an adverse childhood experience. *North Carolina Medical Journal*, *79*(2), 124–126. doi.org/10.18043/ncm.79.2.124

Kinniburgh, K. J, Blaustein, M., Spinazzola, J., & Van der Kolk, B. A. (2005). Attachment, self-regulation, and competency. *Psychiatric Annals*, *35* (5), 424–430.

Kuypers, L. (2011). The zones of regulation. *Think Social Publishing*.

Liang, C. T. H., & Rivera, L. (2017). Psychological approaches to working with vulnerable children. In. F. Beachum & F. Obeakor (Eds.), *Improving educational outcomes of vulnerable children: Starting from the bottom* (pp. 117–144). Oakleaf Books.

Liang, C. T. H., Gutekunst, M. H. C., Kohler, B.A., Rosenberger, T., Mui, V. W., Williams, K., & Safi, J. M. (2023a). The Formation and Functions of School-Based Trauma Leadership Teams: A preliminary qualitative study. *Psychology in the Schools*.

Liang, C. T. H, Gutekunst, M. H. C., Liu, L., Rosenberger, T., & Kohler, B. A. (2023b). Formative evaluation of peace spaces in a middle school: Teacher perceptions and student usage. Psychology in the Schools. doi.org/10.1002/pits.23045

Liang, C. T. H., Liu, L., Rocchino, G., H., Kohler, B., & Rosenberger, T. (2021). Trauma-informed care training for educators: Some preliminary evidence. *Journal of Prevention and Health Promotion*, *1*(2), 240–263. doi.org/10.1177/2632077020972038

Losen, D. J., & Martinez, P. (2020). *Lost opportunities: How disparate school discipline continues to drive differences in the opportunity to learn*. Center for Civil Rights Remedies at the Civil Rights Project, UCLA. www.civilrightsproject.ucla.edu/research/k-12-education/school-discipline/lost-opportunities-how-disparate-school-discipline-continues-to-drive-differences-in-the-opportunity-to-learn/Lost-Opportunities-REPORT-v17.pdf

Madigan, D. J. & Kim, L. (2020). Does teacher burnout affect students? A systematic review of its association with academic achievement and student-reported outcomes. *International Journal of Educational Research*, *105*, 101174. doi.org/10.1016/j.ijer.2020.101714

Mallett, C. A. (2014). Youthful offending and delinquency: The comorbid impact of maltreatment, mental health problems, and learning disabilities. *Child and Adolescent Social Work Journal*, *31*, 369–392. doi.org/10.1007/s10560-013-0323-3

Marchbanks III, M. P., Blake, J. J., Booth, E. A., Carmichael, D., Seibert, A. L., & Fabelo, T. (2015). The economic effects of exclusionary discipline on grade retention and high school dropout. In D. J. Losen (Ed.), *Closing the school discipline gap: Equitable remedies for excessive exclusion* (pp. 59–74). Teachers College Press.

Mendelson, T., Tandon, S. D., O'Brennan, L., Leaf, P. J., & Ialongo, N. S. (2015). Brief report: Moving prevention into schools. The impact of a trauma-informed school-based intervention. *Journal of Adolescence*, *43*, 142–147. doi.org/10.1016/j.adolescence.2015.05.017

Miller, R. T., Murnane, R. J., & Willett, J. B. (2008). Do teacher absences impact student achievement? Longitudinal evidence from one urban school district. *Educational Evaluation and Policy Analysis*, *30*(2), 181–200. doi.org/10.3102/0162373708318019

Miu, A. C., Szentágotai-Tătar, A., Balazsi, R., Nechita, D., Bunea, I., & Pollak, S. D. (2022). Emotion regulation as mediator between childhood adversity and psychopathology: A meta-analysis. *Clinical Psychology Review*, *93*, 1–11. doi.org/10.1016/j.cpr.2022.102141

Nadeem, E., & Ringle, V. A. (2016). De-adoption of an evidence-based trauma intervention in schools: A retrospective report from an urban school district. *School Mental Health*, *8*(1), 132–143. doi.org/10.1007/s12310-016-9179-y

National Association of School Psychologists (2016). *Creating trauma-sensitive schools: Brief tips & policy recommendations*. Retrieved from www.nasponline.org/x53285.xml

National Child Traumatic Stress Network. (n.d.). *Trauma-informed schools for children in K-12: A system framework*. www.nctsn.org/sites/default/files/resources/fact-sheet/trauma_informed_schools_for_children_in_k-12_a_systems_framework.pdf

Newman, L., Wagner, L., Knokey, A. M., Marder, C., Nagle, K., Shaver, D., & Schwarting, M. (2011). *The post-high school outcomes of young adults with disabilities up to 8 years after high school: A report from the National Longitudinal Transition Study-2 (NLTS2)*. (NCSER 2011-3005). Menlo Park, CA: SRI International. Retrieved from www.nlts2.org/reports/

Noltemeyer, A. L., Ward, R. M., & McLoughlin, C. (2015). Relationships between school suspension and student outcomes: A meta-analysis. *School Psychology Review*, *44*(2), 224–240. doi.10.17105/spr-14-0008.1

Oswald, D. P., Coutinho, M. J., Best, A. M., & Singh, N. N. (1999). Ethnic representation in special education: The influence of school-related economic and demographic variables. *The Journal of Special Education*, *32*(4), 194–206.

Owens, A. (2018). Income segregation between school districts and inequality in students' achievement. *Sociology of Education*, *91*(1), 1–27. doi.org/10.1177/0038040717741180

Pechtel, P., & Pizzagalli, D. A. (2011). Effects of early life stress on cognitive and affective function: An integrated review of human literature. *Psychopharmacology*, *214*, 55–70.

Perfect, M. M., Turley, M. R., Carlson, J. S., Yohanna, J., & Saint Gilles, M. P. (2016). School-related outcomes of traumatic event exposure and traumatic stress symptoms in students: A systematic review of research from 1990 to 2015. *School Mental Health*, *8*(1), 7–43. doi.org/10.1007/s12310-016-9175-2

Pierce, H., Jones, M. S., & Gibbs, B. G. (2022). Early adverse childhood experiences and exclusionary discipline in high school. *Social Science Research*, *101*, 102621. doi.org/10.1016/j.ssresearch.2021.102621

Porche, M. V., Costello, D. M., & Rosen-Reynoso, M. (2016). Adverse family experiences, child mental health, and educational outcomes for a national sample of students. *School Mental Health*, *8*(1), 44–60. doi.org/10.1007/s12310-016-9174-3

Pressley, T. (2021a). Factors contributing to teacher burnout during COVID-19. *Educational Researcher*, *50*(5), 325–327. doi.org/10.3102/0013189X211004138

Reinbergs, E. J., & Fefer, S. A. (2018). Addressing trauma in schools: Multi-tiered service delivery options for practitioners. *Psychology in the Schools*, *55*(3), 250–263. doi.org/10.1002/pits.22105

Skiba, R. J., Horner, R. H., Chung, C. G., Rausch, M. K., May, S. L., & Tobin, T. (2011). Race is not neutral: A national investigation of African American and Latino disproportionality in school discipline. *School Psychology Review*, *40*(1), 85–107. doi.org/10.1080/02796015.2011.12087730

Souers, K. V. M., & Hall, P. (2018). *Relationship, responsibility, and regulation: Trauma-invested practices for fostering resilient learners*. ASCD.

Sporleder, J., & Forbes, H. T. (2016). *The trauma-informed school*. Boulder, CO: Beyond.

Sugai, G., & Horner, R. H. (2009). Responsiveness-to-intervention and school-wide positive behavior supports: Integration of multi-tiered systems of approaches. *Exceptionality*, *17*(4), 223–237.

Walkley, M., & Cox, T. L. (2013). Building trauma-informed schools and communities. *Children & Schools*, *35*(2), 123–126.

Webster, E. M. (2022). The impact of adverse childhood experiences on health and development in young children. *Global Pediatric Health*, *9*, 1–11. doi.org/10.1177/2333794X221078708

Weist, M. D., & Evans, S. W. (2005). Expanded school mental health: Challenges and opportunities in an emerging field. *Journal of Youth and Adolescence*, *34*, 3–6.

Wenz-Gross, M., Yoo, Y., Upshur, C. C., & Gambino, A. J. (2018). Pathways to kindergarten readiness: The roles of Second Step Early Learning curriculum and social-emotional, executive functioning, preschool academic and task behavior skills. *Frontiers in Psychology*, *9*, 1886. doi.org/10.3389/fpsyg.2018.01886

Wolpow, R., Johnson, M. M., Hertel, R., & Kincaid, S. O. (2016). *The heart of learning and teaching: Compassion, resiliency, and academic success*. Office of Superintendent of Public Instruction.

PART THREE

# PREVENTION WITH EMERGING ADULTS

# 8 Ecological and Developmental Approaches to Reducing Substance Use and Related Harms among Emerging Adults

Ellen L. Vaughan, Evelyn Claire Williams, Micheal Garza, and Lauren E. Adams

> The point is that in almost every instance of our lives, our social lives, we are, if we pay attention, in the midst of an almost constant, if subtle, caretaking .... This caretaking is our default mode and it's always a lie that convinces us to act or believe otherwise. Always.
>
> —Ross Gay, *The Book of Delights*

> What if joy is not only entangled with pain, or suffering, or sorrow, but is also what emerges from how we care for each other through those things?
>
> —Ross Gay, *Inciting Joy*

Substance use (SU) is a prevalent and pervasive public health problem. Developmentally, SU initiation often starts in adolescence with peak prevalence during emerging adulthood (Substance Abuse and Mental Health Services Administration [SAMHSA], 2022). Prevention of substance use disorders (SUDs) is critical from childhood through emerging adulthood and has the potential to reduce the risk for initiation of use, harmful use, and the development of SUD. Young people are at particularly high risk, with engagement and escalation of SU increasing subsequent risk for SUD. Results from the National Epidemiologic Survey on Alcohol and related conditions found that the lifetime prevalence of alcohol use disorder (AUD) is 29% and drug use disorder (DUD) is 9.9% (Grant et al., 2015, 2016). For those who are 18–29 years of age, the lifetime prevalence of AUD and DUD is a startling 37% and 14.2%, respectively. Narrowing in, 26.7% of young adults meet the criteria for AUDs in the past year, with about 20% in the mild to moderate range. Prevalence for past-year DUD is 8.3% for this age group. Persistent SU in emerging adulthood is an important target for prevention research and intervention development.

The aim of this chapter is to discuss approaches to prevention research and practice that address the problems of SU/SUD in emerging adult populations. We will draw from the Institute of Medicine's (IOM) scope and definitions of prevention, as described by O'Connell and colleagues (2009). Thus, the populations that would benefit from prevention efforts spans from those who have no detectible risks or symptoms of the disorder to those who may have diagnosable mental health concerns that warrant reduction of risk (e.g., reducing the risk of escalating severity or a return to previous levels of symptoms). Additionally, when considering types of prevention, we will use IOM's definitions of *universal, selected*, and *indicated* prevention. *Universal* prevention targets the population at large without attention to the level of risk for a particular problem. *Selected* prevention targets those populations known to be at increased risk. For emerging adult populations, this might be college students who are members of fraternities or sororities or students with a parental history of SUD. *Indicated* prevention targets those populations who are symptomatic. For example, indicated prevention might target emerging adults who are engaging in extensive SU and experiencing harmful consequences of their use, such as academic problems.

This chapter will first discuss SU and SUD in emerging adult populations, including ecodevelopmental and multicultural frameworks for prevention. This section draws from the developmental literature and utilizes up-to-date epidemiologic data that are readily available from the Monitoring the Future Study (https://monitoringthefuture.org/results/). Accessing publicly available data allows prevention practitioners to identify population specific SU rates as well as the trends in SU epidemiology. From there, we will describe risk and protective factor research and intervention development for emerging adults. These approaches will primarily describe our own research with Latinx emerging adults and broader populations of college students. Finally, we will discuss future directions in SU/SUD prevention that attend to diverse groups of emerging adults. An overarching goal is to describe our work in a way that allows mental health and psychology practitioners to develop and implement prevention targeting SU in emerging adult populations in their own practice and work settings.

## 8.1 Emerging Adulthood

Originally proposed by Arnett in 2000, emerging adulthood is a term referring to the developmental stage between the ages of 18 and 25 years (Arnett, 2000). Developmentally, emerging adults can be understood as those who have not yet reaching adulthood, but are no longer adolescents; thus, they are in transition between two developmental periods (Arnett, 2007, 2015). Arnett has expanded the concept of emerging adulthood outside of its use as a specific developmental reference point to include a broader developmental theory (Arnett, 2015). Specifically, he contends that a set of five distinguishing features characterize the period of emerging adulthood in the United States (Arnett, 2015). It is these features that capture the general sense of growth, flexibility, and unpredictability that set this period apart from the broader experience of adulthood. For example, the sense of "in-between" inherent to this period captures the general experience of not yet being an adult p. 9. The graduation to "adulthood" is considered to be gradual and includes milestones, coined the "Big Three" of accepting responsibility, financial independence, and independence in decision-making (Arnett, 2015, p. 15).

The period of emerging adulthood is often associated with a pronounced engagement in, and cultural acceptance of, alcohol and other drug use (SAMHSA, 2022). SU considerations are further heightened by the impacts of college attendance associated with this age range. Though not all emerging adults attend college, enrollment at a university is associated with an increase in the use of alcohol and other substances (Hartzler & Fromme, 2003). In considering prevalence rates, some of the most recent data suggest that the annual prevalence of use of any illicit drug (i.e., marijuana, amphetamines, hallucinogens, cocaine, narcotics other than heroin, sedatives, and tranquilizers) was similar for college (46%) and noncollege emerging adults (45%) (Schulenberg et al., 2021). These similarities are also seen with annual prevalence for marijuana use between college students (44%) and noncollege individuals (43%), specifically. As has been historically documented, differences for riskier drinking correlates, including binge drinking (five or more drinks in the past two weeks) and high intensity drinking (10 or more drinks in the past two weeks) between college youth and noncollege youth, were similar (Schulenberg et al., 2021). When examining prevalence rates for emerging adults compared to other developmental periods, more broadly, individuals aged 18–25 years demonstrate higher rates of binge drinking behavior, alcohol use, illicit drug use, and marijuana use in the past month and past year (SAMHSA, 2022).

While broad and extensive discourse exists concerning what risk factors are specifically responsible for the increased rates of risky SU for emerging adults (see Stone et al., 2012), unique predictors associated with emerging adults include the relevance of greater freedom and less social control (i.e., social standards or norms that influence behavior; Stone et al., 2012). For example, moving out of the parent's home has been found to be associated with an increased risk of SU concerns for emerging adults (White et al., 2006, 2008). Additionally, an important component of receiving a SUD diagnosis involves the criteria of clinical impairment or disruptions to functionality. Arnett (2015) offers that the cultural acceptance of riskier SU behaviors, coupled with less significant consequences, associated with emerging adulthood is an important contributing risk factors. Overall, emerging adulthood includes relevant developmental contributions to SU risk factors.

## 8.2 Prevention from Ecodevelopmental and Multicultural Perspectives

### 8.2.1 Ecodevelopmental Models

Ecodevelopmental models of prevention have been widely used in prevention research and practice (O'Connell et al., 2009). Ecodevelopmental theory integrates the multiple social-ecological systems in which an individual is developing (Szapocznik & Coatsworth, 1999). This theory – first called structural ecosystems theory (SET) – was developed as an explanatory framework for risk and protective factors for adolescent SU (Szapocznik & Coatsworth, 1999). SET integrates social-ecological theory, developmental theory, and social interactions (Ortega et al., 2012; Szapocznik & Coatsworth, 1999). Ecodevelopmental theories also help mental health practitioners and communities identify and focus on the specific populations they aim to serve.

Risk and protective factors related to SU/SUD for an individual can be understood through social-ecology theory, specifically, Bronfenbrenner's ecological theory (1979), which views the individual as developing in multiple, interrelated contexts. Often represented in concentric circles, this model is comprised of the microsystem (the immediate social settings/contexts and the individual's relationships within said contexts, such as with family and peers), the mesosystem (the overlap of microsystems, such as parental involvement in the adolescent's school), the exosystem (where members of the individual's mesosystem engage, but the individual does not participate directly, such as a caregiver's stressful work environment that influences their availability and quality of care for their adolescent), the macrosystem (the philosophical and social ideas and practices of a culture or subculture), and the chronosystem (the life changes and other temporal dimensions of the spheres; Berk, 2019; Ortega et al., 2012). Ecodevelopmental theory sees individuals as developing and growing within the demands of their social contexts, which are constantly changing over time (Ortega et al., 2012).

Ecodevelopmental approaches to prevention view social interactions as a mechanism through which individuals experience risk and protection from relationship patterns across contextual levels of their social ecology (Ortega et al., 2012). Ecodevelopmental models of prevention, therefore, emphasize things like family functioning, caregiver-youth and peer-peer communication about SU, school and community support, caregiver/parenting practices and knowledge on SU, family and community culture, and school and community policies on SU (Ortega et al., 2012). Though primarily focused on adolescents, these ecodevelopmental principles can be applied to emerging adulthood and the primary contexts in which they are developing.

### 8.2.2 Multicultural Models

Ecodevelopmental frameworks for prevention often attend to culture and context. Attending to the cultural and contextual influences on SU is critical when mental health practitioners develop programs and interventions for the emerging adults in their workspace or community. In this section, we aim to go a step further to explicitly address multiculturalism and social justice as integral to prevention research and practice. In counseling psychology and prevention science, concepts such as social justice and multicultural orientations (MCOs) are central tenants in research and practice (American Psychological Association, 2002, 2014, 2017; Davis et al., 2018; Sue, 2001; Wong et al., 2017).

Within counseling and counseling psychology, one of the most recognizable multidimensional models of multicultural competence is known as the tripartite model of cultural competence (Sue, 2001; Sue et al., 2009). The model posits three essential cultural characteristics when working with diverse groups. Professionals should engage in self-awareness and explration of one's own cultural identities and how they can influence our experiences, beliefs, and biases toward diverse groups, pursue knowledge of others' diverse cultural upbringings/backgrounds, and, finally, utilize skills that are culturally sensitive when developing and delivering interventions.

Scholarship has begun to focus on multiculturalism in counseling, a shift from multicultural competence (Sue, 2001; Sue et al., 1992, 2009) to help therapists better understand and build their MCO (Davis, 2018; Watkins et al., 2019). This framework consists of three factors. *Cultural humility is* the openness to listen and the willingness to reflect and understand others' diverse identities. *Cultural comfort* is the feelings that occur before, during, and after the intervention when discussing culturally sensitive information, and *cultural opportunities* refer to professionals exploring cultural content when it presents itself. The MCO perspective stems from language seen in the seminal Multicultural Counseling Competencies (Sue et al., 1992); however, it stresses the clients' cultural experiences to strengthen the working alliance (Davis, 2018; Watkins, et al., 2019). While these models are largely focused on what is happening in a counseling relationship, these concepts can also be used in prevention research and practice.

A recent multicultural perspective on prevention, adapted from the racial–cultural framework (Wong et al., 2013), delineates the three components that comprise the multicultural social justice framework (MSJF) for prevention research and practice (Wong et al., 2017). Component one targets the *constructs* (i.e., theories and research) that help address prevention outcomes within diverse populations. These include identifying social inequities, recognizing how cultural constructs translate into risk and protective factors, and uncovering unique beliefs and attitudes tied to the client's cultural identities. The second component, *populations*, refers to carefully considering the most underserved groups, as well as applying an intersectional lens. The third component, *intervention*, points to the content that interventions should highlight when working with diverse groups. This component relies on creating culturally focused prevention interventions through collaboration with community stakeholders, improving access to resources, and participating in macro-level interventions that further promote multiculturalism and social justice for those who find themselves most underserved and underrepresented (Wong et al., 2017). In a practice, this might include bringing together people from various groups including the population one aims to deliver the prevention programming for, professionals from other disciplines to inform the development of the program (i.e., student affairs or public health professionals), and other critical community stakeholders. Involvement of multiple stakeholders from development through implementation of the program would be consistent with the MSJF framework for prevention.

## 8.3 Risk and Protective Factor Research

Risk and protective factor research with emerging adult populations has been less prevalent when compared to adolescent populations but is showing growth. Since the seminal Hawkins, Catalano, and Miller (1992) article on adolescent risk and protective factors for SU, there has been growth in research aimed at understanding SU in emerging adulthood. Much of this work has focused on college students. For example, Stone and colleagues (2012) conducted a review of risk and protective factors for SU among emerging adults. These authors noted broad categories of risk and protective factors related to what they call "fixed markers of risk", (p. 749) such as race/ethnicity, "contextual factors", (p. 756) such as norms or substance availability, "individual and interpersonal factors", (p. 756) such as family relations, education, or religiosity. Notably, a number of these risk and protective factors are related to developmental processes associated with emerging adulthood. For example, college attendance increases the risk of being in environments where SU is prevalent. Prevention research in this area has moved toward an intersectional lens, with respect to diverse groups of emerging adults, as well as considering the varied contexts in which emerging adults are situated (e.g., college).

To illustrate, next we will review a series of studies we conducted which address correlates of SU among Latinx emerging adults. We will frame these examples using principles from Wong and colleagues (2017) MSJF for prevention. Specifically, our work in this area has focused on cultural constructs as potential risk and protective factors and on understanding risk and protective factors within populations. This can be done in a number of ways including data collection targeting a specific population, as well as utilizing large datasets and narrowing into a specific subsample, including testing group differences within subsamples. The examples we will share are primarily from large datasets that include subsamples of Latinx emerging adults. From these studies, we tested associations among known risk and protective factors, as well as cultural factors among Latinx emerging adults, broadly, and Latinx college students. Practitioners might review the relevant literature in these areas as they set out to develop prevention for their setting and collaborate with local researchers to collect data to understand the population they aim to serve.

Two studies were conducted using a sample of college students from a large university. Wong and colleagues' (2017) MSJF principles of disaggregating data and using an intersectional lens can be applied to these studies. Further, these studies attend to important constructs embedded within ecodevelopmental models of prevention (e.g., family factors). The first study investigated a sex by ethnicity interaction on drinking behavior, followed by multigroup structural equation modeling to investigate group differences in the interrelationships among family drinking, peer drinking, values about the acceptability of drinking, and alcohol use (Corbin et al., 2008). In this sample of White and Latinx college-bound students, family drinking more strongly influenced personal values about drinking for Latinx than for White students. Latinas perceived that they had fewer same-sex family members who were drinkers, which was correlated with less permissive attitudes about drinking. Moreover, these less permissive attitudes were related to lower levels of drinking behaviors. In addition, Latinas perceived less drinking among their same-sex peers than Latinos, which, in turn, led to less permissive attitudes about drinking and fewer drinking behaviors. Together, these results indicate that, among Latinx students, it may be important to attend to the intersections of a student's Latinx identity, as well as their gender or sex at birth to understand alcohol use.

A second study tested the longitudinal relationships between academic and social motives/behaviors and alcohol use/problems among college students (Vaughan et al., 2009). This study employed a multigroup analysis to test race/ethnicity as a moderator of these longitudinal relationships. Results indicated that during the fall of their sophomore year in college, academic motives/behaviors were significantly and inversely related to alcohol use for Latinx students, but not for Asian American students. Specific to social motives/behavior, White and Latinx had stronger positive associations between social motivations and behaviors and alcohol use than Asian American students across time. Racial/ethnic differences in academic and social motives/behaviors and alcohol use problems also emerged. Stronger academic motives/behaviors during the fall of freshman year were associated with fewer drinking problems for Latinx than for White and Asian American students. This study is important because it attends to established risk and protective factors for alcohol use (e.g., social and academic motivations) and identifies important group differences in how these factors influence alcohol use.

Another national dataset that allows for testing correlates of SU among subgroups of college students is the American College Health Association's revised National College Health Assessment (NCHA). From these data, we conducted three studies testing associations among risk and protective factors and SU among Latinx college students (Gonzalez & Vaughan, 2022; Vaughan et al., 2015, 2018). In our first study, we were interested in whether the college environment would change the relationship between alcohol use norms and alcohol use (Vaughan et al., 2015). We specifically tested institution type (Hispanic Serving Institution [HSI] versus not) as a moderator of the relationship between the perception of alcohol use quantity by peers and quantity of alcohol use. The NCHA data allowed us to access a large sample from multiple institutions, thereby tapping students from HSIs. Results revealed that students at HSIs consumed fewer drinks than their counterparts at non-HSIs but did not differ regarding their estimation of peer consumption. This estimation of peer drinking is highly correlated with personal consumption and is central to many prevention efforts with college students. Institution type moderated the relationship between perceived consumption by others and personal alcohol consumption. The relationship between the perception of others' drinking and personal drinking was stronger for students attending non- HSIs. Future research might attend to the factors that reduce risk for students at HSIs such as the climate of the institution with respect to representation of Latinx faculty and culturally affirming or the school's proximity to familial supports. Hypotheses might include a more culturally affirming environment, as well as different life circumstances, such as attending a college closer to home.

A second study using the NCHA addressed whether gender moderated the association between SU norms (perceptions of others' use) and SU (Vaughan et al., 2018). Specifically, we tested two models addressing alcohol use and marijuana use. The rationale for this study stems from previous research suggesting gender differences in SU among Latinx college students and emerging adults (Corbin et al., 2008; Paschall et al., 2005; Raffaelli et al., 2007). The results of this study found similar positive associations between social norms about use and both alcohol and marijuana use outcomes. However, the association was stronger for men than for women. There are several potential reasons for this difference. It is possible that the influence of gender norms on SU impacts the perceptions of others' use and, thereby, impacts personal use. Also, some research suggests that when students are asked about the use of "typical" college students, they may not be referencing groups to which they belong (Lewis & Neighbors, 2007). These authors found that the "typical" college student is likely to be viewed as male and White, suggesting the need to test group-specific norms as correlates of SU among Latinx students.

A third study using the NCHA data tested group differences in SU between Latinx domestic college students and Latinx international students (Gonzalez & Vaughan, 2022). Latinx international students as a group have been understudied. In this study, international students had higher rates of alcohol use than domestic students but had similar rates of cigarette and other drug use. Risk and protective factors were also tested as correlates of alcohol use and binge drinking among the Latinx international students. Among Latinx international students, women had lower rates of drinking than men. Additionally, those who were members of fraternities or sororities had higher rates of drinking than non-members. Finally, students who reported a history of cigarette and marijuana use also had higher rates of drinking. To conclude, while Latinx international students had higher rates of alcohol use than their domestic counterparts, the correlates of drinking such as participation in a fraternity or sorority, other SU, and year in school, parallel those of domestic Latinx students.

Building upon the aforementioned studies with college student samples, we will also review three studies with a sample of Latinx emerging adults that include both college-attending and noncollege-attending participants. These studies have focused on contextual and cultural factors related to SU using data from the National Longitudinal Student of Adolescent to Adult Health (Add Health; Harris, 2018). The first study tested a Latinx subgroup as a moderator of the relationships between family and peer language usage and alcohol use behaviors (Vaughan et al., 2013). We found that the Latinx subgroup moderated the relationship between language usage and alcohol use. For Cuban emerging adults, those who spoke Spanish or half Spanish and half English with their family had reduced odds of any alcohol use in the past year. With respect to language usage with peers, Puerto Rican emerging adults who spoke Spanish reported fewer binge drinking days than their Mexican counterparts. In another study, two dimensions of religiosity (public and private) were tested as protective factors for binge drinking and marijuana use among Latino emerging adults (Escobar & Vaughan, 2014). Public religion was associated with reduced odds of binge drinking and marijuana use. These results suggest that religiosity may be an important cultural construct to consider in prevention research.

In a third study, latent class regression was used to identify relationships between gender roles and binge drinking among Latinx emerging adults (Vaughan et al., 2014). Three dimensions of gender roles were included as independent variables: personal masculinity, social masculinity, and femininity. Personal masculinity reflects characteristics such as independence and leadership. Social masculinity reflects more competitive and aggressive characteristics. Finally, femininity was characterized by traits such as being warm or affectionate. Three patterns of relationships emerged. In two of three classes, gender roles were associated with binge drinking. In the "Protective Personal Masculinity Class," personal masculinity was associated with lower odds of binge drinking. In the "Mixed Masculinity Class," personal masculinity was associated with lower odds of binge drinking, while social masculinity increased the odds of binge drinking. Female participants, born outside the United States, and those with greater English language usage were more likely to be in the "Mixed Masculinity Class." These results underscore the important role that gender roles play in binge drinking for emerging adults.

Taken together, these studies underscore the relevance of Latinx culture in SU behaviors during emerging adulthood. The influence of family remains important, religion reduced the odds of SU, and gender roles were linked to binge drinking, but in different ways for men and women born outside of the United States. The results bring to light the within-group diversity in the Latinx population and identify potential targets for prevention efforts in research and practice. Consistent with the MSJF, we were able to leverage large datasets to investigate cultural constructs as potential risk and protective factors and disaggregate data to better understand correlates of SU within the Latinx emerging adult population. Such studies represent the building blocks for development of culturally focused prevention efforts with Latinx emerging adults.

## 8.4 Intervention Development Studies

In this section of the chapter, we will describe the development of two interventions to target emerging adults. Several prevention models are aimed at reducing SU, largely alcohol use, among college students (Cronce & Larimer, 2011). The college setting represents an important context for SU and is often associated with excessive alcohol use and related harms. For students, the developmental transition from high school into college is often characterized by an increase in alcohol use and associated alcohol-related harms (Fromme et al., 2008; National Institute on Alcohol Abuse and Alcoholism [NIAAA], 2007; Vicary & Karshin, 2002). This increase in SU coincides with several developmental transitions associated with emerging adulthood, such as increases in independence and exploration of identities and opportunities (Arnett, 2015). Emerging adulthood is an opportune time for prevention interventions. The two interventions described later include a parent-based intervention to reduce alcohol-related sexual assault and a cognitive-behavioral intervention for students with SU problems. The development of both interventions draws from the extant research on the problems of alcohol-related sexual assault and SU in the college context as well as clinical and practice observations by the authors regarding gaps in practice and research in the college context. Thus, the clinical and practice observations serve as a motivation to fill in gaps with intervention research.

### 8.4.1 Parent-Based Intervention for Sexual Assault

Sexual assault is pervasive on college campuses and represents critical alcohol-related harm (NIAAA, 2007). Indeed, it is estimated that at least 50% of sexual assaults on campus are alcohol-involved – when the perpetrator and/or the victim were using alcohol (Abbey, 2002; Abbey et al., 2011). Colleges and universities are tasked with the implementation of prevention programming to reduce the costs, both monetary and personal, of student alcohol use and related sexual assaults (Perkins, 2002). A variety of prevention programming is targeted at incoming first-year students across the nation's campuses, and considerable variation exists in the extent to which the programming is based on empirical evidence. Empirically based models of prevention for drinking are often delivered individually to high-risk students (e.g., Brief Alcohol Screening and Intervention for College Students [BASICS]; Dimeff et al., 1999) or universally through online venues (e.g., Alcohol.edu; MyStudentBody.com). Likewise, sexual assault prevention on campus has increasingly employed bystander intervention models (Banyard, 2011; Banyard et al., 2004; McMahon & Banyard, 2011). These programs aim to teach community members to identify high-risk situations for sexual assault and to provide them with tools for intervening.

There is growing interest in prevention efforts that involve parents. The impetus for using parent-based intervention lies in the accumulating research evidence that links family and parenting behaviors to SU, not just in adolescence, but into the college years (Wetherrill & Fromme, 2007). Peer influences have dominated the prevention research during the transition from adolescence to emerging adulthood. However, there is a growing literature on the persistence of parental influence in emerging adult development. That is, from an ecodevelopmental perspective, the relationships between parents and emerging adults continue to impact development and engagement in risk behaviors. For example, among college students, parental monitoring and support have been linked to less frequent drinking (Wetherrill & Fromme, 2007) and fewer sexual behaviors (Wetherill et al., 2010). Other parenting factors, such as attitudes, are also associated with alcohol use (Abar et al., 2009; Abar & Turrisi, 2008).

The intervention model described in this chapter is grounded in ecodevelopmental theories that emphasize family communication and relationships

(Ortega et al., 2012; Szapocznik & Coatsworth, 1999). Communication occurs in the context of interactional processe between different family subsystems (e.g., mother–daughter). Ways of interacting are learned and yield recurring patterns of interaction over time. From this perspective, it is reasonable to expect that parents may need to shift their communication styles to address risks that are pervasive on college campuses, such as alcohol use and sexual assault. However, existing parent-based interventions have largely targeted alcohol use outcomes with less focus on sexual victimization.

Guided by the empirical research on risk and protective factors, several parent-based interventions have been developed to reduce risky drinking and related consequences. The format of these interventions has been to provide parents with psychoeducation in a non-facilitated format, such as a handbook (Doumas et al., 2013; Turrisi et al., 2001) or in an online format (LaBrie et al., 2014). More recent parent-based interventions have used in-person forums. Specifically, LaBrie and colleagues (2016) conducted an in-person parent-based intervention surrounding drinking norms. Results assessed student outcomes and found that students whose parents attended this intervention drank less frequently and were less likely to engage in binge drinking. To our knowledge, this intervention represents the only intervention to be conducted with parents of college students in person but does not address the connection between alcohol use and sexual assault. Testa et al., 2010 developed and tested an intervention, wherein mothers were provided with a booklet with information on alcohol use and college dating and instructed to talk with their daughters about the content. Results showed that those in the intervention condition reported lower rates of incapacitated rape. Together, these studies suggest that parent-based intervention may be effective in reducing alcohol and sexual-assault-related outcomes during the transition into college. However, Testa and colleagues' study did not involve an in-person component and only targeted mothers and daughters. Much of the prevention work in this area now aims to target the larger community and often uses bystander intervention models that encourage action by the whole university community.

Bystander intervention is based upon the premise that community members can be given the tools to intervene in high-risk situations to reduce risk of sexual assault (Banyard, 2011). Bystander intervention has grown considerably in the college context as a way to reduce the occurrence of sexual assault on campus (Mabry & Turner, 2016). Research has pointed to the importance of bystanders in being active participants to intervene in situations where there is high risk for sexual violence (Banyard et al., 2007; McMahon & Banyard, 2011). Given parents' influence in the lives of college students, they may be an important source of information on how to address high-risk situations and to engage in bystander behavior. Further, bystander intervention is innovative in the parent–child context, as it provides a way for parents and students to have conversations about high-risk behavior that reduces defensiveness by talking about intervening in high-risk situations in the college environment.

To address the problem of alcohol-related sexual assault, we conducted a series of studies aimed at developing a parent-based intervention (Vaughan et al., 2017; Vaughan, 2018). To this end, we developed a single-session group intervention to be delivered to parents when they visited our larger university campus for their child's first-year orientation. The structure of the group intervention was divided into three parts. The first third of the group included a discussion and sharing of campus-specific data on the role that alcohol plays in college life, sexual assault on campus (including campus definitions of consent and who is able to give and get consent for sexual behavior), and the principles of bystander intervention. In the second third of the intervention, group facilitators shared and discussed strategies for communication about alcohol and consent for sex. Finally, in the last third of the intervention, group facilitators shared common scenarios that happen on campus involving alcohol use and risk for sexual assault. The aim of the final part of the intervention was to discuss the application of bystander intervention to these scenarios as well as strategies for effective communication with their incoming college student about how to intervene in high-risk situations.

Results from a pilot study indicated that parents experienced changes in their beliefs about alcohol use and a person's ability to give consent for sexual activity (Vaughan et al., 2017). Parents also reported increases in self-efficacy in talking with their teens about consent for sexual activity. Results from the pilot study were used for a larger trial that compared the group with a control condition, which was a group that simply asked parents to talk about the concerns they had for their students as they transitioned into college. For the larger trial, our research team implemented a number of changes in the measurement of outcomes. Specifically, our measurement of self-efficacy in talking about sexual assault was high at the outset, especially for parents of daughters. However, it was less clear if parents would report high rates of efficacy in specifically talking about consent for sexual behavior. Future directions in this area include further refinement of measurement, virtual delivery of the intervention to increase participation from diverse groups of parents, and methods of recruitment of students at follow-up. Overall, the results are promising, but further data analysis and intervention refinement are warranted.

### 8.4.2 CBT for Mild to Moderate SUD

At the outset of this chapter, we noted the high prevalence of emerging adults with mild to moderate SUD. Interventions that target these emerging adults are needed to prevent escalation of use to more severe, persisting SUD. To address the specific needs of college students, a strong empirical base exists for individual prevention efforts delivered on campuses (Cronce & Larimer, 2011). These efforts are developmentally and contextually focused and typically target risky, but not dependent, alcohol use. Few research studies have examined more intensive models of treatment for students who meet the criteria for a SUD or are in recovery, and it is not clear the extent to which practitioners in college counseling centers engage in work around SU problems that would not need a higher level of care (i.e., inpatient care). This represents a critical gap in knowledge as well as practice. Colleges and universities are the center of many emerging adults' lives and, thus, are the optimal place for a broad range of prevention services, spanning from universal through selected prevention models.

Cognitive behavioral therapy (CBT) has empirical support for treating mental health concerns, including SUD (Carroll, 2000; Carroll et al., 2006; Magill & Ray, 2009). A particular area in need of further research is testing the efficacy of a CBT model for college students with active SUD and for students in recovery. Such models would retain the core aspects of CBT (e.g., functional analysis, skills training, and relapse prevention) while addressing developmental concerns, such as identity and career exploration and navigating SU on campus. For example, a counselor might explore whether sober activities are available and identify ways to cope with high-risk collegiate events, such as parties or tailgating. The goal of our research was to develop a CBT protocol for college students with mild to moderate SUD. The impetus for developing such an intervention was to address a gap in service for those students whose needs go beyond existing universal and selected prevention programming to indicated prevention for those who meet criteria for mild to moderate SUD, but do not require more intensive treatment that would exclude them from higher education.

We adapted an existing CBT intervention for students with mild to moderate SUD. The intervention was comprised of eight sessions and utilized the basic approaches of CBT, such as functional analysis, worksheets, role-play, and assigned homework (Carroll, 2000; Kadden et al., 2003). Adaptation included intentional tailoring to address the specific context of college and emerging adulthood as a developmental context. For example, an initial presentation of the CBT model to the client included descriptions of drinking and SU specific to the college context. Other session content included coping, refusal and other communication skills, decision-making and problem-solving, planning for relapse and high-risk situations, and identifying social supports. In addition, the intervention was explicitly a harm reduction model over an abstinence model. That is, interventionists and clients set goals for SU collaboratively.

This aforementioned project is still in the data collection phase. Evaluation of the intervention includes assessments at baseline, posttreatment, and follow-up (at three and six months). It is important to note that assessment of outcomes includes not just measures of SU, but also measures of therapeutic alliance, fidelity to the intervention model, and mental health outcomes, such as overall psychological distress, SU problems, and recovery capital.

## 8.5 Conclusions and Future Directions

The aim of this chapter was to describe approaches to prevention with emerging adult populations using ecodevelopmental and multicultural frameworks for our work. To this end, we discussed risk and protective factor research, as well as the initial development of interventions aimed at reducing the risk for alcohol-related sexual assault and escalation of SU problems. Overall, engagement in prevention research spans risk/protective factor research and intervention development. As authors, we identify as researchers and practitioners. Thus, the aim of the chapter is to also describe our work in a way that can be applied by students, practitioners, and researchers in the development and implementation of prevention in their own work settings.

There are several future directions for the work described here. Specifically, the intervention development research is being conducted on predominantly White campuses. Preliminary results are promising, but future work should attend to whether these interventions would work with diverse groups of college students. For example, the research supporting parent-based interventions has largely been conducted without attention to the diverse identities that college students hold. Applying the MSJF (Wong et al., 2017) to understanding risk and protective factors for alcohol-related sexual assault would be an important avenue to understanding what interventions might look like in diverse groups of college students. Our risk and protective factor research on Latinx emerging adults may indicate that attending to cultural constructs such as gender roles might be important when developing a parent-based intervention for Latinx emerging adults. Similarly, the CBT intervention was built for flexibility to incorporate contextual and cultural factors, such as identity development, but could likewise benefit from applying the MSJF to develop and test interventions for diverse groups of emerging adults.

## References

Abar, C., & Turrisi, R. (2008). How important are parents during the college years? A longitudinal perspective of indirect influences parents yield on their college teens' alcohol use. *Addictive Behaviors*, *33*(10), 1360–1368. doi.org/10.1016/j.addbeh.2008.06.010

Abar, C., Abar, B., & Turrisi, R. (2009). The impact of parental modeling and permissibility on alcohol use and experienced negative drinking consequences in college. *Addictive Behaviors*, *34*(6–7), 542–547. doiorg.proxyiub.uits.iu.edu/10.1016/j.addbeh.2009.03.019

Abbey, A. (2002). Alcohol-related sexual assault: A common problem among college students. *Journal of Studies on Alcohol*, Supplement 14, 118–128. doi.org/10.15288/jsas.2002.s14.118

Abbey, A. (2011). Alcohol's role in sexual violence perpetration: Theoretical explanations, existing evidence and future directions. *Drug and Alcohol Review*, *30*(5), 481–489. doi.org/10.1111/j.1465-3362.2011.00296.x

American Psychological Association. (2002). Guidelines on multicultural education, training, research, practice, and organizational change for psychologists. *American Psychologist*, *58*(5), 377–402. doi.org/10.1037/0003-066x.58.5.377

American Psychological Association. (2014). Guidelines for prevention in psychology. *American Psychologist*, *69*(3), 285–296. doi.org/10.1037/a0034569

American Psychological Association. (2017). *Multicultural guidelines: An ecological approach to context, identity, and intersectionality.* www.apa.org/about/policy/multicultural-guidelines.pdf

Arnett, J. J. (2000). Emerging adulthood: A theory of development from the late teens through the twenties. *American Psychologist*, *55*(5), 469–480. doi.org/10.1037/0003-066X.55.5.469

Arnett, J. J. (2007). Emerging adulthood: What is it, and what is it good for? *Child Development Perspectives*, *1*(2), 68–73. doi.org/10.1111/j.1750-8606.2007.00016.x

Arnett, J. J. (2015). *Emerging adulthood: The winding road from the late teens through the twenties* (2nd ed.). Oxford University Press.

Banyard, V. L. (2011). Who will help prevent sexual violence: Creating an ecological model of bystander intervention. *Psychology of Violence*, *1*(3), 216–229. https://psycnet-apa-org.proxyiub.uits.iu.edu/doi/10.1037/a0023739

Banyard, V. L., Moynihan, M. M., & Plante, E. G. (2007). Sexual violence prevention through bystander education: An experimental evaluation. *Journal of Community Psychology*, *35*(4), 463–481. doi.org/10.1002/jcop.20159

Banyard, V. L., Plante, E. G., & Moynihan, M. M. (2004). Bystander education: Bringing a broader community perspective to sexual violence prevention. *Journal of Community Psychology*, *32*(1), 61–79. dx.doi.org.proxyiub.uits.iu.edu/10.1002/jcop.10078

Berk, L. (2019). *Exploring child and adolescent development.* Pearson Education, Inc.

Bronfenbrenner, U. (1979). *The ecology of human development.* Harvard University Press.

Carroll, K. M. (2000). *A cognitive-behavioral approach: Treating cocaine addiction* (Vol. 1). US Department of Health and Human Services, National Institutes of Health, National Institute on Drug Abuse.

Carroll, K. M., Easton, C. J., Nich, C., Hunkele, K. A., Neavins, T. M., Sinha, R., Ford, H. L., Vitolo, S. A, Doebrick, C. A., & Rounsaville, B. J. (2006). The use of contingency management and motivational/skills-building therapy to treat young adults with marijuana dependence. *Journal of Consulting and Clinical Psychology*, *74*(5), 955–966. doi.org/10.1037/0022-006X.74.5.955

Corbin, W. R., Vaughan, E. L., & Fromme, K. (2008). Ethnic differences and the closing of the sex gap in alcohol use among college-bound students. *Psychology of Addictive Behaviors*, *22*(2), 240–248. doi.org/10.1037/0893-164X.22.2.240

Cronce, J. M., & Larimer, M. E. (2011). Individual-focused approaches to the prevention of college student drinking. *Alcohol Research & Health*, *34*(2), 210–221. https://proxyiub.uits.iu.edu/login?qurl=https%3A%2F%2Fwww.proquest.com%2Fscholarly-journals%2Findividual-focused-approaches-prevention-college%2Fdocview%2F912154914%2Fse-2%3Faccountid%3D11620

Davis, D. E., DeBlaere, C., Owen, J., Hook, J. N., Rivera, D. P., Choe, E., Van Tongeren, D. R., Worthington, E. L., & Placeres, V. (2018). The multicultural orientation framework: A narrative review. *Psychotherapy*, *55*(1), 89–100. doi.org/10.1037/pst0000160

Dimeff, L. A. (Ed.). (1999). *Brief alcohol screening and intervention for college students (BASICS): A harm reduction approach*. Guilford Press.

Doumas, D. M., Turrisi, R., Ray, A. E., Esp, S. M., & Curtis-Schaeffer, A. K. (2013). A randomized trial evaluating a parent based intervention to reduce college drinking. *Journal of Substance Abuse Treatment*, 45(1), 31–37. doi.org/10.1016/j.jsat.2012.12.008

Escobar, O. S., & Vaughan, E. L. (2014). Public and private religiosity and substance use among Latino emerging adults. *Substance Use and Misuse*, *49*(10), 1317–1325. doi .org/10.3109/10826084.2014.901384

Fromme, K., Corbin, W. R., & Kruse, M. I. (2008). Behavioral risks during the transition from high school to college. *Developmental Psychology*, *44*(5), 1497–1504. doi .org/10.1037/a0012614

Grant, B. F., Goldstein, R. B., Saha, T. D., Chou, S. P., Jung, J., Zhang, H., Pickering, M. S., June Ruan, W., Smith, S. M., Huang, B., & Hasin, D. S. (2015). Epidemiology of DSM-5 alcohol use disorder: Results from the National Epidemiologic Survey on Alcohol and Related Conditions III. *JAMA Psychiatry*, *72*(8), 757–766. doi .org/10.1001/jamapsychiatry.2015.0584

Grant, B. F., Saha, T. D., Ruan, W. J., Goldstein, R. B., Chou, S. P., Jung, J., Zhang, H., Smith, S. M., Pickering, R. P., Huang, B., & Hasin, D. S. (2016). Epidemiology of DSM-5 drug use disorder: Results from the National Epidemiologic Survey on Alcohol and Related Conditions-III. *JAMA Psychiatry*, *73*(1), 39–47. doi.org/10.1001/jamapsychiatry.2015.2132

Gonzalez, P. D. & Vaughan, E. L. (2022). Substance use among Latinx international and domestic college students. *Journal of Ethnicity in Substance Abuse*, *21*(1), 230–252. doi.org/10.1080/15332640.2020.1747037

Hartzler, B., & Fromme, K. (2003). Heavy episodic drinking and college entrance. *Journal of Drug Education*, *33*(3), 259–274. doi.org/10.2190/2L2X-F8E1-32T9-UDMU

Harris, K. M. (2018). *The National longitudinal study of adolescent to adult health (add health), waves I & II, 1994–1996; wave III, 2001–2002; wave IV, 2007–2009; wave V, 2016–2018*. Chapel Hill, NC: Carolina Population Center, University of North Carolina at Chapel Hill.

Hawkins, J. D., Catalano, R. F., & Miller, J. Y. (1992). Risk and protective factors for alcohol and other drug problems in adolescence and early adulthood: Implications for substance abuse prevention. *Psychological Bulletin*, *112*(1), 64–105. doi .org/10.1037/0033-2909.112.1.64

Kadden, R., Carroll, K., Donovan, D., Cooney, N., Monti, P., Abrams, D, Litt, M. & Hester, R. (2003). Cognitive-behavioral coping skills therapy manual. US Government Printing Office.

LaBrie, J. W., Earle, A. M., Boyle, S. C., Hummer, J. F., Montes, K., Turrisi, R., & Napper, L. E. (2016). A parent-based intervention reduces heavy episodic drinking among first-year college students. *Psychology of Addictive Behaviors*, *30*(5), 523–535. dx.doi.org/10.1037/adb0000187

LaBrie, J. W., Napper, L. E., & Hummer, J. F. (2014). Normative feedback for parents of college students: Piloting a parent based intervention to correct misperceptions of students' alcohol use and other parents' approval of drinking. *Addictive Behaviors*, *39*(1), 107–113. doi.org/10.1016/j.addbeh.2013.08.036

Lewis, M. A., & Neighbors, C. (2007). Optimizing personalized normative feedback: The use of gender-specific referents. *Journal of Studies on Alcohol and Drugs*, *68*(2), 228–237. doi.org/10.15288/jsad.2007.68.228

Mabry, A., & Turner, M. M. (2016). Do sexual assault bystander interventions change men's intentions? Applying the theory of normative social behavior to predicting bystander outcomes. *Journal of Health Communication*, *21*(3), 276–292. dx.doi.org/10.1080/10810730.2015.1058437

Magill, M., & Ray, L. A. (2009). Cognitive-behavioral treatment with adult alcohol and illicit drug users: A meta-analysis of randomized controlled trials. *Journal of Studies on Alcohol and Drugs*, *70*(4), 516–527. doi.org/10.15288/jsad.2009.70.516

Monitoring the Future (n.d.). *Results*. https://monitoringthefuture.org/results/

McMahon, S., & Banyard, V. L. (2011). When can I help? A conceptual framework for the prevention of sexual violence through bystander intervention. *Trauma, Violence, & Abuse*, *13*(1), 3–14. doi.org/1524838011426015

National Institute on Alcohol Abuse and Alcoholism. (2007).*What colleges need to know now: An update on college drinking research* (NIH Publication No. 07-5010). www.collegedrinkingprevention.gov/1College_Bulletin-508_361C4E.pdf

O'Connell, M. E., Boat, T. & Warner, K. E. (2009). *Preventing mental, emotional, and behavioral disorders among young people: Progress and possibilities*. The National Academies Press.

Ortega, J., Huang, S., & Prado, G. (2012). Applying ecodevelopmental theory and the theory of reasoned action to understand HIV risk behaviors among Hispanic adolescents. *Hispanic Health Care International: The Official Journal of the National Association of Hispanic Nurses*, *10*(1), 42–52. doi.org/10.1891/1540-4153.10.1.42

Paschall, M. J., Bersamin, M., & Flewelling, R. L. (2005). Racial/ethnic differences in the association between college attendance and heavy alcohol use: A national study. *Journal of Studies on Alcohol*, *66*(2), 266–274. doi.org/10.15288/jsa.2005.66.266

Perkins, J. H. W. (2002). Surveying the damage: A review of research on consequences of alcohol misuse in college populations. *Journal of Studies on Alcohol*, *s14*, 91–100. doi.org/10.15288/jsas.2002.s14.91

Raffaelli, M., Stone, R. A. T., Iturbide, M. I., McGinley, M., Carlo, G., & Crockett, L. J. (2007). Acculturation, gender, and alcohol use among Mexican American college students. *Addictive Behaviors*, *32*(10), 2187–2199. doi.org/10.1016/j.addbeh.2007.02.014

Schulenberg, J. E., Patrick, M. E., Johnston, L. D., O'Malley, P. M., Bachman, J. G., & Miech, R. A. (2021). *Monitoring the future national survey results on drug use, 1975–2020: Volume II, College students and adults ages 19–60.* http://monitoringthefuture.org/pubs.html#monographs

Stone, A. L., Becker, L. G., Huber, A. M., & Catalano, R. F. (2012). Review of risk and protective factors of substance use and problem use in emerging adulthood. *Addictive Behaviors*, *37*(7), 747–775. doi.org/10.1016/j.addbeh.2012.02.014

Substance Abuse and Mental Health Services Administration. (2022). *2018–2020 National survey on drug use and health substate age group tables* (2018–2020 Substate Estimates of Substance Use and Mental Illness, Issue). www.samhsa.gov/data/sites/default/files/reports/rpt35976/NSDUH%20Substate%20Region%20Estimates%20by%20Age%202020/NSDUH%20Substate%20Region%20Estimates%20by%20Age%202020/2020NSDUHsubstateAgeGroupTabs041222.pdf

Sue, D. W. (2001). Multidimensional facets of cultural competence. *The Counseling Psychologist*, *29*(6), 790–821. doi.org/10.1177/0011000001296002

Sue, D. W., Arredondo, P., & McDavis, R. J. (1992). Multicultural counseling competencies and standards: A call to the profession. *Journal of Counseling & Development, 20*(2), 64–88. dx.doi.org/10.1002/j.2161-1912.1992.tb00563.x

Sue, S., Zane, N., Nagayama Hall, G. C., & Berger, L. K. (2009). The case for cultural competency in psychotherapeutic interventions. *Annual Review of Psychology, 60*, 525–548. doi.org/10.1146/annurev.psych.60.110707.163651

Szapocznik, J., & Coatsworth, J. D. (1999). An ecodevelopmental framework for organizing the influences on drug abuse: A developmental model of risk and protection. In *Drug abuse: Origins & interventions* (pp. 331–366). American Psychological Association.

Testa, M., Hoffman, J. H., Livingston, J. A., & Turrisi, R. (2010). Preventing college women's sexual victimization through parent-based intervention: A randomized controlled trial. *Prevention Science, 11*(3), 308–318. dx.doi.org/10.1007/s11121-010-0168-3

Turrisi, R., Jaccard, J., Taki, R., Dunnam, H., & Grimes, J. (2001). Examination of the short-term efficacy of a parent intervention to reduce college student drinking tendencies. *Psychology of Addictive Behaviors, 15*(4), 366–372. doi.org/10.1037/0893-164X.15.4.366

Vaughan, E. L. (2018, August). Prevention of substance use disorders and alcohol-related sexual assault. In S. M. Hage & K. Raczynski (Chairs), *Interdisciplinary dialogue on prevention – Invitation for collaborative action across psychology*. Symposium conducted at the 2018 American Psychological Association Convention, San Francisco, CA.

Vaughan, E. L., Chang, T. K., Escobar, O. S., & de Dios, M. A. (2015). Enrollment in Hispanic serving institutions as a moderator of the relationship between drinking norms and quantity of alcohol use among Hispanic college students. *Substance Abuse, 36*(3), 314–317. doi.org/10.1080/08897077.2014.932887

Vaughan, E. L., Corbin, W. R., & Fromme, K. (2009). Academic and social motives and drinking behavior. *Psychology of Addictive Behaviors, 23*(4), 564–576. doi.org/10.1037/a0017331

Vaughan E. L., Kratz, L. M., Escobar, O. S., & Middendorf, K. G. (2013). Latino subgroup as a moderator of the relationship between language usage and alcohol use in a national sample of Latino emerging adults. *Journal of Latina/o Psychology, 1*(3), 182–194. doi.org/10.1037/a0033384

Vaughan, E. L., Limas E. F., Chase, A. Gonzalez, P. D., McKean Blackwell, N., Klann, E., & Zounlome, N. (2017, June). *Results of a pilot study of a parent – Based prevention group to address alcohol related sexual assault among college students*. Poster presented at the 2017 Research Society on Alcoholism, Denver, CO.

Vaughan E. L., Wong, Y. J., & Middendorf, K. G. (2014). Gender roles and binge drinking among Latino emerging adults. *Psychology of Addictive Behaviors, 28*(3), 719–726. doi.org/10.1037/a0037406

Vaughan, E. L., Wright, L., Cano, M. A., & de Dios, M. A. (2018). Gender as a moderator of descriptive norms and substance use among Latino college students. *Substance Use & Misuse, 53*(11), 1840–1848. doi.org/10.1080/10826084.2018.1441305

Vicary, J. R., & Karshin, C. M. (2002). College alcohol abuse: A review of the problems, issues, and prevention approaches. *The Journal of Primary Prevention, 22*(3), 299–331. doi.org/10.1023/A:1013621821924

Watkins, C. E., Hook, J. N., Owen, J., DeBlaere, C., Davis, D. E., & Van Tongeren, D. R. (2019). Multicultural orientation in psychotherapy supervision: Cultural humility, cultural comfort, and cultural opportunities. *American Journal of Psychotherapy, 72*(2), 38–46. doi.org/10.1176/appi.psychotherapy.20180040

Wetherill, R. R., & Fromme, K. (2007). Perceived awareness and caring influences alcohol use by high school and college students. *Psychology of Addictive Behaviors*, *21*(2), 147–154. doi.org/10.1037/0893-164X.21.2.147

Wetherill, R. R., Neal, D. J., & Fromme, K. (2010). Parents, peers, and sexual values influence sexual behavior during the transition to college. *Archives of Sexual Behavior*, *39*(3), 682–694. dx.doi.org/10.1007/s10508-009-9476-8

White, H. R., Fleming, C. B., Kim, M. J., Catalano, R. F., & McMorris, B. J. (2008). Identifying two potential mechanisms for changes in alcohol use among college-attending and non-college-attending emerging adults. *Developmental Psychology*, *44*(6), 1625–1639. doi.org/10.1037/a0013855

White, H. R., McMorris, B. J., Catalano, R. F., Fleming, C. B., Haggerty, K. P., & Abbott, R. D. (2006). Increases in alcohol and marijuana use during the transition out of high school into emerging adulthood: The effects of leaving home, going to college, and high school protective factors. *Journal of Studies on Alcohol*, *67*(6), 810–822. doi.org/10.15288/jsa.2006.67.810

Wong, Y. J., Maffini, C. S., & Shin, M. (2013). The racial-cultural framework. *The Counseling Psychologist*, *42*(1), 13–54. doi.org/10.1177/0011000012470568

Wong, Y. J., Vaughan, E. L., & Klann, E. M. (2017). The science and practice of prevention from multicultural and social justice perspectives. In M. Israelashvili & J. L. Romano (Eds.), *The Cambridge handbook of international prevention science* (pp. 107–132) Cambridge University Press. doi.org/10.1017/9781316104453.007

# 9 Building Action from Awareness Movements

Conlin Bass

> What mental health needs is more sunlight, more candor, more unashamed conversation.
>
> —Glenn Close (2010)

## 9.1 The Bandana Project Beginnings

While I was in middle school, I noticed that my mom was spending more and more evenings out on our front porch. She was usually talking to my uncle on the phone. The calls when he was sober typically went better than others. Part of a boisterous, tight-knit, Irish Catholic family, my uncle was always quick to crack a clever joke – sometimes at your expense – but always with a loving twinkle in his eye. Though always funny to be around, I knew he was sad a lot of the time; I failed to fully grasp what his experience of depression and addiction was really like. Typically a "sharer" with my friends, I chose not to express my thoughts about what was going on with friends. No one else was talking about similar struggles in their family lives. If I were to bring it up, I intuitively knew that those I loved would be unfairly judged.

At the start of my freshman year of high school, my uncle took his own life. Our entire extended family was devastated. In telling friends what had happened, I started to hear that other people had family members who had died by suicide, or that so-and-so was on medication for their anxiety, and so on. My scope of how many people were affected in some way by mental illness broadened. After accompanying my family to a slew of suicide prevention and mental health awareness walks throughout high school, it became clear that nobody lives a life unaffected by mental illness and/or suicide in some way.

The social stigma associated with mental illness, or really anything outside of "normal" on the spectrum of neurodiversity, I realized, was pervasive and poisonous. The hushed tones and judgment dished out when talking about it seemed to prevent so many people from feeling heard, seeking help, or accessing acceptable help. I started talking openly with my friends about these frustrations and learned the value of solidarity and support from sharing these experiences. In doing so, I learned that a surprising number of my friends saw therapists for a variety of mental health experiences, including one of my close friends, who I will call Kayla.

Just before my senior year of high school, Kayla's boyfriend called me with the news that she had ended her life earlier that day. When the school year began, the school administration's public response to her passing left many students confused and distraught and did not offer adequate support or transparency to facilitate healing. Throughout the year, our friend group met with administrators to work towards policies that would make mental health a priority in the district and to make resources for those struggling more accessible and appropriate. After the year passed and not much changed, I grew angry. I was angry that another person in my life was gone to suicide, and I was angry at how isolated those with mental illness are made to feel.

I went to college avidly searching for community and for outlets to dismantle the stigma surrounding mental illness, understand the brain better, and help normalize how common being anything other than "well" is. After committing my studies to neurobiology, I happened to walk by a student organization with the tagline, "Stop the stigma against mental illness!" – the National Alliance on Mental Illness, University of Wisconsin–Madison chapter. During my freshman year, I learned of a friend's professor whose son had died by suicide. In support of that professor, students wore white bandanas (Dan's BP, UW-River Falls). This simple display of solidarity sparked the beginning of my decision to found the BP, which broadened the scope of this idea. Students would tie a lime-green bandana to their backpack, a color known to be associated with mental health awareness. Given a campus imperative to lessen intimidating social barriers to accessing resources, those lime-green-clad students could also serve as peer supports for anyone who may be in or near a crisis.

## 9.2 The Bandana Project Today

The BP began as a college campus-wide mental health awareness and suicide prevention program. To be involved, students and staff members tie a lime-green bandana to their backpack, bag, purse, and so on, which signifies to others that they carry resource cards. These resource cards provide compiled campus-specific, local, and national mental health/suicide prevention information, and brief prompts to help make conversations about mental health easier to start. They were created in coordination with University Health Services and various other campus stakeholders engaged in student wellness. Not only do participants agree to be a vehicle for these resources, but they also take a pledge that details their commitment to be a nonjudgmental source of support for and have open, honest, and affirming conversations about mental health with their peers, friends, and family. All members also access a brief (four-minute long) video explaining the premise of the project, what it takes to be involved, and why the program is important. The BP members are asked to display stigma-free solidarity; initiating a peer-to-peer connection may be less intimidating or stigmatizing than going to institutional resources available on campus.

Just over six years later, the initiative has been implemented at over fifty campuses, with membership at each ranging from 50 to 5,000 students/staff (usually dependent on the overall size of the campus). Each chapter of this program is led by a handful of dedicated student leaders, all of whom have a vested interest in mental health promotion, peer support, and suicide prevention on campus. The program is received enthusiastically and embraced quickly by students, staff, and members of the campus' mental health systems, even while individual campuses have widely varied mental health provisions.

With this momentum, the BP became a formal organization, offering additional programming elements, novel services, and resources to its members, and deepening its impacts in reducing stigma and equipping members to be more supportive. Today, the BP helps groups (from college campuses, community groups, high schools, senior living communities, businesses, and even medical settings) adapt the basic components of this initiative to their context and expand from there. With customizable templates to help with every step of establishing a chapter, a group can launch the program in their area within the span of a month. Typically, this implementation process involves compiling any mental health resources in an area which are responsive to the needs of the population being served, gathering all relevant stakeholders to build a sustainable structure around the program, and creating deeper opportunities for collaboration and alignment among mental health systems. Educational modules and various resource collections have been developed and are offered through the program to college students and staff members of the BP; some components are targeted specifically toward BP chapter leadership to assist with their advocacy efforts. These modules consist of a brief video or series of videos (all under 15 minutes long), a suite of accompanying educational tools, infographics, and resources for anyone nearing or experiencing a mental health crisis.

## 9.3 Mental Health, Mental Illness, Suicide, and Mental Health Services on College Campuses

College-aged individuals in the United States (typically 18–24 years old) are at significantly disproportionate risk of mental illness and suicide (Pedrelli et al., 2015). This may be due to a variety of reasons. It is a time often marked by novel stressors, significant life changes/transitions, and complex or lacking social relationships and settings. Mental health concerns are more likely to arise or be exacerbated during this developmental period; roughly three-quarters of mental illnesses begin by age 24 and influence educational attainment, employment, relationships, and mortality, all of which have their own health effects (Eisenberg et al., 2012). In fact, just under two-thirds of college students report symptoms of at least one mental health concern; a disproportionate amount of these students are indigenous, and students of color receive mental health treatment at lower rates (Lipson et al., 2022). This increased risk of distress is also not benign. A recent study found that over 12% of undergraduate students experienced suicidal ideation, and just under 6% seriously considered suicide over the course of an academic year (Oh et al., 2021). Worse, over 1,100 students die by suicide annually (Applebaum, 2006).

Statistics aside, in meetings with the BP team, students, staff, and mental health providers on campuses often express that the frequency and intensity of mental health concerns and stressors seem to be – at the very least anecdotally – increasing year-to- year. Universities attempt to meet this dire public and mental health problem with professional counseling, crisis services, and other supports. Even so, these services are strapped for personnel and funding and are offered inconsistently based on the type, size, and location of the school. For example, the JED Foundation reports that under two-thirds of colleges can offer their students psychiatric services (JED Foundation, 2016).

The discrepancy between mental health service availability and student need is indeed concerning, especially when considering scant access to, acceptability, and use of these services. Most students do not receive professional mental health treatment during their time at college, and treatment options themselves are highly variable between institutions (Lipson et al., 2015). There are many explanations for this trend aside from a lack of availability, and the following are some of the most frequently studied: self and perceived public stigma about mental illness or getting help, poor expectations of quality of care (Zivin et al., 2009), lack of knowledge of or orientation to available resources (Drum & Denmark, 2012), belief that one's social network is enough support, and different (and in some cases, culturally influenced) attitudes about getting help for mental health (Eisenberg et al., 2007). It turns out that approximately 80% of students who need help with their mental health will not access professional services but will first talk about mental illness and suicide with peers or faculty (Eisenberg et al., 2012). Understanding how and why someone may first seek informal, or nonprofessional, support is key to the BP programming; growing literature supporting various frameworks around help-seeking behavior informs updates to BP educational content regarding peer support (Magaard et al., 2017).

The BP first seeks to destigmatize help-seeking behavior, helping to make the idea of accessing any mental health resource less daunting. It goes on to influence social norms surrounding mental health, illness, and suicide, facilitating conversations about what's going on "upstairs." The project provides students and staff a unique opportunity to support the mental health of their peers and contribute to suicide prevention efforts on campuses, bolstering what is available through formal campus structures. This is particularly the case when institutional, professional resources may not have the capacity or reach to meet people where they are struggling or offer sufficient ongoing support for student mental health needs. The BP's members can provide tangibly helpful information, tools, and strategies to peers, effectively preventing and navigating mental health crisis situations.

## 9.4 Supporting Evidence, Theories, and Frameworks

The college student demographic group provides a promising target for intervention. There are over 18.4 million students on college campuses in the United States. It is easier to access students through their institutions in comparison with the general population of the same age, and, as mentioned previously, most symptoms of mental illness will emerge during the college years (Census Bureau, 2019). The large proportion of college students that will struggle with their mental health creates a notable public health burden, highlighting the need for prevention, intervention, and postvention when it comes to mental illness and suicide. While students will mostly likely go to their peers and faculty with mental health concerns and decisions, a 2016 study found that over half of all students and staff do not feel equipped to do any of the following: recognize when someone is nearing a mental health crisis, approach the person about their concerns, or refer someone to mental health resources (Albright & Schwartz, 2016). In light of the previous discussion, a clear need exists for widespread implementation of subclinical or nonprofessional, social network-based mental health promotion and suicide prevention efforts on college campuses.

As such, the BP its chapters, and the programming offered through these means approach suicide prevention, mental health promotion and literacy/education within the universal, selective, and indicated (USI) prevention framework (Goldsmith et al., 2002). The educational modules operate within this broader framework because they may be applied to a variety of different school contexts; the barriers to getting help for, and the actual incidence of, mental illnesses also vary significantly by individual characteristics of different schools (Ketchen Lipson et al., 2015). The programming elements comprise a component of a universal prevention in that they are available to all members of a campus that has a BP chapter, and they broadly promote student mental health and related information. They also facilitate easier access to campus and national resources by educating students about what is available and where. The BP's content encourages the creation of destigmatizing infrastructure and messaging to prevent, inform, and respond to mental health concerns and crises. Highlighting existing resources in the BP educational modules and on the BP website can also drive campuses to improve the quality and number of resources offered to students.

The modules are selective in that the targeted audience has already shown particular interest and investment in supporting the mental health of their peers and learning more about what that looks like, given their involvement in the BP. The wider student body at participating campuses also maintains access to the material, increasing the chances that someone not already tuned into this movement may do so.

Lastly, the educational modules of the BP address indicated populations through their salient presentation of situations and crisis resources specific to college students who may be struggling. For those in positions with more direct opportunity to support, tangible gatekeeper intervention education and tools are taught to them so they may intervene with students who may be having thoughts of, a desire, or plans to die by suicide. This education also includes providing material and training specific to each of the most common barriers to seeking professional help listed earlier.

Literature and frameworks contributing to the BP's approach to destigmatization of mental illness and suicide, peer support, and mental health promotion/suicide prevention have grounded the information and language present in the existing BP educational modules. The different types of stigma associated with mental illness and suicide and interventions to reduce them have been increasingly studied over the last two decades. Fox et al. (2018) have proffered the mental illness stigma framework (MISF) as a way for researchers and interventionists to describe and classify how these stigmas affect those with mental illness. This work builds on foundational stigma literature (see Corrigan & Watson, 2002; Hatzenbuehler et al., 2013; Link & Phelan, 2001) and offers ways of framing language to address different dimensions of stigma in the modules. For example, the welcome video module describes the differences between self- versus perceived public stigma, specifically as applied to college students' likelihood of accessing mental health care. This informational content, in combination with portraying what it can be like to have a mental illness or to be suicidal, has been shown to reduce associated stigmas (Morgan et al., 2018). Statements like, "recovery from mental illness is possible and happens in big and small ways every day," are also frequently included as affirmative and validating sentiments that reduce stereotyping and prejudice against those with mental illness (Corrigan & Bink, 2016).

Pescosolido et al.'s (2008) framework integrating normative influence on stigma (FINIS) is also helpful for a synthesis of a wealth of literature conceptualizing which and to what degree various social factors influence the stigma associated with mental illness and, relatedly, help-seeking attitudes and behaviors. An example of how this framework influences stigma at the macro-level is ensuring that the emotional tone of the BP's messaging is positive, warm, and relatable. This is especially important when demonstrating the lived experience of those with chronic or ongoing mental illness, as well as those with experiences of crisis and engagement with resources. Additional BP content offers suggestions for bettering infrastructure and standardizing policies around mental health, which can instill considerable and lasting changes in social norms regarding mental illness and suicide. All the educational modules emphasize and reiterate a sense of BP community and shared responsibility to talk openly about mental health and to intervene in mental health crises, a social network intervention at the meso-level. Members and their social networks may then be more likely to disclose mental health concerns, help-seeking, and provide support.

The connectedness framework of suicide prevention in college settings integrates foundational theories, concepts, and literature related to interpersonal and social factors that may put someone at increased risk of suicide (Whitlock et al., 2013). This framework posits that someone's perceived sense of connection to their campus community, as well as that community's sense of shared well-being and responsibility for those struggling with mental health, is driving factor that can be protective (or lead to higher suicide risk if lacking or absent). A person's perceptions of the quality of their social connections can influence their ability to buffer stressors that would be a detriment to their mental health, attitudes toward and likelihood of getting help, and knowledge of resources available (Chronister et al., 2015; Cohen, 2004).

Generally, the BP and its members serve to make social support much more salient and visible by mass visualization of green bandanas on backpacks and, thus, improve peers' perceptions of the amount of social support available to them. The connectedness framework and related area of literature were further incorporated into each of the educational modules in varying ways, dependent on their focus.

Before the creation of the BP educational modules, no formal or uniform orientation/training was offered to members of the BP. This led to inconsistent representations of what the initiative was, varied expectations of members' role in being involved, and a lack of a sense of cohesive community among members and between BP chapters. First and foremost, the Welcome Video module filled this gap in the BP's programming and solidified the initiative as a multicampus, grassroots movement. Though this module has the shortest video (~4 minutes) and the smallest amount of additional content, user testing with faculty and students indicates an appreciation and use of the informational, easy-to-understand, and positively framed content for daily application.

The BP is first a simple awareness movement, and relatively minimal expectations exist for those involved. The lower level of commitment and investment to participate makes it more likely for students and staff to join the initiative. However, the inclusion of the BP pledge, a commitment of all incoming members, makes participants more likely to engage with both additional related content and the broader goals and programming of the initiative overall (Hill & Thompson-Hayes, 2017). As such, the BP is an engaging means to mobilize preliminarily engaged students in peer support efforts, giving them basic understandings of mental illness, suicide, and knowledge about how to get help that may prepare them to be a resource. There is also content presented in the modules which normalizes having a mental health concern or illness, in the form of a summary of recent findings from the national Healthy Minds Study detailing how many students deal with mental health concerns, illness, and suicidal thoughts, ideation, and intent while in college (Eisenberg et al., 2020). Some of this information might be difficult for some students to reflect on and/or may stir up emotions related to mental illness or crises. All the videos are preceded by a content warning, and they all link directly to a wide array of resources on the BP website (Bentley, 2017). These content warnings and resource compilations also increase knowledge of supports available, and their robust descriptions reduce intimidation related to not knowing what a particular support may be like for someone to access.

Sometimes used as a nebulous, ill-defined concept in similar programs, stigma is clearly defined (as requested by participants). Self and public stigma are clarified, which nuances definitions of stigma present in similar mental health promotion programs. The different types of stigma are presented along with a compelling visual display of how the vast majority of college students would not judge someone for getting help for their mental health, a refute of commonly held perceived public stigma. In another effort to reduce the barrier of stigma related to help-seeking in the module, supportive and affirmative phrases like "let's find help together," "you are not alone," and "you matter" are presented by graphics representing BP members (Corrigan & Bink, 2016). This graphic also incorporates the connectedness framework, implicating that a community-wide imperative to support the mental health of peers in help-seeking can indeed work to prevent suicide.

## 9.5 The Bandana Project Educational Opportunities

The following resources were particularly informative for guiding the creation of the BP educational modules: the CDC's "Technical Package of Politics, Policies, and Programs for Suicide Prevention" (Stone et al., 2017), the Suicide Prevention Resource Center's "Guide for Effective Suicide Prevention" (SPRC, 2020), and the JED Foundation's "Campus Mental Health Action

Planning" document (JED Foundation, 2011). These recommendations contributed a host of evidence-based suggestions for the module's mental health promotion and suicide prevention educational content, messaging, and accompanying educational tools. These resources, along with a review of relevant literature, existing programming, and media, were central to orient the modules according to well-researched principles of peer support and gatekeeper suicide prevention programming (definition to follow). Though informational and educational, the BP educational modules are not described or offered as formal training or certification in gatekeeper suicide prevention. Again, while the basic premise of the BP intentionally does not demand a large amount of commitment, the educational opportunity was developed for members who can and want to do more.

Mental health initiatives that employ peers to support other peers' mental health are an effective way to improve the social integration of those with mental illness and to support their recovery (Davidson et al., 1999; Repper & Carter, 2011). Peer-to-peer interventions also improve mental health outcomes and reduce incidence of mental health crises (Tsong et al., 2019). Further, peers are typically more likely to disclose more sensitive information to peers over mental health professionals (assuming many view mental health concerns to be sensitive in nature), partially because of a shared experience and perspective with the peer.

Specifically for the college campus setting, there is increasing recognition that peer support programs to prevent suicide must be implemented at the scale that other health-related programs have been. Even today, tremendous, relatively un-tested capacity exists for such programs to prevent suicides (Catanzarite & Robinson, 2013). The BP leaders, members, and associated faculty have expressed that an unmet need occurs in this area as well. Peer-led suicide prevention and mental health promotion efforts, what the BP educational modules at hand help facilitate, have demonstrated efficacy in improving knowledge about suicide, perceived capability of handling a crisis, and the chances that someone will actually intervene (Byrom, 2018; Samuolis et al., 2020). Mental health-oriented peer support programs can also work to reduce stigmas associated with mental health challenges and with getting help (Mental Health Association of San Francisco, 2020).

Further, the existing BP educational modules – and opportunity to develop more – could do much to introduce many students to and increase the likelihood that they will access more in-depth trainings in suicide prevention and mental health promotion, education, and awareness programs. Given the brevity of these modules, it is recommended that within the module students access other programs like Question, Persuade, Refer (QPR Institute, 2022), and/or Mental Health First Aid (MHFA, 2022). Increasing mental health literacy can be a promising precursor to increasing help-seeking and mental health intervention (Kelly et al., 2007). Even with the BP education modules' brevity, shorter term gatekeeper-style trainings have been shown to be effective in increasing interpersonal suicide prevention skills (Cross et al., 2010).

Many of the programs like MHFA and QPR rely on the gatekeeper prevention model, mentioned earlier (Hawgood et al., 2022). This is the prevailing model of suicide prevention efforts on campuses (and in many other contexts), which has been supported by a growing body of research in the United States and internationally (Isaac et al., 2009). A gatekeeper suicide prevention model refers to the idea that nonprofessionals, in this case BP members on campuses, have a role in responding to and intervening in a mental health crisis. These gatekeepers, including students, staff, and faculty in the campus setting, are often better positioned to intervene due to the higher likelihood of informal disclosure of mental health concerns or crises to nonprofessionals first (Mitchell et al., 2013). Common elements of all gatekeeper training, including the information in the modules, are recognizing when someone might be in distress, providing education about how to respond to what is recognized, and discussing referral to professional resources afterward.

The educational modules highlight risk factors and warning signs of suicide in everyday situations and conversations (American Foundation for Suicide Prevention, 2020). Presenting risk factors and warning signs have been shown to increase knowledge and recognition of suicidal crises, but not increase stigmatization of those near/in crisis (Van Orden et al., 2006). The modules cover how to respond to these warning signs and risk factors, including the following steps: acknowledging what a BP member has noticed that concerns them about the other person, listening actively, offering statements of encouragement and support, clarifying if vaguely concerning statements are said by who is struggling, and then directly asking about suicide if it is thought that the person is considering ending their life (Quinnett, 2012; Spencer-Thomas, 2019).

The modules go on to discuss what crisis resources are available through the BP website, but also they provide general information about the different types of professional resources that are typically available for additional help on a given campus. The modules also suggest that the BP member accompanies the person struggling to the helping resource or attempts to ensure that they indeed access professional help. Different ideas are offered for what any BP member may do to show continued support, interest, and investment in the other person's mental health state and how to go about getting professional help.

Despite it being the most widely used model for suicide risk recognition and intervention, evidence in support of gatekeeper training and education is relatively limited. However, encouraging evidence has been collected to varying degrees in certain contexts (Isaac et al., 2009). Indelicato et al. (2011) found that implementing gatekeeper prevention training in a university setting increased participants' likelihood and capability (both perceived and actual) of intervening in a crisis. This work is supported by another campus-based study that found shorter and longer term increases in knowledge about suicide and related resources, conversations, and intervention practices following the introduction of QPR suicide prevention training (Mitchell et al., 2013). Similarly, a US Air Force–conducted, multifaceted suicide prevention effort that focused on stigma reduction and peer support (drawing on many of the same bodies of literature and programming referenced earlier) showed a decline in risk and incidence of suicide (Knox et al., 2003). Clearly, gatekeeper prevention is a feasible model to more widely proliferate mental health crises intervention practices and information into peer support contexts.

To bolster these effects, it is well known that catering to clearly defined groups/audiences can improve suicide prevention knowledge and comfort in relevant situations following brief training (Cimini et al., 2014). This module's gatekeeper prevention content is specific to members of the BP; for example, a BP member-to-peer intervention is modeled via text conversation. The viewer is encouraged to review and select responses based on a bank of response options, which increases the interactivity of the module and promotes learning of the content (Tannenbaum, 2000). In the video, this interaction is also modeled via text messages to increase applicability to the modern viewer's day-to-day life, as well as their (perceived and actual) capability of being a mental health resource for peers (Cross et al., 2011). The interaction is also modeling a prevention scenario, wherein peers arrive at a positive outcome, successfully intervening and getting professional help; incorporating this information has been shown to increase both perceptions of support available and perceptions about the likelihood of an intervention succeeding (Petrova, 2015). There are a multitude of potential avenues for tailoring informational and training content specifically to the various audiences the BP reaches, as described earlier.

Inclusion of this type of text message-based interaction is unique among existing programming, as well as a few other components of BP programming. Though risk factors and warning signs are frequently presented in similar programs, many of these programs do not typically include a theory or theories to explain what might drive someone to die by suicide. Feedback from BP members has indicated that they are interested in at least a brief explanation of this "why" question. Because of this interest, a commonly held theory of why someone may die by suicide is presented to take away some of the mystery around a suicidal individual's mental state and to explain it in an easily digestible way. This information also presents the opportunity to identify where BP members may more directly work against the drivers presented, sometimes even just by having their bandana on their backpack. It is further suggested that overt statements of support should be expressed to make it clear to the person in crisis that they are not a burden and are cared for in their community. Other gatekeeper intervention trainings only fleetingly address lethal means reduction and restriction (if at all); when it has been addressed, it has been shown to be effective in increasing confidence in suicide interventions and means reduction skills (Rosen et al., 2020).

Overall, the BP programming is further distinct in its commitment to the de-stigmatization of mental illness, suicide, and getting help. A goal of the organization is to reduce stigma associated with and to describe how normal it is to experience suicidal ideation, intent, or planning, by increasing knowledge of and empathy toward a suicidal individual's possible mental state. There are portions of the program dedicated to destigmatizing language around suicide, reducing implications of judgment, and being more supportive with word choice (Sommer-Rotenberg, 1998). Statistics that normalize having mental health concerns and the potential of handling mental health crises in oneself and others while in college are also threaded through the BP's content. Along with these statistics, the most common barriers to intervening are portrayed as natural initial reactions to these types of difficult, emotionally charged situations. However, this potential discomfort is then couched in an examination of stigma and is reframed to encourage BP members to both recognize how stigma is at play in these situations, which can be helpful for moving past it (Monteith et al., 2020). Members are encouraged to use the actual word "suicide" when asking directly if someone is considering killing themselves. Through various forms, common misconceptions and myths about suicide are presented and then discounted, explaining with sound evidence what the reality of the situation may be.

In addition to approaching suicide prevention interventions with a stigma reduction lens, the BP serves a younger population, namely, college students. The educational modules are distinct in their timeliness/relevance of commonly experienced situations and related resources offered. They walk through the pros and cons of a texting conversation about a mental health crisis; being in person for these conversations is preferred (there is a higher likelihood of the person in crisis responding, and the bystander may be able to more tangibly intervene). However, many of these conversations do happen over text message, and preliminary feedback from the various advisory teams (see later in this chapter) suggests that inclusion of an example of this form of communication is preferred. Feedback also suggested the inclusion of a play-by-play of what to expect when 9-1-1 is called with a mental health emergency, given that this is not typically included in suicide prevention trainings (NAMI, 2018). NAMI's "Navigating a Mental Health Crisis" guide is one of the additional resources that is part of a module, in addition to a crisis safety plan template inspired by Brown and Stanley's worksheet (2008).

The educational modules and additional resources brevity is both an asset and a detriment; existing suicide prevention trainings are usually longer (at least 45 minutes, and sometimes over multiple days). Though certainly worthwhile to take these trainings when time and budget allow, key gatekeeper suicide prevention knowledge and skills should still be available in brief and affordable formats. This provides more widespread access to vital, lifesaving information for many college students. Further, other trainings usually only address situations that have already progressed to a crisis and do not typically assert that crisis and general mental health resources can be accessed prior to any emergency intervention. Again, the BP programming is best offered as a compliment to other such trainings, so that the widest range of peer support and prevention training options are available to interested BP members.

A common challenge with *all* gatekeeper prevention strategies is that their effectiveness wanes over time, typically even after just 3–6 months (Shtivelband et al., 2015). To this end, Shtivelband et al. (2015) found several strategies that may prolong training effects, including having gatekeepers do the following: (a) connect with their peers to normalize intervention knowledge, behavior, and confidence; (b) learn more about mental illness, suicidality, and prevention efforts; (c) collaborate with one another to raise awareness. Training that is accessible and convenient is more likely to stick, and providing reminders about the content through ongoing communication keeps gatekeepers engaged in this effort. Offering opportunities to update and bolster programming with additional information also prolongs training effects, as well as accounting for accountability and accreditation after completing a training. The larger BP programming accomplishes most, if not all, of these components, and the accompanying educational tools offered alongside the video aid in continued learning. Access is provided 24/7 through the BP website, and the module can be revisited whenever a refresher is needed (which is also encouraged by the organization regularly). All the BP's content is also intended to be accessible/disability compliant (Web Accessibility Initiative, 2020).

## 9.6 Meeting the Moment: The Bandana Project and the Diversity of Students on Campus

Part of the BP's content is intended to give members – but particularly chapter leaders – ideas, templates, and resources for creating more equitable, positive, lasting change in campus-based mental health promotion and suicide prevention efforts. This information is targeted specifically toward BP members, who have identified themselves as student leaders in peer-based support; their collective capacity for group suicide prevention efforts can be leveraged for tangibly impactful change in health equity and social justice for this population. The creation of this type of content was specifically requested by end users and was primarily guided by personal and other BP members' experiences in implementing change on college campuses in this sphere.

Prior to joining the BP, many members already have an active willingness to perform such advocacy activities, but perhaps lack the structure and/or community to feel empowered doing so. Student and staff efforts to improve mental health systems on campuses are most effective when they comprehensively address factors at multiple levels of the socioecological model (SEM, including the societal, community/institutional, relationship, and individual levels; CDC, 2021), which is used to organize the content within parts of the educational modules (Caine, 2013). To this end, the BP suggests the involvement of diverse sets of stakeholders in prevention efforts, creating changes in norms regarding mental health help-seeking, and working to instill a campus culture and community of mutual support and inclusion (Caine et al., 2018; Whitlock et al., 2013).

Progressing through each level of an adapted version of the SEM, the module suggests activities/actions that BP leaders and members can take to improve, bolster, or start various aspects of suicide prevention and mental health promotion on their campus. Though available through sources like the Suicide Prevention Resource Center (SPRC, 2020), this type of vital suicide prevention and mental health promotion content is not included in any other programs or training of this type. The educational modules reference recommendations and insights from the JED Foundation's Campus Mental Health Action Planning guide (JED Foundation, 2011), a highly useful resource. An example of how these resources were incorporated is a suggestion to implement mental health training for all students and faculty on campus, usually recognized as a much-needed effort on any given campus.

Student life today looks very different than what many readers may remember. This is especially the case after the COVID-19 pandemic transformed what campus structures can be and how those attending any form of higher education experience this time period. The BP advocates that its chapters work to make sure that students' basic needs and supports like stable access to housing, food, safety, financial security, and other highly important social determinants of mental health are met (Compton & Shim, 2015). Many campuses do not meet these most basic necessities for all of its students (Romo, 2018). The BP members should thus be attuned to the resources available for the wide array of people and mental health experiences on their campus. Further, certain populations of students face these struggles more frequently than others due to historical and ongoing oppressive structures in academia that disproportionately affect Black and Brown, queer, trans, nonbinary students, and those of lower socioeconomic status. For these groups, the burden of both mental illness, suicidal ideation, and suicide is consistently elevated, as well as their likelihood of dropping out of college (which is also often associated with negative mental and other health outcomes) (Assari, 2018; Seale & Givens, 2019). A progressive organization working to make mental health systems more just and equitable is Project LETS, a powerful peer-run advocacy group (Project LETS, 2022). As part of their mission statement, they note that it is the responsibility of all mental health organizations to be anti-racist, inclusive, repair past harms in this area, and prevent future harms from disproportionately affecting oppressed groups.

Another suggested way for BP members to support students' mental health and prevent suicide comes in the form of analyzing and implementing more comprehensive means reduction practices, policies, and precautions on their campus. This is also a component of the SPRC's "Comprehensive Approach to Suicide Prevention" that is sometimes overlooked in campus-based prevention programming (SPRC, 2020). Specifically, campuses are encouraged to assess how physical structures may be altered to reduce their capacity to be a means to die by suicide (i.e., examining if bridges and buildings have tall barriers and/or nets). Members are also given advice to ensure that any mental health trainings offered on campuses address means restriction specifically. It is also suggested that viewers analyze campus norms, behaviors, and activities that contribute to higher suicide risk (i.e., norms around drinking habits and other risk-taking behaviors, activities, and attitudes).

This SPRC proposal is followed by a recommendation that campuses either introduce or more outwardly communicate messaging about amnesty policies. An amnesty policy is a provision that, if students were to be engaging in underage drinking or related behavior, the student(s) will not face punitive measures in mental health crisis situations if emergency services are accessed. Not only does this policy create a culture of trust and communal responsibility for the well-being of others, but it also provides a way for professional mental health services to still be accessed when necessary rather than not being accessed due to a fear of punishment (Carpenter, 2016).

The implementation of a norm-changing, destigmatizing, and positive mental health promotion/suicide prevention messaging campaign on campuses is particularly supported by the Connectedness Framework put forth by Whitlock et al. (2013). This type of campaign can run the gamut from postering, tabling, and advertising efforts to speaking in front of student organizations and academic departments, among others, to help reduce stigmas associated with mental illness, help-seeking, and suicide (Silk et al., 2017). Anecdotally, positive and accurate messages that emphasize empowerment, agency, and emotional strength in seeking help can do wonders to make students feel more comfortable doing so. This expanded help-seeking has been seen in a variety of campus contexts; improvements in campus mental health climates via widespread efforts to be more supportive of mental health can help students take that leap to services, if they are needed (Stein et al., 2016). This effort and messaging campaign should seek to spread the BP and a given campus' mental health and suicide prevention resource cards to every physical and virtual space on campus. Including as many student organizations and other groups on campus as possible in outreach efforts (e.g., Greek life, athletics, student government, academic concentrations, academic departments, and faculty groups) will help increase awareness of the BP and resources available to a diverse population. It will also help establish the initiative at a given university and improve the program's visibility beyond the visual cue of the lime-green bandanas already plentiful on backpacks.

Case examples of mental health advocacy that has been accomplished by BP chapters include a three-pronged proposal for improvement of mental health service provision: increased funding to mental health services, more comprehensive, culturally sensitive, and suicide prevention-oriented health screening practices, and more transparent reporting of mental health-related data collected on campus. Another BP recommendation is the creation of an official suicide prevention coordinator staff position and a task force or council to drive sustainable efforts in the area. A longer term transition from police as responders to trained mental health crisis intervention personnel to address mental health crises situations is also advised in the module. In advance of a full transition to mental health crisis responders, the BP module suggests greater collaboration be facilitated between mental health professionals and police or a more rigorous training of police/campus safety in crisis intervention in the meanwhile. Generally speaking, the BP thrives on a campus where its leadership and membership collaborate with many groups around campus.

## 9.7 Tips for Starting This Movement

For any campus interested in starting a chapter of the BP, it is recommended that they first reach out to the BP website and request our comprehensive start-up guide. This guide will walk groups through first steps and give tips and ideas for practical development and adaptation. First, it is particularly important to identify a passionate group of students interested in creating a campus peer support community. From there, figuring out what local resources they see as needed, or what to highlight of what already exists, is a great place to start planning. After this, bringing all relevant campus and community partners to the table makes sure the movement is well ingrained, supported, and aligned across campus. This final step ultimately helps create a sustainable structure around the program, identify gaps, and make strategic goals and plans,. Staff members of the BP are available for consultation before and after these initial steps.

## 9.8 Evaluating the Impact

To date, no formal public health evaluation has been performed for the BP and ongoing evaluation is a goal of the organization moving forward. Any evaluation process for the BP should be user-centered, participatory, and multifaceted, involving both participants in the program and those leading it. This inclusive process will help ensure the acceptability, accessibility, and quality of the programming (World Health Organization, 2016). The BP's current proposed evaluation framework and toolkit were created by Stephanie Vazquez, MPH (Vazquez, 2021). The outcomes measured by this evaluation include reducing self- and public stigma related to mental illness and suicide, increasing help-seeking attitudes and behaviors, and increasing the likelihood and self-perceived capability of BP members to distribute resources and to intervene in mental health crises. After distributing prepopulated surveys for participating campuses, chapters would submit synthesized results to the BP yearly.

## 9.9 Continuing the Momentum

The BP is a program whose mission is to reduce the perceived and actual stigmas associated with having a mental illness, a (suicidal) crisis, or getting help for either, as well as to increase education about, awareness of, and ability to use basic prevention skills and resources relevant to common peer-to-peer situations. The members are involved in a mental health awareness program that proliferates crisis and noncrisis mental health supports and are thus uniquely well positioned to act as inspiring agents of change and pillars of support if given the context, information, and access to tools to do so. A recent effort to have this initiative become part of a different organization called SAVE (Suicide Awareness Voices of Education, 2022) will help push this movement past awareness and flesh out the resources it can offer individual chapters.

No one lives a life unaffected by mental health concerns, illness, and suicide, which is an unfortunate reality made worse by the intense stigmas that surround this universal experience. One bandana at a time, the BP loosens this stigma's grip on campus mental health climates. While this positive change starts with bandanas on backpacks, the further directions for the BP provide the opportunity for this change to go much farther, sweeping through college campuses and beyond. Through an impossible-to-miss, lime-green symbol, the

BP shows communities that it is okay to struggle with mental health. It is a simple beacon to open a conversation about mental illness and suicide, personal strength, agency, resilience, and self-love.

## References


Albright, G., & Schwartz, V. (2016). *Are campuses ready to support students in distress?* http://go.kognito.com/rs/143-HCJ-270/images/HiEd_WP_080817_HigherEdSurveyWhitePaper.pdf

American Foundation for Suicide Prevention. (2020, January 24). *Risk factors and warning signs of suicide.* https://afsp.org/risk-factors-and-warning-signs

Applebaum P. S. (2006). Law & psychiatry: "depressed? Get out!": Dealing with suicidal students on college campuses. *Psychiatric Services 57*(7), 914–916. doi.org/10.1176/ps.2006.57.7.914

Assari S. (2018). Multiplicative effects of social and psychological risk factors on college students' suicidal behaviors. *Brain Sciences, 8*(5), 91. doi.org/10.3390/brainsci8050091

Bentley, M. (2017). Trigger warnings and the student experience. *Politics, 37*(4), 470–485. doi.org/10.1177/0263395716684526

Brown, G., & Stanley, B. (2008). *Patient safety plan template.* http://suicidesafetyplan.com/Home_Page.html

Byrom, N. (2018). An evaluation of a peer support intervention for student mental health. *Journal of Mental Health, 27*(3), 240–246. doi.org/10.1080/09638237.2018.1437604

Caine E. D. (2013). Forging an agenda for suicide prevention in the United States. *American Journal of Public Health, 103*(5), 822–829. doi.org/10.2105/AJPH.2012.301078

Caine, E. D., Reed, J., Hindman, J., & Quinlan, K. (2018). Comprehensive, integrated approaches to suicide prevention: Practical guidance. *Injury Prevention, 24*(Suppl 1), i38–i45. doi.10.1136/injuryprev-2017-042366

Carpenter, T. (2016). Advocating for a comprehensive and mandatory medical amnesty/Good Samaritan Policy on the University of Tennessee, Knoxville Campus. *Baker Scholar Projects, 6.* https://trace.tennessee.edu/utk_bakerschol/38

Catanzarite, J. A., & Robinson, M. D. (2013). Peer education in campus suicide prevention. *New Directions for Student Services, 2013*(141), 43–53. doi.org/10.1002/ss.20039

CDC. (2021, January 28). *The social-ecological model: A framework for PREVENTION |violence Prevention|Injury Center|CDC.* www.cdc.gov/violenceprevention/about/social-ecologicalmodel.html

Chronister, J., Chou, C. C., Kwan, K. L., Lawton, M., & Silver, K. (2015). The meaning of social support for persons with serious mental illness. *Rehabilitation Psychology, 60*(3), 232–245. doi.org/10.1037/rep0000038

Cimini, M. D., Rivero, E., Bernier, J., Stanley, J., Murray, A., Anderson, D., Wright, H., & Bapat, M. (2014). Implementing an audience-specific small-group gatekeeper training program to respond to suicide risk among college students: A case study. *Journal of American College Health, 62*, 92–100. doi.org/10.1080/07448481.2013.849709

Close, G. (2010, March 18). Mental illness: The stigma of silence. *Huffington Post.* www.huffpost.com/entry/mental-illness-the-stigma_b_328591

Cohen, S. (2004). Social relationships and health. *The American Psychologist, 59* (8), 676–684. doi.org/10.1037/0003-066X.59.8.676

Compton, M., & Shim, R. (2015). The social determinants of mental health. *FOCUS, 13*(4), 419–425. doi.org/10.1176/appi.focus.20150017

Corrigan, P., & Bink, A. (2016). The stigma of mental illness. *Encyclopedia of Mental Health.* doi.org/10.1016/B978-0-12-397045-9.00170-1

Corrigan, P., & Watson, A. (2002). Understanding the impact of stigma on people with mental illness. *World Psychiatry: Official Journal of the World Psychiatric Association (WPA), 1*(1), 16–20.

Cross, W., Matthieu, M. M., Lezine, D., & Knox, K. L. (2010). Does a brief suicide prevention gatekeeper training program enhance observed skills? *Crisis, 31*(3), 149–159. doi.org/10.1027/0227-5910/a000014

Cross, W., Seaburn, D., Gibbs, D., Schmeelk-Cone, K., White, A. M., & Caine, E. D. (2011). Does practice make perfect? A randomized control trial of behavioral rehearsal on suicide prevention gatekeeper skills. *The Journal of Primary Prevention, 32*(3–4), 195–211. doi.org/10.1007/s10935-011-0250-z

Davidson, L., Chinman, M., Kloos, B., Weingarten, R., Stayner, D., & Tebes, J. K. (1999). Peer support among individuals with severe mental illness: A review of the evidence. *Clinical Psychology: Science and Practice, 6*(2), 165–187. doi.org/10.1093/clipsy.6.2.165

Drum, D., & Denmark, A. (2012). Campus suicide prevention: Bridging paradigms and forging partnerships. *Harvard Review of Psychiatry, 20*(4), 209–221. doi.org/10.3109/10673229.2012.712841

Eisenberg, D., Golberstein, E., & Gollust, S. E. (2007). Help-seeking and access to mental health care in a university student population. *Medical Care, 45*(7), 594–601. doi.org/10.1097/MLR.0b013e31803bb4c1

Eisenberg, D, Hunt, J, & Speer, N. (2012). Help seeking for mental health on college campuses: Review of evidence and next steps for research and practice. *Harvard Review of Psychiatry, 20*(4), 222–232.

Eisenberg, D., Ketchen Lipson, S., & Heinz, J. (2020). The health minds study, 2020 report. https://healthymindsnetwork.org/wp-content/uploads/2021/02/HMS-Fall-2020-National-Data-Report.pdf

Fox, A. B., Earnshaw, V. A., Taverna, E. C., & Vogt, D. (2018). Conceptualizing and measuring mental illness stigma: The mental illness stigma framework and critical review of measures. *Stigma and Health, 3*(4), 348–376. doi.org/10.1037/sah0000104

Goldsmith S. K., Pellmar, T. C., Kleinman, A. M., & Bunney, W. E., Institute of Medicine (US) Committee on Pathophysiology and Prevention of Adolescent and Adult Suicide. (2002). Programs for Suicide Prevention. In *Reducing suicide: A national imperative.* National Academies Press. www.ncbi.nlm.nih.gov/books/NBK220931/

Hatzenbuehler, M. L., Phelan, J. C., & Link, B. G. (2013). Stigma as a fundamental cause of population health inequalities. *American Journal of Public Health, 103*(5), 813–821. doi.org/10.2105/AJPH.2012.301069

Hawgood, J., Woodward, A., Quinnett, P., & De Leo, D. (2022). Gatekeeper training and minimum standards of competency. *Crisis, 43*(6), 516–522. doi.org/10.1027/0227-5910/a000794

Hill, M., & Thompson-Hayes, M. (2017). *From awareness to commitment in public health campaigns: The awareness myth.* Lexington.

Indelicato, N., Mirsu-Paun, A., & Griffin, W. (2011). Outcomes of a suicide prevention gatekeeper training on a university campus. *Journal of College Student Development, 52*(3), 350–361. doi.org/10.1353/csd.2011.0036

Isaac, M., Elias, B., Katz, L. Y., Belik, S. L., Deane, F. P., Enns, M. W., Sareen, J., & Swampy Cree Suicide Prevention Team (2009). Gatekeeper training as a preventative intervention for suicide: A systematic review. *Canadian Journal of Psychiatry. Revue Canadienne de Psychiatrie, 54*(4), 260–268. doi.org/10.1177/070674370905400407

JED Foundation. (2011). *Campus mental health action plan.* https://sprc.org/sites/default/files/resource-program/CampusMHAP_Web%20final.pdf

JED Foundation. (2016). *Psychiatric times: The crisis in college and university mental health.* www.jedfoundation.org/psychiatric_times_the_crisis_in_college_and_university_mental_health/

Kelly, C. M., Jorm, A. F., & Wright, A. (2007). Improving mental health literacy as a strategy to facilitate early intervention for mental disorders. *The Medical Journal of Australia, 187*(S7), S26–S30. doi.org/10.5694/j.1326-5377.2007.tb01332.x

Ketchen Lipson, S., Gaddis, S. M., Heinze, J., Beck, K., & Eisenberg, D. (2015). Variations in student mental health and treatment utilization across U.S. colleges and universities. *Journal of American College Health, 63*(6), 388–396. doi.org/10.1080/07448481.2015.1040411

Knox, K. L., Litts, D. A., Talcott, G. W., Feig, J. C., & Caine, E. D. (2003). Risk of suicide and related adverse outcomes after exposure to a suicide prevention programme in the U.S. Air Force: Cohort study. *BMJ (Clinical Research* ed.), *327*(7428), 1376. doi.org/10.1136/bmj.327.7428.1376

Link, B., & Phelan, J. (2001). Conceptualizing stigma. *Annual Review of Sociology, 27*(1), 363–385. doi.org/10.1146/annurev.soc.27.1.363

Lipson, S. K., Zhou, S., Abelson, S., Heinze, J., Jirsa, M., Morigney, J., Patterson, A., Singh, M., & Eisenberg, D. (2022). Trends in college student mental health and help-seeking by race/ethnicity: Findings from the national healthy minds study, 2013–2021. *Journal of Affective Disorders, 306*, 138–147.

Magaard, J. L., Seeralan, T., Schulz, H., & Brütt, A. L. (2017). Factors associated with help-seeking behaviour among individuals with major depression: A systematic review. *PLOS ONE, 12*(5), e0176730. doi.org/10.1371/journal.pone.0176730

Mental Health Association of San Francisco. (2020). *Peer support.* www.mentalhealthsf.org/what-is-peer-support/

Mental Health First Aid. (2022). *Mental health first aid: About us.* www.thenationalcouncil.org/about-us/

Mitchell, S. L., Kader, M., Darrow, S. A., Haggerty, M. Z., & Keating, N. L. (2013). Evaluating Question, Persuade, Refer (QPR) suicide prevention training in a college setting. *Journal of College Student Psychotherapy, 27*(2), 138–148. doi.org/10.1080/87568225.2013.766109

Monteith, L. L., Smith, N. B., Holliday, R., Dorsey Holliman, B. A., LoFaro, C. T., & Mohatt, N. V. (2020). "We're afraid to say suicide": Stigma as a barrier to implementing a community-based suicide prevention program for rural veterans. *The Journal of Nervous and Mental Disease, 208*(5), 371–376. https://journals.lww.com/jonmd/Fulltext/2020/05000/_We_re_Afraid_to_Say_Suicide___Stigma_as_a_Barrier.3.aspx

Morgan, A. J., Reavley, N. J., Ross, A., Too, L. S., & Jorm, A. F. (2018). Interventions to reduce stigma towards people with severe mental illness: Systematic review and meta-analysis. *Journal of Psychiatric Research, 103*, 120–133. doi.org/10.1016/j.jpsychires.2018.05.017

NAMI. (2018). *Navigating a mental health crisis*. https://nami.org/Support-Education/Publications-Reports/Guides/Navigating-a-Mental-Health-Crisis

Oh, H. Y., Marinovich, C., Jay, S., Zhou, S., & Kim, J. H. J. (2021). Abuse and suicide risk among college students in the United States: Findings from the 2019 Healthy Minds Study. *Journal of Affective Disorders*, *282*, 554–560. doi.org/10.1016/j.jad.2020.12.140

Pedrelli, P., Nyer, M., Yeung, A., Zulauf, C., & Wilens, T. (2015). College students: Mental health problems and treatment considerations. *Academic Psychiatry: The Journal of the American Association of Directors of Psychiatric Residency Training and the Association for Academic Psychiatry*, *39*(5), 503–511. doi.org/10.1007/s40596-014-0205-9

Pescosolido, B., Martin, J., Lang, A., & Olafsdottir, S. (2008). Rethinking theoretical approaches to stigma: A framework integrating normative influences on stigma (FINIS). *Social Science & Medicine*, *67*(3), 431–440. doi.org/10.1016/j.socscimed.2008.03.018

Petrova, M., Wyman, P. A., Schmeelk-Cone, K., & Pisani, A. R. (2015). Positive-themed suicide prevention messages delivered by adolescent peer leaders: Proximal impact on classmates' coping attitudes and perceptions of adult Support. *Suicide and Life-Threatening Behavior*, *45*(6), 651–663. doi.org/10.1111/sltb.12156

Project LETS. (2022). *Project LETS: About. https://projectlets.org/about*

QPR Institute. (2022). *Question, Persuade, Refer: What is QPR?* https://qprinstitute.com/about-qpr

Quinnett, P. (2012). *QPR gatekeeper training for suicide prevention: The model, rationale and theory*. https://qprinstitute.com/uploads/main/QPR-Theory-Paper-Master-Final-2019.pdf

Repper, J., & Carter, T. (2011). A review of the literature on peer support in mental health services. *Journal of Mental Health*, *20*(4), 392–411. doi.org/10.3109/09638237.2011.583947

Romo, V. (2018). *Hunger and homelessness are widespread among college students, study finds*. www.npr.org/sections/thetwo-way/2018/04/03/599197919/hunger-and-homelessness-are-widespread-among-college-students-study-finds

Rosen, M. R., Michael, K. D., & Jameson, J. P. (2020). CALM gatekeeper training is associated with increased confidence in utilizing means reduction approaches to suicide prevention among college resident assistants. *Journal of American College Health*, 1–8. Advance online publication. doi.org/10.1080/07448481.2020.1756825

Samuolis, J., Harrison, A. J., & Flanagan, K. (2020). Evaluation of a peer-led implementation of a suicide prevention gatekeeper training program for college students. *Crisis*, *41*(5), 331–336. doi.org/10.1027/0227-5910/a000638

Seale, S., & Givens, T. (2019). *The state of mental health in college students today*. https://higheredconnects.com/the-state-of-mental-health-in-college-students-today/

Shtivelband, A., Aloise-Young, P. A., & Chen, P. Y. (2015). Sustaining the effects of gatekeeper suicide prevention training. *Crisis*, *36*(2), 102–109. doi.org/10.1027/0227-5910/a000304

Silk, K. J., Perrault, E. K., Nazione, S. A., Pace, K., & Collins-Eaglin, J. (2017). Evaluation of a social norms approach to a suicide prevention campaign. *Journal of Health Communication*, *22*(2), 135–142. doi.org/10.1080/10810730.2016.1258742

Sommer-Rotenberg D. (1998). Suicide and language. *CMAJ: Canadian Medical Association Journal = journal de l'Association medicale canadienne*, *159*(3), 239–240.

Spencer-Thomas, S. (2019). *How to ask someone about suicide.* www.nami.org/Blogs/NAMI-Blog/September-2019/How-to-Ask-Someone-About-Suicide

Stein, B. D., Sontag-Padilla, L., Ashwood, J. S., Woodbridge, M. W., Eberhart, N. K., May, L., Seelam, R., Briscombe, B., Mendelsohn, J. D'Amico, E. J., Jaycox, L. H., Osilla, K. C., & Burnam, M. A. (2016). *Campus climate matters: Changing the mental health climate on college campuses improves student outcomes and benefits society.* RAND Corporation.

Stone, D. M., Holland, K. M., Bartholow, B. N., Crosby, A. E., Davis, S. P., & Wilkins, N. (2017). *Preventing suicide: A technical package of policies, programs, and practice.* https://stacks.cdc.gov/view/cdc/44275

Suicide Prevention Resource Center. (2020). *Effective suicide prevention: Getting started.* Suicide Prevention Resource Center. www.sprc.org/effective-suicide-prevention

Suicide Prevention Resource Center. (2020). *Evidence-based prevention.* Suicide Prevention Resource Center. www.sprc.org/keys-success/evidence-based-prevention

Suicide Prevention Resource Center. (2020). *Reduce access to means of suicide.* www.sprc.org/comprehensive-approach/reduce-means

Suicide Awareness Voices of Education. (2022). *SAVE: What we do.* https://save.org/what-we-do/

Tannenbaum, R. (2000). Theoretical foundations of multimedia. *Ubiquity, 2000.* doi.org/10.1145/347634.347643

Tsong, Y., Young, J. T., Killer, J. D., Takemoto, M. A., & Compliment, B. (2019). Suicide prevention program on a diverse college campus: Examining the effectiveness of a peer-to-peer model. *Journal of College Student Psychotherapy*, *33*(2), 131–144. doi.org/10.1080/87568225.2018.1434716

US Census Bureau. (2019, June 04). *More than 76 million students enrolled in U.S. Schools.* www.census.gov/newsroom/press-releases/2018/school-enrollment.html

Van Orden, K. A., Joiner, T. E., Jr., Hollar, D., Rudd, M. D., Mandrusiak, M., & Silverman, M. M. (2006). A test of the effectiveness of a list of suicide warning signs for the public. *Suicide & Life-Threatening Behavior*, *36*(3), 272–287. doi.org/10.1521/suli.2006.36.3.272

Vazquez, Stephanie Nickole, "The Bandana Project: Program Evaluation Plan" (2021). *Public Health Theses.* 2103. https://elischolar.library.yale.edu/ysphtdl/2103

Web Accessibility Initiative (WAI). (2020). *Making audio and video media accessible.* Web Accessibility Initiative. www.w3.org/WAI/media/av/transcripts/.

Whitlock, J., Wyman, P., & Barreira, P. (2013). *Connectedness and suicide prevention in college settings: Directions and implications for practice.* www.selfinjury.bctr.cornell.edu/perch/resources/connectedness-suicide-prevent.pdf

World Health Organization. (2016). *Availability, accessibility, acceptability, quality infographic.* www.who.int/gender-equity-rights/knowledge/aaaq-infographic/en/

Zivin, K., Eisenberg, D., Gollust, S. E., & Golberstein, E. (2009). Persistence of mental health problems and needs in a college student population. *Journal of Affective Disorders*, *117*(3), 180–185. doi.org/10.1016/j.jad.2009.01.001

# 10 Best Practices in Building Comprehensive Strategies to Prevent Sexual Violence for College-Age Students

Patricia Cook-Craig

It always seems impossible until it's done.

—Nelson Mandela

## 10.1 Overview

Just weeks before earning my master of science degree in social work (MSSW), I started my practice career at an agency that operated a dual domestic violence shelter and sexual assault programming. It was there that I began what would become a lifelong pursuit, helping others find safety – safety in their relationships, in the places they called home, and in their communities. It was also there that I really began to understand the psychological and physical costs when a person's safety is compromised. I was humbled by the experiences of working with individuals trying to work their way back to a place of safety. But as much as I recognized the importance of that work, year-over-year and across agencies and cities, I became equally frustrated that the rates of sexual violence and domestic violence were getting worse. Then one day, I found myself in a conference, "Imagining a World Without Sexual Assault," and I realized that I believe it could be possible. I just did not know how. I resolved that there was only one thing to do, and it was then I decided to return to get a Ph.D. in social work with the goal of getting ahead of the problem.

This path led me to focus on research and evaluation of programs that prevent violence before it occurs. Soon after obtaining my Ph.D. in social work, I began working with state and local partners to engage in evidence-based program design and evaluation to learn what works to prevent violence, and most of my research in this area has focused on prevention of sexual violence for high school and college populations. While there is still so much more work to do, I have seen such transformation in the field of sexual violence as we build a base of knowledge about what works to get ahead of the problem. We have gone from struggling to define what constitutes violence prevention to measuring when it has been prevented. Campuses once fearful of acknowledging the existence of assault and rape now have laws and road maps in place that guide their design of prevention strategies. The chapter that follows is designed to outline what we have learned about best practices to build campus-based programs.

## 10.2 The History of Campus Responses to Violence Prevention

Since the 1970s, the landscape of violence prevention efforts on college campuses has evolved considerably. This evolution is commonly traced back to Title IX of the Educational Amendments Act of 1972, which first prohibited discrimination on the basis of sex by any educational institution receiving federal financial benefits (The Education Amendments Act of 1972, 20 U.S.C. Đ 1681–1688 (1972)). This legislation was the first federal recognition that campuses had a responsibility to address sexual harassment, including sexual violence (White House Task Force to Protect Students from Sexual Assault, 2014). Building off of this foundation in 1990, the Jeanne Clery Disclosure of Campus Security Policy and Campus Crime Statistics Act (Clery) (20 U.S.C. §1092(f)) was passed in an effort to ensure that campuses collected data about and disclosed incidents of sexual and dating violence. This act requires campuses receiving federal funding to collect and report violence-related data, including rape and sexual assault, forcible and non-forcible sex crimes, domestic violence, dating violence, stalking, and hate crimes. It further requires campuses to provide timely warnings when incidences have taken place.

It was the 2005 reauthorization of the landmark legislation, the Violence Against Women Act (first enacted in 1994), that augmented early legislation focused on sexual violence surveillance and intervention by earmarking funding for prevention programming (National Network to End Domestic Violence [NNEDV], 2017). The first federal legislation that paid specific attention to promoting sexual violence prevention on college campuses was the 2013 Campus Sexual Violence Elimination (SaVE) Act requiring campuses to provide primary prevention and awareness training to all students and employees (Violence Against Women Reauthorization Act (42 USC §13,701)). In 2014, the White House, under the Obama Administration, launched the *It's On Us* campaign (www.itsonus.org/) and provided a campus toolkit highlighting research evidence that demonstrated the link between bystander prevention strategies and violence reduction on college campuses (White House Task Force to Protect Students from Sexual Assault, 2014).

While legislative action has moved toward the promotion of inclusive strategies to prevent campus violence, a much more compelling reason exists to engage in effective prevention programming designed to reduce rates of sexual violence on college campuses. Despite legislative focus on increasing sexual violence prevention programming, rates of sexual violence remain alarmingly high, even taking into account the problem of underreporting. According to the 2022 National Intimate Partner and Sexual Violence Survey (NISVS) that was based on 2016/2017 data, one in four women reported an attempted or completed rape, and one in nine men reported being made to penetrate someone in their lifetime. More than 80% of females and just under 80% of males reported they were first raped before the age of 26 (Basile et al., 2022).

Rates of sexual violence vary among demographic groups. Racial and ethnic minorities are at heightened risk of sexual violence. Based on 2010 NISVS data, lifetime prevalence of violence was greater among non-Hispanic Black, non-Hispanic Native American/Alaskan Native, and non-Hispanic multiracial women. Lifetime prevalence was greater for Hispanic and non-Hispanic multiracial men (data were insufficient to estimate rates of non-Hispanic Native populations) (Basile et al., 2022).

Although limited national data exist, available analyses of the prevalence of sexual violence show that gender identity and sexual orientation also impact risk of violence. According to 2010 estimates of NISVS data, gay men and bisexual individuals had higher lifetime rates of sexual violence than did heterosexual persons (Walters et al., 2013). A 2022 study of sexual violence experienced by LGBQ community college students also found higher rates of violence for LGBQ students compared to their heterosexual peers (Pottera et al., 2022). Transgendered persons also have higher lifetime rates of sexual violence (James et al., 2016).

Persistently high rates of sexual violence have contributed to its identification as a public health crisis. The mandate is clear: Campuses must work to prevent sexual violence on their campuses in ways that protect ALL students. The most effective way to meet this mandate is not as simple. This chapter will review best practices in the design of campus responses to this prevention challenge. This discussion begins with a description of the public health model (Mercy et al., 1993) that may be a useful framework to aid in designing a comprehensive prevention response. The chapter then examines best practices for employing each step of the model. Strategies for integrating social justice and social inclusion are also discussed. Finally, key recommendations for a robust campus sexual violence effort are reviewed.

## 10.3 Planning Comprehensive Sexual Violence Prevention Using the Public Health Model

With the recognition that research has demonstrated that one time, or episodic, violence prevention strategies are not effective at preventing violence (DeGue et al., 2014), a growing body of research and technical assistance is designed to help practitioners build a comprehensive strategy to address violence on their campuses (Basile, 2015; Campus Technical Assistance and Resource Project, 2017; Dills et al., 2016). The cornerstone of building a comprehensive violence prevention strategy is a planning team that can invest time and expertise into creating a sexual violence prevention plan that will drive the selection, implementation, and evaluation of their sexual violence programming.

A team-guided planning approach to campus prevention activities allows for the ability to connect campus and population-specific risk of violence to strategies that will address that violence. It also allows for ongoing use of surveillance and evaluation data to gauge the success of prevention strategies in promoting behaviors that increase safety and decrease rates of violence. Dills et al. (2016) recommend that prevention planning teams are multidisciplinary in nature, involve a wide array of active participants, and work to reinforce a visible and consistent prevention message across the campus.

Equally as important to a well-thought-out prevention team is a framework that guides their decision-making as they assess need, choose strategy(ies), guide implementation, and monitor outcomes. Used appropriately, the framework can guard against drift away from strategies designed to achieve desired prevention outcomes. The most commonly used framework is the four-step public health model. The four steps include (a) problem identification or surveillance; (b) identification of risk and protective factors; (c) development, implementation, and evaluation of programs; and (d) evaluation and assurance of widespread adoption (McMahon, 2000; Mercy et al., 1993). Best practices for successful negotiation of each phase of the public health model are highlighted in the following sections.

### 10.3.1 Step 1: Problem Identification/Surveillance

The first step of the public health model has been called both problem identification (CDC, n.d.) and surveillance (McMahon, 2000; Mercy et al., 1993). The purpose of this stage is to gather and analyze data that will focus planning efforts to create a comprehensive sexual violence prevention effort on campus. Two goals of this step are to (a) examine the unique way in which sexual violence is experienced on the campus(es) where programming will be delivered and (b) assess the campus(es) organizational capacity to deliver a comprehensive prevention effort.

#### 10.3.1.1 Assessing Sexual Violence on Campus

The design of a comprehensive sexual violence prevention strategy should begin with a review of campus-specific data. These data can then be used to define the population(s) that will be the focus of campus prevention strategies. In sexual violence prevention programming, the intended populations can be universal, targeted/selected, or indicated. Universal strategies are intended for the general population. Target/selected strategies are intended for populations who are considered at heightened risk of violence victimization or perpetration. Indicated strategies are designed to prevent further violence for populations who have already experienced victimization/perpetration (CDC, 2004).

The primary method that campuses use to assess sexual violence on campus is through the use of already existing or secondary data. Several types of publicly available data can be triangulated to better understand how violence is experienced on campus including campus demographic data, annual campus safety report data, and campus climate surveys.

**CAMPUS DEMOGRAPHICS.** Campus demographics can provide useful information on the student population that can guide the type of prevention programming offered. Demographic data can give you both a profile of the student population and the geographic boundaries of the student population. Campus student profiles report individual student demographics such as age, race, ethnicity, and gender identity. Campus profiles can also tell the planning team something about the nature of campus life. Important variables to consider include the ratio of students living on and off campus, the ratio of students taking in-person classes versus online-only classes, and the type of campus activities that students participate in such as Greek organizations, student groups, and athletics. Both where student live and the type of classes they take may inform the method of prevention program delivery, with in-person programming working better for on-campus populations and online delivery better for commuter and online-only students. In addition, some campus activities may heighten the risk of alcohol use, which has been associated with a greater risk of sexual violence (Abbey et al., 2001; Basile et al., 2021; Norris, 2008).

**CAMPUS SAFETY DATA.** In response to Clery Act (20 U.S.C. §1092(f)) reporting requirements, campus safety data are publicly available on federally funded campus websites and are updated annually. Annual security reports (ASRs) can be useful in helping to understand which types of sexual violence are more prevalently reported on campus. In addition, the reports are required to include where the violence occurred, including if it was at an on- or off-campus college facility or in a residence hall. Universities and colleges with multiple campuses report each campus separately. This reporting process can allow for the contextualization or adaptation of sexual violence prevention strategies based on where violence occurs. Included in ASRs are annual data for the past three years on the number of incidences of sexual assault (including rape, fondling, incest, and statutory rape), domestic violence, dating violence, and stalking. While ASR reports can be useful data to help understand the nature of sexual violence reported on college campuses, they also must be interpreted with caution as they do not include incidences of violence that are not reported or that occur in some off-campus settings. The actual incidences of violence are therefore historically underreported and should not be used to estimate rates of violence among college students (Clery Center for Security on Campus, 2018).

**CAMPUS CLIMATE SURVEYS.** Campus climate surveys can be a very useful tool to assist the planning team in getting broader data on sexual violence experiences in college and on student perceptions about campus responses to violence (Krause et al., 2019). Campus climate surveys are not required in statute to be conducted at all institutions receiving federal funding, but their use has grown in popularity since they were recommended by the Obama Administration (Krause et al., 2019; White House Task Force to Protect Students from Sexual Assault, 2014). Recommended domains for inclusion in the survey include experiences with sexual harassment, coerced sexual contact, sexual assault victimization and perpetration, intimate partner violence victimization, sexual harassment, school climate related to sexual harassment and sexual assault prevention, and school connectedness (Krebs et al., 2016). The lack of universal adoption of campus climate surveys can be a limitation for a campus that has not yet adopted the practice, but for those who have access to the data, it can provide the most complete picture available about what students are experiencing on campus and their trust in professionals to address the issue.

Research on the use of campus climate surveys suggests that much work needs to be done to improve their usefulness. In a systematic review of 107 campus climate survey reports, Krause et al. (2019) found that campuses self-select which domains they include and methodologies they use on their climate surveys, rather than following the recommendations for instrument development and data collection design recommended by the Obama White House Task Force to Protect Students from Sexual Assault (2014), after pilot testing the methodology for validity (Krebs et al., 2016). Recent VAWA changes include the 2022 Reauthorization Act signed into law as part of the Consolidated Appropriations Act 2022, which will require federally funded campuses to administer a universal Campus Climate Survey that will standardize and increase campus climate data collection activity (Consolidated Appropriations Act, 2022 [USC 117–103, 2022]).

#### 10.3.1.2 Assessing Organizational Capacity

Literature on campus sexual violence prevention planning clearly argues that in order to successfully implement a comprehensive sexual violence prevention plan, the campus as an organization must be assessed for its capacity to deliver selected strategies (Baker et al., 2021; Wasco & Zadnic, 2013).

Table 10.1 *Organizational capacity needed for comprehensive sexual violence prevention*

| Capacity domain | Literature on assessing and building capacity |
|---|---|
| Campus climate | Wasco and Zadnic (2013) |
| Collaboration/partnerships/relationships | Dills et al. (2016); Klein-Jiminez et al. (2018); Veto Violence (2020) |
| With referral services | Dills et al. (2016) |
| With other prevention programs | Dills et al. (2016) |
| Data/evaluation | Veto Violence (2020) |
| Institutionalization of prevention | Dills et al. (2016) |
| Knowledge of sexual violence | Wasco and Zadnic (2013) |
| Leadership | Klein-Jiminez et al. (2018); Veto Violence (2020); Wasco and Zadnic (2013) |
| Prevention team/workgroup/committee | Dills et al. (2016) |
| Programs address multiple forms of violence | Dills et al. (2016) |
| Readiness | Wasco and Zadnic (2013) |
| Resources | Klein-Jiminez et al. (2018); Veto Violence (2020) |
| Skills/expertise | Veto Violence (2020) |
| Staffing | Klein-Jiminez et al. (2018); Veto Violence (2020) |
| Dedicated to prevention | Dills et al. (2016) |
| Well-trained | Dills et al. (2016) |
| Standardized training | Dills et al. (2016) |
| Structure/processes | Klein-Jiminez et al. (2018) |
| Support for campus-wide prevention efforts | Wasco and Zadnic (2013) |
| Sustainability | Dills et al. (2016) |
| Use of trauma-informed approach | Dills et al. (2016) |

While assessing sexual violence on campus is typically done through a review of existing or secondary data, organizational capacity assessment data typically must be collected by the planning team. This is usually accomplished through either surveys or interviews of key stakeholder to identify gaps in capacity that must be addressed. The literature on assessing organizational capacity identifies several domains of needed organizational capacity to support comprehensive sexual violence prevention. These domains are summarized in Table 10.1.

### 10.3.2 Step 2: Identification of Risk and Protective Factors

A common problem when developing sexual violence prevention programs is the lack of either clarity or congruence between the outcomes a campus hopes to achieve and the types of strategies that a campus selects to implement. Step 2 of the public health model encourages prevention planning teams to clarify the outcomes that they are working to achieve (Mercy et al., 1993). Two frameworks have proven useful in facilitating the selection of target program outcomes in sexual violence prevention.

The first framework is the socioecological model (Dahlberg & Krug, 2002). In their review of the roots of violence, Dahlberg and Krug (2002) concluded "No single factor explains why some individuals behave violently toward others or why violence is more prevalent in some communities than in others" (p. 286). Rather, researchers have found that violence occurs across four levels of the socioecology (Heise, 1998; Moylan & Jovorka, 2020; Tolan & Geurra, 1994). Building on the work of Bronfenbrenner (1979), the socioecological model posits that violence exists at the individual level, at the relationship level, in our communities, and in society. While, historically, sexual violence prevention strategies primarily addressed sexual violence at the individual and relationship levels, Dills et al. (2016) highlight the CDC recommendation that strategies target reducing rates of violence at the population level. Reviews of best practices for campus-based prevention recommend selecting a strategy(ies) that is designed to address multiple levels of the socioecology (CDC, 2014; Dills et al., 2016).

A second framework used to formulate sexual violence prevention strategies is risk and protective factor theory (Hawkins, Catalano, & Miller, 1992). As applied to sexual violence, this framework posits that identifiable factors exist that increase the likelihood that violence will occur. These factors are called risk factors. Risk factors for both victimization and perpetration at each level of the socioecology have been identified in the literature (Bonar et al., 2022). The framework further suggests that identifiable factors exist that mitigate the likelihood of violence. These factors are called protective factors. While much less is known about protective factors that act to prevent violence on college campuses, a few have been identified in the literature (Bonar et al., 2022). Examples of protective factors that may help prevent violence among college students include empathy (Bonar et al., 2022; Tharpe et al., 2013) and perceived and actual social support (Bonar et al., 2022) although researchers are unified in their call for additional research to identify and validate protective factors that prevent college sexual violence.

Using these frameworks and the data gathered in Step 1 of the public health model, prevention planning teams can map out how risk is experienced on campus, determine what levels of the socioecology are best to intervene at to prevent sexual violence, and assess what inequities exist on campus. By clarifying intended outcomes, the prevention team can assess potential sexual violence prevention strategies to determine if they are designed to mitigate risk of violence at a desired level of the socioecological model. Examples of campus-based sexual violence strategies that address each level of the socioecological model can be found in the research literature (Basile, 2015; Moylan & Jovorka, 2020) and technical assistance packages (DeGue, 2014; Dills et al., 2016).

### 10.3.3 Step 3: Development and Evaluation of Programs

It is not until Step 3 of the public health model that campuses begin the strategy selection process, which when selected must be tested to demonstrate whether or not they are effective (Mercy et al., 1993). The identification of a population(s) on which to focus one's prevention efforts and the selection of intended outcomes for change in Steps 1 and 2 of the public health model helps guide decision-making related to which prevention strategy(ies) to implement on campus. It is now well understood from sexual violence prevention research that any campus response to prevent sexual violence must be comprehensive in order to be effective (Basile, 2015; DeGue, 2014). So, in order to develop an effective campus response to sexual violence, the planning team must consider what criteria establish a program or strategy as comprehensive. The most commonly used criteria for comprehensivity were published in 2003 by Nation and colleagues. Their review of prevention research identified nine characteristics of effective prevention programs including using multiple components to be *comprehensive*, employing *varied teaching methods*, offering *sufficient dosage*, emanating from a *theory-driven* justification, establishing *positive relationships* with peers/adults, offering elements that are *appropriately timed* to foster behavior change, ensuring *sociocultural relevance*, having an embedded *outcome evaluation*, and using *well-trained staff* for its delivery (p. 452). Prevention planning teams can use these criteria as either a guide for the development of new programs or to establish a rubric for vetting existing ones.

## 10.4 Selecting Evidence-Based/Evidence-Informed Strategies

A growing body of evidence on what works to prevent sexual violence has changed the conversation on available evidence-informed or evidence-based strategy(ies). Several systematic literature reviews and meta-analyses of research on sexual violence prevention programs are available (Brecklin & Forde, 2001; DeGue et al., 2014; Dills et al., 2016; Katz & Moore, 2013; McMahon et al., 2019; Newlands & O'Donohue, 2016; Vladutiu et al., 2011). These reviews say as much about what has not been found to be effective at reducing rates of violence as what has. Many open questions still remain about which programs work for which populations, and much more research needs to be done to understand what works to prevent campus sexual violence (McMahon et al., 2019; Newlands & O'Donohue, 2016). The incomplete nature of the state of the research does not, however, absolve universities from their federal and ethical obligation to, "employ the prevention programs with the strongest empirical support" (Newlands & O'Donohue, 2016, p. 8).

## 10.5 Types of Campus-Based Prevention

In 2016, the CDC published a technical package for selecting sexual violence prevention strategies recommending five domains of strategies called STOP SV. The first strategy type is *Promoting Social Norms That Protect Against Violence.* Both individuals and communities can endorse norms that discourage acceptance of violence. Social norms promotion strategies for college campuses include bystander programs and mobilization of campuses communities, such as coaches, teams, and Greek organizations that can promote prevention-focused social norms. Bystander strategies also capitalize on the use of persons who might witness the violence who can be trained to intervene and potentially stop violent acts before they occur (Dills et al., 2016).

The second strategy type is *Teaching Skills to Prevent Violence.* This type of campus-based prevention focuses on the relationship level of the socioecological model. Skills development strategies for college campuses include programs that teach students about healthy sexuality, affirmative consent, and healthy relationships as well as programs that promote socioemotional learning (Dills et al., 2016).

The third strategy type is *Providing Opportunities to Empower and Support Girls and Women.* Women have historically experienced higher rates of sexual violence than men, and as such, this strategy is focused on building community and societal structures that support gender equality. Campus-based strategies to provide these opportunities include leadership training and programming that empowers women to improve confidence in pursuing opportunities and improve earning potential (Dills et al., 2016).

The fourth strategy type is *Creating Protective Environments.* This strategy type is designed to impact the community level of the socioecological model by promoting policies and changing or enhancing the physical environment to reduce the likelihood that violence will occur. Campus-based strategies to foster protective environments include the development of campus policies that include clear, strong codes of conduct that do not tolerate violence, policies that reduce alcohol access, easy-to-navigate information on policies and reporting procedures, and prevention messaging that follow students from entry through their college years (Dills et al., 2016). McMahon and colleagues (2022) recommend assessment of four aspects of the built environment of college campuses for their contribution to the promotion or prevention of sexual violence. The first aspect, active guardianship and monitoring, refers to the use of increased monitoring using safety features (such as lighting) or through bystanders such as faculty, staff, and students. The second aspect, organization and investment, refers to addressing spatial disorganization that could increase the likelihood for violence, for example, investing in immediate removal of misogynist graffiti. The third aspect, sense of ownership and access to power, refers to students' values about the use of their environment including shared identity, involvement, care, and pride. The fourth aspect, placement and mix of health spaces, refers to the location and amount of places that have a positive impact and places that have a negative impact on students' health.

The fifth strategy type is *Supporting Victims/Survivors to Lessen Harms* (Dills et al., 2016). While the push for campus-based sexual violence prevention efforts is focused on primary prevention, many students will come to campus having already experienced sexual violence. Just under half (49%) of female rape victims and over half (56.6%) of male rape victims were first raped under the age of 18 (Basile et al., 2022). In addition, even students with the most sophisticated primary prevention programming campuses will still experience violence. For these reasons, campuses must also put into place secondary and tertiary prevention programming to support and lessen harm for victims of sexual violence. Campus-based strategies for this type of strategy include confidential, coordinated services using a trauma-informed approach for victims of violence (American College Health Association, 2020; Dills et al., 2016), training for faculty and staff to ensure they can make appropriate referrals and engage in supportive conversations, and participation in holding perpetrators accountable both through campus policies and cooperation with off-campus authorities (Dills et al., 2016).

Reviewing existing campus policies for their impact on victims of violence is also important. For instance, campus policies requiring compelled disclosure of sexual assaults by faculty and staff, while intended to improve reporting, have been scrutinized in the literature for their potential negative unintended consequences for victims of violence. Some potential increased harm includes discounting consent of the victim to report, increased mistrust and potential for re-traumatization (Holland et al., 2018).

## 10.6 Key Implementation Considerations When Selecting an Existing Strategy

Two key considerations are important in the selection and implementation of an existing prevention strategy on a college campus. The first is matching strategy selection with capacity to deliver the strategy as designed. Selecting a particular prevention strategy because it is comprehensive, has a solid basis of evidence of effectiveness, and/or addresses risk factors that the campus is dedicated to reducing is of little use if the campus does not have the resources, training, or expertise to successfully guide implementation. Strategy selection should involve a review of all four factors: comprehensiveness, ability to shift desired outcomes, evidence base of effectiveness, and campus organizational capacity needed to deliver all components of the strategy.

The second important question to consider is whether a potential strategy has a well-defined, feasible adaptation strategy. The assessment of how sexual violence is experienced on any particular campus will demonstrate the unique characteristics of the population of students on campus and the campus culture. This often necessitates adapting the strategy to local culture and target student groups. As Nations et al. (2003) argue, a comprehensive prevention strategy should have sociocultural relevance. One way to ensure this is to design an adaptation strategy for implementers to follow so that they can adapt the strategy without compromising the strategy's essential elements or theory of change.

## 10.7 Evaluating Campus-Based Prevention Strategies

Whether the violence prevention strategy(ies) that the planning team chooses for their campus is or are evidence-based, evidence-informed, or home-grown, it is important to design an evaluation plan to track whether the strategy is impacting the outcomes identified in Step 2. Best practice is to continually evaluate rates of victimization and perpetration along with changes in risk and protection factors (Newlands & O'Donohue, 2016). Tracking rates of violence may prove to be difficult due to resource or cost constraints, however. In cases when annual surveillance of rates of violence on campus is not possible, it is minimally critical to track whether the essential elements of the strategy impact short and intermediate outcomes such as lowering a risk factor, improving a protective factor, or training students to engage in a desired new behavior.

Participatory evaluation models are very helpful in aligning the selection, implementation, and evaluation of campus sexual violence strategies. Participatory evaluation has been defined as "… applied social research that involves a partnership between trained evaluation personnel and practice-based decision makers, organization members with program responsibilities, or people with a vital interest in the program" (Cousins & Earl, 1992, pp. 399–400). They allow evaluators to work alongside stakeholders throughout the entire process (Cousins & Whitmore, 1998; Wandersman, 2019). Participatory evaluation models also aid in ensuring that evaluation data will be used for program improvement (Cox et al., 2009).

An often-used participatory evaluation model in the sexual violence field *is Empowerment Evaluation* (EE) (Campbell et al., 2004; Cook-Craig et al., 2014; Cox et al., 2009; Noonan & Gibbs, 2009). The definition of EE is "the use of evaluation concepts, techniques, and findings to foster improvement and self-determination" (Fetterman, 1996, p. 4). Three facets of EE are particularly useful in designing and implementing a campus violence prevention plan. First, as a member of the planning team, the evaluator can assist the team to do assessments, literature reviews, and program reviews prior to any implementation of programs to be evaluated. Second, EE fosters ownership of all stakeholders in program evaluation, which can result in shared ownership of findings. Third, EE operates from a continuous improvement paradigm that promotes the use of evaluation data to make changes or adaptations to program implementation if needed to achieve desired results.

### 10.7.1 Step 4: Assuring Adoption of What Works

The final step in the public health model asks campuses to engage in dissemination of what they have learned (Mercy et al., 1993). One of the keys to building best practices in sexual violence prevention is sharing implementation lessons and program evaluations across campuses to build a bank of knowledge about what works. Miller and Shinn (2005) identified four challenges that inhibit communities from disseminating lesson learned in their prevention work. These challenges include lack of capacity, lack of values congruence between organizations and programs, bias that promotes programs labeled evidence-based over indigenous practices, and a lack of attention to the complexity of adopting new practices. DeGue (2014) emphasizes the importance of campuses sharing lessons learned across multiple channels such as conferences and networks of college administrators and prevention staff, as well as through scientific publications, as important components to building an evidence base for sexual violence prevention programs. To ensure the most learning possible, campuses should be transparent in sharing what did not work for them along with what did.

## 10.8 Promoting Social Inclusion in Campus Sexual Violence Prevention Work

Historically, the movement to end sexual violence has been criticized for its lack of attention to the disproportional victimization of marginalized populations (Brubaker et al., 2017; Coulter et al., 2017; Smith & Pick, 2015), the lack of prevention strategies that are socioculturally relevant for persons of diverse identities (DeGue et al., 2014), and the lack of research establishing evidence of program effectiveness for diverse populations (McCauley et al., 2019). The result is that "our work often centers the experiences of White, heterosexual, cisgender women and our systems reify the power of privileged groups" (McCauley et al., 2019, p. 1907). When campus responses to and research on sexual violence do strive for sociocultural relevance, they often fail to take into account the intersectional nature of identity (Iverson, 2017).

The failure to ensure inclusivity in campus sexual violence prevention responses has at its worst done damage to populations they seek to help (McMahon et al., 2020; Parks et al., 2018). For example, in their study of historically minoritized college students, McMahon et al. (2020) found that when students evaluated bystander sexual violence prevention programming they reported microaggressions and elements of the programs that were racist, homophobic, and transphobic in their design. At the institutional level, Iverson's (2017) study of campus sexual violence policies on 22 campuses demonstrated a pattern of heterosexism, genderism, and ableism. The policies also failed to discuss the intersection of race and ethnicity in students' experience of sexual violence or to take into account religious accommodations.

In order to promote social inclusion, working through the development of a campus sexual violence prevention response must address the intersectional nature of students' complex identities and work to dismantle exclusionary practices in each step of the public health model. First, it is important to ensure that the selection of the planning team is built using an intersectional lens that values the diversity of identity of its members. In addition to membership based on diverse individual identity, McMahon and colleagues (2021) suggest the adoption of a "Whole School Approach" in which campus sexual violence responses are planned in active participation with students, parents, staff, faculty, administrators, and community members, each with an integral role to play in the success of preventing violence on campus. In addition, guidance on how to prevent sexual violence on college campuses recommends the inclusion of members who approach the problem using multiple disciplinary lenses to address the complex nature of how to prevent sexual violence (Dills et al., 2016; Prevention Institute & NSVRC, 2021).

In Step 1 of the public health model that is focused on assessment of the problem, it is important to prioritize efforts to address gaps in available data to understand the extent of sexual violence on campus. Even when triangulating multiple sources of available data, there is a lack of surveillance on how sexual violence is experienced by different groups, often those who are more vulnerable to it. While no easy solutions exist to address data gaps, McMahon and colleagues (2019) advocate for modification of surveillance tools, such as campus climate surveys, to be more inclusive. In the meantime, in cases where data are not available to fully examine the extent of the experience and risk of sexual violence for students on campus, the planning group should strive to collect data through the use of surveys or focus groups that could work to fill these gaps.

In addition, campus climate surveys provide a snapshot of students' experiences with campus responses to sexual violence. These data provide the opportunity to explore what actions campuses can take to ensure that their response is equitable and inclusive. Some suggestions for dialogue and action include exploring whether the environment is safe for authentic expression, whether indirect forms of oppression exist in the culture, and if policies are created and applied equitably (Prevention Institute & NSVRC, 2021).

In Step 2 of the public health model, the planning team evaluates risk and protective factor research across the socioecological model, which can then be used to inform strategy selection to achieve intended outcomes. In order to have a more complete picture of risk of sexual violence on campus, the data and research from Steps 1 and 2 must be considered together. Persons with different backgrounds experience risk of sexual violence at different rates. In addition, intersectionality recognizes that an individual is an intersection of many social identities including race, class, ability, gender, sexuality, and socioeconomic status, among others, each of which can influence risk of violence (Dills et al., 2019).

In Step 3 of the public health model, the planning team selects/develops campus prevention strategies, implements, and evaluates them. Taken together, the literature seems to promote both culturally specific sexual violence prevention strategies for targeted populations and evidence-based strategies, which at present tend to be designed and tested on universal populations. One frame for negotiating program selection that promotes social inclusion is selecting programming that is either culturally grounded or has undergone deep-structure adaptation (Parks et al., 2018). When there is a clear understanding of the cultural background of a targeted population, a campus has the opportunity to design the prevention strategy with components that "evolve from the world-views, values, beliefs, and behaviors of the populations that the program is intended to serve" (Parks et al., 2018, p. 19). Often this may not be possible, particularly if the plan is to deliver the intervention to multiple or universal audiences. In this case, Parks and colleagues (2018) recommend deep-structure adaptation of evidence-based programming. This adaptation strategy requires partnership with members of cultural communities for whom the strategy is being adapted to serve. This adaptation partnership can help ensure that the delivery of the strategy can both adhere to essential program components while ensuring that core values, stressors, and coping styles of the population are taken into consideration.

With respect to sexual violence prevention strategies that are deemed evidence-based, the planning team must take time to critically assess the research that establishes the strategy as "evidence-based," assessing for which students the program has been found effective with in preventing violence. In their systematic review of sexual violence prevention strategies, DeGue and colleagues (2014) found few evidence-based prevention programs that are designed for diverse groups. McCauley and colleagues (2019), in their examination of the intersectional nature of sexual violence research, found that studies designed to establish evidence of effectiveness of college sexual violence prevention programs are not evaluated for their impact on diverse student samples.

Because only a small number of evidence-based sexual violence prevention program for college campuses are evaluated on students of all identities, the planning team has an obligation to assess whether available strategies are socioculturally relevant to students on their campus. This may mean that time and resources will need to be allocated to the adaptation of a selected prevention strategy to intended student populations that will receive the strategy. In addition, any strategy delivered to a student population for which there is little or no evidence of effectiveness for that population should be evaluated as it is delivered on campus to assess outcomes for that population.

Step 4 of the public health model calls for efforts to ensure widespread adoption of what works. Since there is an the absence of a comprehensive catalogue of culturally relevant evidence-based programs, three strategies are suggested for fostering a discussion of what works and for whom in campus sexual violence sexual prevention. These include sharing: (a) home grown or promising programs designed for targeted populations, (b) deep-structure cultural program adaptations of existing evidence-based programs, and (c) evaluation results of the impact of programs on diverse populations. As mentioned earlier, DeGue (2014) suggests sharing across multiple channels including both through publications and networking with colleagues.

In addition, a key recommendation for campus planning teams is that they connect sexual violence prevention strategies with other prevention programs on campus. Using an intersectionality frame, the California Coalition Against Sexual Assault (2017) outlined the connections between the movement to end sexual violence and the movements for LGBTQ equality, racial justice, economic justice, transformative justice, immigrant justice, reproductive rights, and health and wellness. By broadening partnerships to include groups promoting equality, equity, and justice, campus sexual violence prevention strategies are naturally challenged to infuse an intersectional lens into their work.

## 10.9 Conclusion

A synthesis of the literature on best practices in campus-based sexual violence prevention points to some key suggestions for success.

### 10.9.1 Make Planning the Plan

With a wealth of literature and guides on programs available, it would be easy to pick program that seems preferable rather than developing a comprehensive campus-based plan. Key activities in planning include the following:

- Build an inclusive planning team.
- Follow a framework such as the public health model (Mecy et al., 1993) to guide the work of the team.

- Connect the selection of a strategy to data that demonstrate how violence is experienced on the campus.
- Be mindful of capacity by selecting a strategy(ies) that is as comprehensive as your capacity will allow.

### 10.9.2 Stay Engaged in the "What Works?" Conversation

Rather than seeing success as getting a program implemented, the "What Works?" framework pushes the planning team to organize discussion and actions around achieving outcomes rather than activity. Key activities in pushing toward agreed-upon outcomes include the following:

- Design the program evaluation consistent with strategy selection before implementation.
- Use an improvement approach to assess evaluation results.
- Do not do it alone. Connect with other campuses, coalitions, state health departments.
- Ultimately the success of a campus-based prevention effort depends on a commitment to comprehensivity.

## References

Abbey, A., Zawicki, T., Buck, P. O., Clinton, A. M., & McAuslan, P. (2001). Alcohol and sexual assault. *Alcohol Research & Health*, *25*(1), 42–51.

Baker, J., Kerr, A., Meyer, A., Wargel, K., Flaspohler, P., Acosta, J. D., Chinman, M., Wanderman, A., Fortson, B., & Tharp, A. (2021). *Self-assessment guide for university prevention programs focused on sexual assault and sexual harassment.* Rand Corporation.

Basile, K. C. (2015). A comprehensive approach to sexual violence prevention. *New England Journal of Medicine*, *372*(24), 2350–2352. doi.org/10.1056/NEJMe1503952

Basile, K. C., Smith, S. G., Kresnow, M., Khatiwada S., & Leemis, R. W. (2022). *The National intimate partner and sexual violence survey: 2016/2017 report on sexual violence*. National Center for Injury Prevention and Control, Centers for Disease Control and Prevention.

Basile, K. C., Smith, S. G., Lui, Y., Lowe, A., Gilmore, A. K., Khatiwada S., & Kresnow, M. (2021). Victim and perpetrator characteristics in alcohol/drug-involved sexual violence victimization in the U.S. *Drug and Alcohol Dependence*, *226*, 108839. doi.org/10.1016/j.drugalcdep.2021.108839

Bonar, E. E., DeGue, S., Abbey, A., Coker, A. L., Lindquist, C. H., McCauley, H. L., Miller, E., Senn, C. Y., Thompson, M. P., Ngo, Q. M., Cunningham, R. M., & Walton. M. A. (2022). Prevention of sexual violence among college students: Current challenges and future directions, *Journal of American College Health*, *70*(2), 575–588. doi.org/10.1080/07448481.2020.1757681

Brecklin, L. R., & Forde, D. R. (2001). A meta-analysis of rape education programs. *Violence and Victims*, *16*, 303–321. doi.org/10.1891/0886-6708.16.3.303

Bronfenbrenner V. (1979). *The ecology of human development: Experiments by nature and design*. Harvard University Press.

Brubaker, S. J., Keegan, B., Guadalupe Diaz, X. L., & Beasley, B. (2017). Measuring and reporting campus sexual assault: Privilege and exclusion in what we know and what we do. *Sociology Compass*, *11*(12), e12543. doi.org/10.1111/soc4.12543

California Coalition Against Sexual Assault [CALCASA]. (2017). *Ending sexual violence: An intersectional approach*. California Coalition Against Sexual Assault.

Campbell, R., Dorey, H., Naegeli, M., Grubstein, L. K., Bennett, K. K., Bonter, F., Smith, P. K., Grzywack, J., Baker, P. R., & Davidson, W. S., II. (2004). An empowerment evaluation model for sexual assault programs: Empirical evidence of effectiveness. *American Journal of Community Psychology*, *34*(3–4), 251–262. doi.org/10.1007/s10464-004-7418-0

Centers for Disease Control and Prevention [CDC]. (2004). *Sexual violence prevention: Beginning the dialogue*. Centers for Disease Control and Prevention.

Clery Center for Security on Campus. (2018). *Understanding Clery statistics*. Clery Center for Security on Campus. Consolidated Appropriations Act, 2022 [USC 117–103, 2022].

Cook-Craig, P. G., Millspaugh, P. H., Recktenwald, E. A., Kelly, N. C., Hegge, L. M., Coker, A. L., & Pletcher, T. S. (2014). From EMPOWER to Green Dot: Successful strategies and lessons learned in developing comprehensive sexual violence prevention programming. *Violence Against Women*, *20*(10), 1162–1178. doi.org/10.1177/1077801214551286

Coulter, R. W. S., Mair, C., Miller, E., Blosnich, J. R., Matthews, D. D., & McCauley, H. L. (2017). Prevalence of past-year sexual assault victimization among undergraduate students: Exploring differences by and intersections of gender identity, sexual identity, and race/ethnicity. *Prevention Science*, *18*(6), 726–736. doi.org/10.1007/s11121-017-0762-8

Cousins, J. B., & Earl, L. M. (1992). The case for participatory evaluation. *Education Evaluation and Policy Analysis*, *14*(4), 397–418. doi.org/10.3102/01623737014004397

Cousins, J. B., & Whitmore, E. (1998). Framing participatory evaluation. *New Directions for Evaluation*, *80*, 5–23. doi.org/10.1002/ev.1114

Dahlberg, L. L., & Krug, E. G. (2002). Violence-a global public health problem. In E. Krug, L. L. Dahlberg, J. A. Mercy, A. B. Zwi, & R. Lozano (Eds.), *World report on violence and health* (pp. 1–56). World Health Organization.

DeGue, S. (2014). *Preventing sexual violence on college campuses: Lessons from research and practice. Part 1: Evidence-based strategies for the primary prevention of sexual violence perpetration* (pp. 2–13). Centers for Disease Control and Prevention Division of Violence Prevention National Center for Injury Prevention and Control. https://stacks.cdc.gov/view/cdc/43896

DeGue, S., Valle, L. A., Holt, M., Massetti, G., Matjasko, J., & Tharp, A. T. (2014). A systematic review of primary prevention strategies for sexual violence perpetration. *Aggression and Violent Behavior*, *19*(4), 346–362. doi.org/10.1016/j.avb.2014.05.004

Dills, J., Fowler, D., & Payne, G. (2016). *Sexual violence on campus: Strategies for prevention*. National Center for Injury Prevention and Control, Centers for Disease Control and Prevention. www.cdc.gov/violenceprevention/pdf/campussvprevention.pdf

Dills, J., Jones, K., & Brown, P. (2019). *Continuing the dialogue: Learning from the past and looking to the future of intimate partner violence and sexual violence prevention.*

National Center for Injury Prevention and Control, Centers for Disease Control and Prevention. www.cdc.gov/violenceprevention/pdf/sv/Continuing-The-Dialogue-508.pdf

Fetterman, D. M. (1996). *Empowerment evaluation: An introduction to theory and practice*. In D. M. Fetterman, S. J. Kaftarian, & A. Wandersman (Eds.), *Empowerment evaluation: Knowledge and tools for self-assessment and accountability* (pp. 3–46). Sage.

Hawkins, J. D., Catalano, R. F., & Miller, J. Y. (1992). Risk and protective factors for alcohol and other drug problems in adolescence and early adulthood: Implications for substance abuse prevention. *Psychological Bulletin*, *112*(1), 64–105. doi .org/10.1037/0033-2909.112.1.64

Heise, L. L. (1998). Violence against women: An integrated ecological framework. *Violence Against Women*, *4*(3), 262–290. doi.org/10.1177/1077801298004003002

Holland, K. J., Cortina, L. M., & Freyd, J. J. (2018). Compelled disclosure of college sexual assault. *American Psychologist*, *73*(3), 256–268. doi.org/10.1037/amp0000186

Iverson, S. V. (2017). Mapping identities: An intersectional analysis of policies on sexual violence. In J. Harris, C. Linder, & W. Wanjuki (Eds.), *Intersections of identity and sexual violence on campus: Centering minoritized students' experiences*. Stylus Publishing, LLC. www.ustranssurvey.org/reports

James, S. E., Herman, J. L., Rankin, S., Keisling, M., Mottet, L., & Anafi, M. (2016). *The report of the 2015 U.S. transgender survey*. National Center for Transgender Equality.

Katz, J., & Moore, J. (2013). Bystander education training for campus sexual assault prevention: An initial meta-analysis. *Violence and Victims*, *28*, 1054–67. doi .org/10.1891/0886-6708.vv-d-12-00113

Kaukinen, C. (2014). Dating violence among college students: The risk and protective factors. *Trauma, Violence, & Abuse*, *15*(4), 283–296. doi.org/10.1177/1524838014521321

Klein-Jiminez, A., Somji, A., Lockhart, S., Huffman, M., Austin, M., & Aragon, V. C. (2018, February 28). *2018 PreventConnect Webinar Series: How to build organizational capacity to support sexual and domestic violence prevention*. ValorUS PreventConnect. www.preventconnect.org/2018/02/how-to-build-organizational-capacity-to-support-sexual-and-domestic-violence-prevention/

Krause, K. H., Woofter, R., Haardörfer, R., Windle, M., Sales, J. M., & Yount, K. M. (2019). Measuring campus sexual assault and culture: A systematic review of campus climate surveys. *Psychology of Violence*, *9*(6), 611–622. doi.org/10.1037/vio0000209

Krebs, C., Lindquist, C., Berzofsky, M., Shook-Sa, B., Peterson, K., Planty, M., Langton, L., & Stroop, J. (2016). *Campus climate survey validation study final technical report*. Bureau of Justice Statistics, U.S. Department of Justice.

McCauley, H. L., Campbell, R., Buchanan, N. T., & Moylan, C. A. (2019). Advancing theory, methods, and dissemination in sexual violence research to build a more equitable future: An intersectional, community-engaged approach. *Violence Against Women*, *25*(16), 1906–1931. doi.org/10.1177/1077801219875823

McMahon, P. M. (2000). The public health approach to the prevention of sexual violence. *Sexual Abuse: A Journal of Research and Treatment*, *12*(1), 27–36. doi .org/10.1023/A:1009559720231

McMahon, S., Banyard, V. L., Peterson, N. A., Cusano, J., Brown, Q. L., & Farmer, A. Y. (2022). Physical spaces for campus sexual violence prevention: A conceptual model. *Journal of Prevention and Health Promotion*, *3*(3), 347–368. doi .org/10.1177/26320770221093641

McMahon, S., Burnam, J., & Banyard, V. L. (2020). Bystander intervention as a prevention strategy for campus sexual violence: Perceptions of historically minoritized college students. *Prevention Science*, *21*(6), 795–806. doi.org/10.1007/s11121-020-01134-2

McMahon, S., Steiner, J. J., Snyder, S., & Banyard, V. L. (2021). Comprehensive prevention of campus sexual violence: Expanding who is invited to the table. *Trauma, Violence, & Abuse*, *22*(4), 843–855. doi.org/10.1177/1524838019883275

McMahon, S., Wood, L., Cusano, J., & Macri, L. M. (2019). Campus sexual assault: Future directions for research. *Sexual Abuse*, *31*(3), 270–295. doi.org/10.1177/1079063217750864

Mercy, J. A., Rosenberg, M. L., Powell, K. E., Broome, C. V., & Roper, W. L. (1993). Public health policy for preventing violence. *Health Affairs*. *12*(4), 7–29. doi.org/10.1377/hlthaff.12.4.7

Moylan, C. A., & Jovorka, M. (2020). Widening the lens: An ecological review of campus sexual assault. *Trauma, Violence, & Abuse*, *21*(1), 179–192. doi.org/10.1177/1524838018756121

Nation, M., Crusto, C., Wandersman, A., Kumpfer, K., Seybolt, D., Morrisey-Kane, E., & Davino, K. (2003). What works in prevention: Principles of effective prevention programs. *American Psychologist*, *58*(6/7), 449–456. doi.org/10.1037/0003-066X.58.6-7.449

Newlands, R., & O'Donohue, W. (2016). A critical review of sexual violence prevention on college campuses. *Acta Psychopathologica*, *2*(2), 1–13. doi.org/10.4172/2469-6676.100040

NNEDV. (2017). *The Violence Against Women Act*. National Network to End Domestic Violence. https://nnedv.org/content/violence-against-women-act/

Noonan, R. K., & Gibbs, D. (2009). Empowerment evaluation with programs designed to prevent first-time male perpetration of sexual violence. *Health Promotion Practice*, *10*(1 suppl), 5S–10S. doi.org/10.1177/1524839908329139

Norris, J. (2008). *The relationship between alcohol consumption and sexual assault victimization*. VAWnet: The National Online Resource Center on Violence Against Women. https://vawnet.org/sites/default/files/materials/files/2016-09/AR_AlcVictimization.pdf

Parks, L. J., Piatt, A., Fulton, D., Lee, D., & Marroquin, J. (2018). *Building bridges to culturally-informed prevention: Summary of findings and recommendations from the California domestic violence and sexual violence prevention initiative*. California Partnership to End Domestic Violence and California Coalition Against Sexual Assault. www.calcasa.org/wp-content/uploads/2019/02/BuildingBridges_021119.pdf

Pottera, S., Moschella, E., Moynihan, M. M., & Smith, D. (2022). Sexual violence among LGBQ community college students: A comparison with their heterosexual peers. *Community College Journal of Research and Practice*, *44*(10–12), 787–803. doi.org/10.1080/10668926.2019.1706668

Prevention Institute & National Sexual Violence Resource Center [NSVRC]. (2021). *A health equity approach to preventing sexual violence*. Prevention Institute and National Sexual Violence Resource Center. www.nsvrc.org/sites/default/files/2021-06/health_equity_approach_to_preventing_sv_final508_0.pdf

Smith, R. A. E., & Pick, L. H. (2015). Sexual assault experienced by deaf female undergraduates: Prevalence and characteristics. *Violence and Victims*, *30*(6), 948–959. doi.org/10.1891/0886-6708.VV-D-14-00057

Tharp, A. T., DeGue, S., Valle, L. A., Brookmeyer K. A., Massetti, G. M., & Matjasko, J. L. (2013). A systematic qualitative review of risk and protective factors for sexual violence perpetration. *Trauma, Violence, & Abuse*, *14*(2), 133–167. doi .org/10.1177/1524838012470031

The Education Amendments Act of 1972, 20 U.S.C. Ð 1681–1688 (1972). www.justice .gov/crt/title-ix-education-amendments-1972

The Jeanne Clery Disclosure of Campus Security Policy and Campus Crime Statistics Act (20 U.S.C. §1092(f)) (1990).

Tolan, P. H, & Guerra, N. G. (1994). *What works in reducing adolescent violence: An empirical review of the field.* Center for the Study and Prevention of Violence.

VetoViolence. (2020). *General capacity assessment for violence prevention resources.* Centers for Disease Control and Prevention Injury Prevention and Control Division of Violence Prevention. https://vetoviolence.cdc.gov/apps/capacity-assessment-tool/#/resources#top

Vladutiu, C. J., Martin, S. L., & Macy, R. J. (2011). College- or university-based sexual assault prevention programs: A review of program outcomes, characteristics, and recommendations. *Trauma, Violence, & Abuse*, *12*(2), 67–86. doi .org/10.1177/1524838010390708

Walters, M. L., Chen J., & Breiding, M. J. (2013). *The National Intimate Partner and Sexual Violence Survey (NISVS): 2010 findings on victimization by sexual orientation.* National Center for Injury Prevention and Control, Centers for Disease Control and Prevention.

Wandersman, A. (2019). Empowerment evaluation: A stakeholder involvement approach. *Health Promotion Journal of Australia*, *30*(2), 137–142. doi.org/10.1002/hpja.243

Wasco, S. M., & Zadnik, L. (2013). *Assessing campus readiness for prevention: Supporting campuses in creating safe and respectful communities.* Pennsylvania Coalition Against Rape.

White House Task Force to Protect Students from Sexual Assault. (2014). *Not alone: The first report of the White House task force to protect students from sexual assault.* White House.

## Suggested Resources

### Campus Sexual Violence Policies

The VAWA Act Clery Act: www.govinfo.gov/content/pkg/FR-2014-10-20/pdf/2014-24284.pdf

### Organizational Capacity Assessment Tools

Prevention Institute. (n.d.). Collaboration multiplier: www.preventioninstitute.org/tools/collaboration-multiplier

General Capacity Assessment for Violence Prevention: https://vetoviolence.cdc.gov/apps/capacity-assessment-tool/#/

### Organizations

Centers for Disease Control and Prevention Injury Prevention and Control Center: www.cdc.gov/violenceprevention/sexualviolence/

It's On Us: www.itsonus.org/about-us/our-story/
The National Sexual Violence Resource Center (NSVRC): www.nsvrc.org
PreventConnect: www.preventconnect.org
Raliance: www.raliance.org/

## Sexual Violence Prevention Programming Guides/Toolkits

American College Health Association. (2020). *Addressing sexual and relationship violence: A trauma-informed approach*. American College Health Association.

Basile, K. C., DeGue, S., Jones, K., Freire, K., Dills, J., Smith, S. G., & Raiford, J. L. (2016). *STOP SV: A technical package to prevent sexual violence*. National Center for Injury Prevention and Control, Centers for Disease Control and Prevention. www.cdc.gov/violenceprevention/pdf/sv-prevention-technical-package.pdf

Campus Technical Assistance and Resource Project. (2017). *Addressing gender-based violence on college campuses: A guide to a comprehensive strategy*. Center for Changing Our Campus Culture.

Centers for Disease Control and Prevention [CDC]. (2014). *Preventing sexual violence on college campuses: Lessons from research and practice*. Centers for Disease Control and Prevention.

Cox, P.J., Keener, D., Woodard, T., & Wandersman, A. (2009). *Evaluation for improvement: A seven step Empowerment Evaluation approach for violence prevention organizations*. Centers for Disease Control and Prevention.

Dills, J., Fowler, D., & Payne, G. (2016). *Sexual violence on campus: Strategies for prevention*. National Center for Injury Prevention and Control, Centers for Disease Control and Prevention. www.cdc.gov/violenceprevention/pdf/campussvprevention.pdf

Miller, R. J., & Shinn, M. (2005). Learning from communities: Overcoming difficulties in dissemination of prevention and promotion efforts. *American Journal of Community Psychology*, *35*(3–4), 169–183. doi.org/10.1007/s10464-005-3395-1

Schwartzman, N. (2020). *Red roll red toolkit: College athletic administrators, coaches and counselors*. Raliance. www.raliance.org/report_posts/roll-red-roll-toolkit-for-college-coaches/

Thomas-Williams, C. O. (2017). *Sidewalks to sexual violence protection: A guide to exploring social inclusion with adults with developmental & intellectual disabilities*. Indiana Coalition Against Domestic Violence. https://icadvinc.org/wp-content/uploads/2019/12/new-sidewalks-to-sexual-violence-prevention.pdf

# 11 College: The Window of Opportunity

Genevieve E. Chandler and Jim Helling

> I feel like a fire fighter called to a burning building, always arriving on the scene too late, after the damage is done. All I can do is try to limit the loss and get everyone out in one piece.
>
> J. Helling (second author, personal communication, April 2016)

Embedded in the Department of Athletics as a sports social worker, athletic counselor, and performance consultant, Jim, the second author, witnessed the fallout from an under resourced and reactive mental health support system. Typically, Jim's referrals were being made after intercollegiate athletes were already missing practices, neglecting assignments, or misusing substances. Jim could see that to thrive students needed support before they ran into difficulty. His experience of too little, too late matched my mantra, "Why wait?" We know the transition to college is predictably stressful for all students and especially for intercollegiate athletes, so why wait to intervene until students are already floundering? This inquiry led to the creation of a general education course, Changing Minds, Changing Lives (CMCL), open to all students, specifically designed to disrupt the stress-to-struggle trajectory upstream of illness and debilitation.

Surveying the scientific literature and drawing on original research, we developed an experiential learning curriculum to meet basic students' psychological needs, buffer predictable stress, and promote health. The wellness curriculum, Changing Minds, Changing Lives (CMCL), is an experiential, strength-based, and skill forward approach to illness prevention. Building a wellness culture around the CMCL-based model changes the campus environment to furnish students with critical experiences of competence, agency, and relatedness that can facilitate autonomy and self-efficacy. Delivering the curriculum at scale alters the trajectory of stress to struggle at the individual level and fortifies psychological resilience at the organizational level by building a culture of wellness in the campus community.

The CMCL model emerged from resilience research and theory development to identify and operationalize a set of essential resilience competencies for college students to facilitate healthy coping, academic success, and personal thriving. Based on translational research, we define resilience as a process of how an individual, group, or a community responds to adversity by utilizing internal attributes, building on existing strengths and cultivating connections to access available resources to meet the challenge and grow from the experience. This evidence-based definition differs from the popular belief that resilience is limited to bouncing back from adversity by pulling yourself up by your bootstraps and soldiering on. That may be a good place to start, but it is neither sufficiently flexible nor skillful to be sustainable. In this chapter, we describe the CMCL model and explain how a strengths-based curriculum of psychological wellness promotion can buffer stress and boost success during life transition. The social determination theory and social–ecological model provide the theoretical framework. To capture the outcome data, our research methods are described. We end with operationalizing the constructs of strength-based teaching, mindfulness practice, expressive writing, and inclusion with recommendations on how to integrate these key constructs in any college course.

## 11.1 Changing Minds, Changing Lives to Promote Health

Changing Minds, Changing Lives is not a typical college curriculum that relies on assigned readings, lectures, and tests to teach students about resilience. Rather than teaching about resilience, CMCL teaches students how to be resilient. The course pedagogy and practices invite and guide students to be resilient by recognizing how they experience the resilience response. The resilience response is a sequence of physiological, affective, cognitive, interpersonal, and behavioral actions that begin with orienting to a salient challenge cue and culminates in focused engagement in purposeful, adaptive action. A resilience response consists of actions to mobilize relevant assets and leverage social connections to navigate adversity. The pedagogy is based on neuroscientific studies of habit formation, neuroplasticity, and learning models. To encourage habit formation, the action components of resilience are taught through repetition of structured activities that call upon students to engage and practice core resilience competencies. Proficiency in the actions emerges from this repetition of small activities over time, a type of nondeclarative or procedural learning (Grigsby & Stevens, 2002). Declarative learning is learning about something so one can name it, analyze it, and describe it. Procedural learning, by contrast, is acquiring the action skills to do something. It is the difference between telling you about what a bicycle is, describing how it works, and getting on a bike. In the CMCL course, we combine both declarative learning of studying resilience theory and reviewing empirical research with procedural learning by practicing the sequence of actions that comprise the resilience response.

The college years provide a window of opportunity for emerging adults to learn new skills to self-regulate and socialize, develop healthy habits, and establish capabilities that can reduce stress and increase success throughout the lifespan. The emerging adult years are a sensitive period for higher cognitive development actively shaped by patterns of response to life challenge. Cortical brain areas associated with integration of self-regulation and meaning-making including executive function, impulse control, emotion modulation, and contextualization, are consolidating functional network connectivity during this period (Taber-Thomas & Koraly, 2015). Preventing stress-related debilitation and facilitating health promotion through successful adaptation to the challenges of emerging adulthood builds a foundation of self-efficacy and self-confidence that generalizes into an identity as a "can-do" person. The CMCL model facilitates this identity transformation through experiences of personal effectiveness in coping and capability in adapting to the challenge of college life.

The CMCL strength-based model is designed to invite students to take charge of their own learning by using their voices through writing, reflecting, and sharing feedback. Every class begins with a check-in to invite each participant's voice to be heard. Participants share a strength that they used in the past week and their experience with a positive practice they have selected from the textbook (Chandler, 2021). Following the check-in, a guided relaxation practice is designed to facilitate presence, receptivity, and neurobiological readiness to learn. Once the group is alert and settled, a bite-sized piece of research is presented with an invitation to write for five minutes to describe their own life experience with the research topic. For example, in the class on leadership, the research presentation covers the history, styles, and characteristics of leaders from autocrats to the servant leaders. In response, students are prompted to write about a leader who has made an impression on them, such as a historical figure, a celebrity, or someone in their life. The majority of students write about a leader in their own life. The writing prompt elicits stories that they then share with each other in small breakout groups. Peer feedback on the writing is structured to be affirmative and focus on strengths of the writing. In sharing the stories and receiving feedback, students discover both similarities and differences in their experience and perspective. Students report feeling respected and welcomed for what they have brought to the group and feel empowered and connected when they see the impact of their feedback on their peers. They can see, hear, and feel the difference that their active self-leadership makes in their own learning experience.

Every class concludes with a reflective ritual in which each individual describes something they learned in the last hour, something they appreciated hearing in class, or a question or suggestion they may have. One student commented,

> I thought I just can outwork things and stand on top of them. The [class] changed that. Now I understand better what resilience means for me. It changed from working out everything to giving just more intention and energy to taking a step back, understand what's happening around me, and realizing what I need to do to cope to overcome the stress.

CMCL has served as a first-year seminar, a senior capstone, and a reorientation course for students on academic probation. In addition to multiple sections open to the general undergraduate population, the colleges of business, engineering, nursing, and natural sciences have offered the course. The Center for Multicultural Student Success and the Honors College have adopted the curriculum to support first-generation students, students of color, and those matriculating from under resourced public schools. In the most recent academic year, over 450 students completed courses employing the CMCL curriculum at our home campus. We also support satellite programs at other institutions. The outcomes have been consistent across schools, levels and majors with 90% of the students highly recommending that every student has an opportunity to take the course. One student commented in 2022: "I learned many strategies to deal with something I [sic] been struggling with this whole year of transition: stress." Another student noted in 2021: "Learning to understand and care for yourself in the presence of others working towards the same goal is beneficial in being happier and more self-sufficient."

CMCL students report two types of beneficial change after completing the course, social–emotional skill development, and personal transformation. Pre- and post-surveys indicate an increase in the ability to cope with stress, improvement in managing emotions, enhanced self-efficacy, and a stronger sense of belonging, all antecedents for persisting and succeeding in college (Hartley, 2011; McNaughton-Cassill et al., 2021; Mrazek et al., 2018). Qualitative data show improved leadership capacity, stronger role engagement, and a greater respect for differences. A consistent pattern in student narratives indicates an increase in competence, agency, and community relatedness:

> This semester has been one of the most difficult ones I had to go through, and this class helped me tremendously in conquering those battles. Understanding to breathe and be compassionate with myself was vital to finishing the semester strong. What happened to me this semester would have prevented me from continuing on. However, this class reinforced my resilience in making sure I have the tools necessary to make it out of whatever situation I am in. I am grateful for all the lessons this course has taught me.

Student feedback from both in-person and remote instructional experiences attributes the wellness learning outcomes to writing and sharing stories, feeling respected by peers and faculty, and using identified strengths in daily life (Chandler et al., 2020).

## 11.2 The Theory behind the Curriculum

CMCL is a theory-grounded, evidence-based curricular approach to wellness promotion that focuses on fostering healthy adaptation to challenge in order to disrupt the stress-to-struggle trajectory and prevent illness. Self-determination theory (Ryan & Deci, 2000) and a social–ecological model of psychological function (Ungar, 2018) are the theoretical bases for the CMCL wellness course. Within self-determination theory, the basic psychological needs of competence, autonomy, and relatedness must be met to facilitate thriving (Ryan & Deci, 2000). In the CMCL curriculum, competence and autonomy increase from exercises that teach practical skills ranging from self-regulation to self-expression. The relaxation practices in each class acquaint students with a range of tools and techniques to modulate arousal, balance emotions, and increase focus. Writing in response to the weekly topic and sharing their stories of success and struggle, along with receiving affirming peer feedback, provides students with the critical connection that boosts the felt sense of relatedness. The social–ecological model that informs our understanding of resilience is based on the assumption that interactions between the individual and the environment significantly shape cognitive, emotional, and behavioral responses (Bronfenbrenner, 1974). Ungar (2018) emphasizes the critical contribution of access to culturally resonant relationships and resources for successful growth, noting "Our success depends on how well others provide us what we need to survive and thrive, and motivation is only a small part of the reason why some people do well, and others do not" (p. 6).

The learning objectives of the CMCL curriculum focus on three core competencies of resilience: active coping, building strengths, and cultivating connections (Chandler et al., 2019). Active coping is being ready to bring skills to bear when they are needed by identifying what skills have worked in the past and learning what new capabilities can be added for the future. Active coping includes emotional self-regulation, decision-making, help-seeking, cognitive reframing, self-compassion, and a growth mindset. Building strengths starts with identifying the individual's top five psychological strengths and developing a plan to use the strengths in their daily life to develop a sense of agency and self-efficacy. Cultivating connections means expressing oneself authentically and listening opening and respectfully to others while learning how to access needed resources.

With a small class size, a high level of classroom interaction with faculty and peers, and multiple immersive learning experiences in the curriculum, CMCL embodies features of high-impact education practices (HIEP; Kuh, 2008). HIEP are known to significantly advance student success and connectedness. HIEP are well suited to practical training in psychosocial wellness with an emphasis on culturally relevant learning. Most resilience training programs consist largely of psychoeducational sessions that are prerecorded or in webinar format. A central aspect relies on addressing deficiencies, focusing on adapting to failure, and employing self-reliant resilience strategies. The CMCL curriculum differs in that it is strength focused, as opposed to deficit, failure-oriented courses, through experiential learning, in-class interactions, and homework practice that engage participants in activities that build new patterns and habits of responding to stress and facilitating growth. CMCL has shown a robust capacity to engage students from diverse backgrounds even those starting with a preference for self-reliant forms of resilience and who are unaccustomed to sharing personal material in a new social environment. One student noted,

> Sharing with others was uncomfortable for me. It's just unnatural to be sharing my personal stories with people I don't know. I learned that even though it felt weird my anxiety was eased because everybody was very open, willing to listen and be supportive.

The social ecology of the CMCL classroom functions as an opportunity structure that elicits expression of latent, implicit, and unrecognized resilience competencies including an interest to be known, connect, and belong.

## 11.3 Resilience Boosts Prevention and Health Promotion

Whether two or seventy-two years old, we all have an inherent drive to thrive. In our individualistic, achievement-oriented culture, we often start to respond to adversity by using our "push through the pain" attitude; we use our grit. Though armoring up and pushing through may be one way to begin, we educate and empower our students to broaden their resilience repertoire, to expand their network of relationships and resources.

The grit approach emerged from studies of elite, top-level performers. Persistence rather than raw talent was found to be the most important individual character trait for highest percentile achievement in a variety of fields (Duckworth & Seligman, 2017). Among the *crème de la crème*, grit will differentiate those who rise to the very top. Little consideration was given to social–ecological factors that determine access to health-promoting and development-facilitating resources. In many instances, access to those facilitative resources, including mentoring relationships, social capital, good schools, or adequate health care, may be the decisive factor that leads to individual success. Why are so few African American athletes found on soccer pitches, tennis courts, ice rinks, lacrosse fields, or in swimming pools? Clearly not for lack of grit or some other character trait. Sociocultural disparities in access to resources likely explain the underrepresentation of top-level Black athletes in these sports. Additionally, character-based models of resilience have a hard time explaining how resilience varies from day to day. Character traits are defined as relatively stable over time, but an individual's resilience frequently varies depending on the situation and the internal and external resources available.

Our ecological approach to thriving began with studying the long-term health effects of early life adversity (Kalmakis & Chandler, 2014, 2015). The adverse childhood experiences (ACEs) study is the research that fundamentally changed our understanding of emotional stress loads, psychological traumatization, and their devastating effects on physical, social, and mental health across the lifespan (Felitti et al., 1998; Wade et al., 2016). Our line of inquiry became: How can we disrupt the trajectory from high early life stress exposure to compromised adult health? Surveying the literature, we found an answer: Build resilience, the inherent drive to thrive characteristic of all living organisms. Missing in the research, however, were two things which became our research and practice foci: first, a useful description of the process of resilience, and second, a protocol to strengthen and elicit resilience responses during times of stress. The process of resilience begins with an internal locus of control, a sense of agency that increases the likelihood of managing stress successfully (Rutter, 2012). Yet, our own internal sense of agency, the "I can do this" attitude, is only the initial step. Though the resilience process is often described as the individual rebounding through their own exertion that is actually a myth. No one is resilient on their own. Our celebrity superstars, our Olympic athletes, and our top politicians have a whole entourage right behind them. Resilience involves an interaction between what we have inside of us and the support of others and the external resources the environment has to offer. For example, an internal attribute may be our curiosity. We may be curious in some accepting, welcoming environments where our curiosity, our interest, and our questioning are encouraged. In other more judgmental, evaluative environments, however, we may be less likely to communicate or even experience our curiosity. Our self-expression and interaction vary depending on the relationships in the current situation and the resources that are available and are culturally resonant.

Though the propensity for resilience may start with genetics and neurobiology, it is greatly influenced by social and environmental factors. Individual variables, such as stress reactivity and personality style, as well as social variables, such as family, friends, and accessible community resources, impact our ability to be resilient. As Ungar (2018) states, "Resilience is not a do-it-yourself endeavor" (p. 14). The good news is that resilience is a process that can be operationalized, taught, and learned (Houston et al., 2017). With practice, the ability to be resilient in managing stress can facilitate changes to central nervous system structure and function that are associated with enhanced emotional regulation (Nechvatal & Lyons, 2013). Thus, we become more adept at recognizing and managing our emotions as we develop our capacity to be resilient.

Though scientific study of resilience began with asking "Who is resilient?" as the science advanced, the question became "What kind of resilience does one have?" This shift from thinking that only a certain few select individuals have resilience to the understanding that everyone is resilient in different ways introduces the idea of being able to build resilience, thereby increasing the capacity to prevent illness and promote health.

In studying resilience in a low-resource high school, the consensus at that time was that resilient adolescents were those with good grades, good attendance, and involvement in extracurricular activities (Chandler, 1999). Researchers assumed that high achievers must be those with the most resilience, so studies focused on identifying common traits found among these successful students. In studying and writing with diverse groups of students in a low-resource high school, however, a very different picture emerged. By contrast, the students in the study sample did not attend school regularly, had jobs after school, and had lower grades. They all, however, wrote stories of being resilient. Their stories of rising to cope with struggle, racism, poverty, and challenge certainly confirmed their belief. Far from lacking resilience, these young people showed resilience in forms unrecognized and even rendered invisible by the prevailing consensus model. The outcome of these studies led to the development of the resilience continuum (Hunter & Chandler, 1999). On one end of the continuum was health-defeating resilience, commonly thought of as health risk behavior, such as hiding emotions or isolating from others or by using whatever resources were available to manage stress such as smoking, drinking, or using illicit drugs. Health-defeating behavior, like drug or alcohol use, often starts as a way to manage stress or emotional pain. No one starts smoking with a plan to have lung cancer or uses drugs to develop endocarditis. When we view health-defeating behaviors as tools to manage stress using the resources available, we are better able to see the hidden resilience behind the risk behavior. When there are more enriched resource options in the community or family environment, then individuals can move up the continuum toward more health-promoting forms of resilience such as supportive social connections, better nutrition, regular exercise, or accessing other culturally relevant resources (Figure 11.1).

The Resilience Continuum adds a different perspective to health defeating behaviors that includes the individual interaction with their environment,

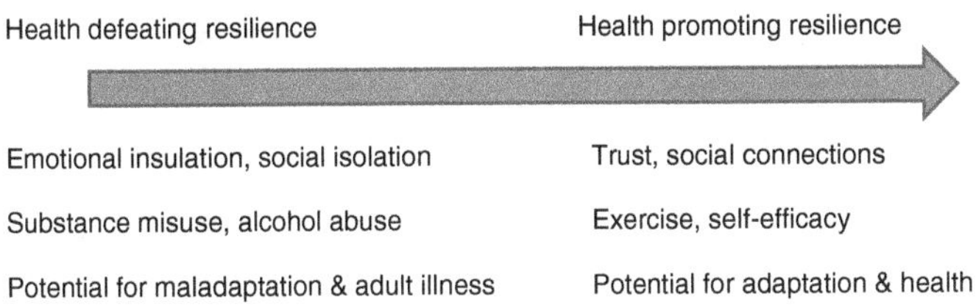


Figure 11.1 Resilience continuum

When considering the individual and their environment then the focus can be on strategies to alter social ecologies, enrich resource environments and teach skills to facilitate movement to more health-promoting resilience behaviors to disrupt the stress to struggle trajectory.

## 11.4 Research Design and Results

Outcome research has been a critical component in developing and refining the CMCL model. Mixed method research design allows us to capture and interpret pre-to-post participant changes. Over the seven years of data collection using a battery of standard instruments and detailed statistical analysis, the results indicate a significant increase in emotional awareness, decision-making, resilience, and sense of belonging (Chandler et al., 2020, 2022). The qualitative data set consists of student writing and final presentations from the course, which include self-assessments of learning outcomes, identification of mechanisms of change, and an evaluation of the personal significance of changes experienced (Chandler et al., 2020, 2022). The qualitative narratives are instrumental in identifying subtleties of change experienced by participants that are not easily measured quantitatively, such as shifts in identity development, role engagement, and leadership capacity. The results indicate that students participating in CMCL experience two kinds of change: skill acquisition and personal transformation (Helling & Chandler, 2019). Alterations in self-schemas emerge from experiences that expand participants' general sense of competence, agency, connectedness, and personal effectiveness. This improvement in general self-efficacy indicates that participants gain practical knowledge of themselves as capable, effective, and responsive young adults. Self-confidence scaffolds persistence by building intrinsic motivation, which is strongly associated with high levels of satisfaction and enhanced performance (Mahoney et al., 2014). A robust positive sense of self equips emerging young adults to meet challenge with confidence and to respond to adversity with flexibility, the hallmarks of resilience. The data indicate that the CMCL pedagogy provides the information, opportunities, resources, and relationships to empower student resilience and a reliable pathway to thriving.

Strength-based teaching, mindfulness practices, expressive writing, and inclusiveness are the key components that make the CMCL curriculum effective in promoting health. These key components can be integrated into any course.

## 11.5 Start with Strength

> It's more efficient and effective to build on strengths rather than try to correct problems
>
> (Luther & Cicchetti, 2000).

The strength-based teaching classroom is a unique gathering place where the instructor locates and affirms the assets and capabilities that each student brings to the table. Identifying strengths contributes to meeting the basic psychological need for competence and lays the groundwork for self-efficacy (Ryan & Deci, 2000). Starting with strengths is a different approach for students who are used to focusing on what they do not know in academic work and what they lack in social–emotional skill. Inviting students to share past positive experience, their success and their abilities build a strength base to grow from. Anchoring in past success is the best way to expand and extend capability by building on the strengths we already possess rather than focusing on where we are deficient. Strengths do not mean armoring up to be tough and invulnerable, but rather operating from a strength base is being open to others' perceptions, open to change, open to vulnerability, and receptive to new ideas. As one student noted, "One thing I learned by listening in class is that you have many ways to cope with situations. I learned by listening that you should never judge anyone."

People learn faster, perform better, and feel more engaged when their strengths are highlighted rather than emphasizing their deficiencies. Evoking strength activates the areas and operations of the brain that are involved with receptivity, openness to change, and positive feelings. Recognizing strengths activates a cycle of self-efficacy in which people attribute agency to themselves as a positive force for change. With both students and faculty trained to focus on what we do not know in order to grow and improve, it does take practice to change our brain, refocus on capabilities, and emphasize what we do well. Changing habits involves working with procedural memory, a specific memory system for actions. Neuroplastic learning and procedural change develop through repetition and recognition of small positive actions in daily life. The use of reflection, visualization, and writing begin to create new neural pathways that grow stronger with practice. Within class, the instructor continuously surveys the classroom landscape for opportunities to highlight student strengths. The instructor models emotional attunement that is expressed nonverbally through facial expressions, eye contact, and gestures. Attuning and responding to students' emotions establishes a sense of affective resonance in the classroom and provides participants with the felt experience of being heard, understood, and seen. Explicit recognition such as thanking a student for sharing a particularly emotive, charged, or perceptive comment contributions invites further engagement. The strength-based pedagogical approach cultivates and holds the classroom as a secure environment in which witnessing takes priority over evaluating, inviting a free flow of ideas and expression. Students respond to the experience of being witnessed in their full humanity by spontaneously bringing more of themselves into view. With faculty modeling acceptance and witnessing, students follow suit, creating a positive feedback loop that rewards joining in and sharing more. One student commented, "This class taught me that when you join in you can get to know one another. When we joined in by sharing our writing we got more comfortable with one another."

As instructors, sometimes we have to look deeply to find the hidden strength that animates a reactive, evasive, or resistant response. For example, when a student misses class or is late submitting an assignment, we ask ourselves what strength that student might be expressing. When we find ourselves unable to locate a ready answer to this question, it moves us to inquire further, to connect with the student, learn more about them, and hear more of their story. Rather than judging students based on their compliance with educational directives, we stay curious about what strengths they have available to build on in their learning journey. One student shared, "Strengths can benefit you any many ways. By knowing your strengths, you can put them in action to helping you overcome situations."

## 11.6 Be Mindful

Learning to be in the moment, to cultivate calm, and to be present is an essential practice in strength-based teaching. Mindfulness is the mental action of noticing the present moment internal and external experience. A brief mindfulness practice, like observing the sensations and movements of breath, is a good beginning. We can direct mindful attention to any activity of daily life to bring ourselves more fully into the present moment, from noticing how our hands are holding our phone to looking up to see a cloud passing overhead.

Though the origin of mindfulness is in spiritual meditative practices, mindfulness is now recognized as a useful psychological skill that can support greater well-being (Kabat-Zinn, 1994). Numerous elite colleges, professional organizations, and Olympic athlete programs provide mindfulness skills training to optimize performance and prepare for competition (Mumford, 2015; Rogers, 2016). Directing mindful attention to the sensory, motor, or cognitive components of experience activates a particular way of being present. This practice can be used in any class to facilitate greater mental clarity, emotional balance, ease, and stability. A student observed, "Knowing how to calm down helps me sleep at night. I follow the same steps we do in class and notice that tension leaves my body."

## 11.7 Expressive Writing

"Writing isn't therapy, but it can be healing," Pat Schneider (2003) observed. Empirical studies have shown a positive relationship between expressive writing and physical and mental health. Substantial peer-reviewed research documents that prompted free writing improve self-awareness, emotional processing, and immune system functioning (Pennebaker, 1997). In the CMCL classroom, the writing process is modeled after the Amherst Writers and Artist method where instructors write and share their stories, along with students, to establish the mutuality and reciprocity that leads to engaged learning (Schneider, 2003). Writing with the students decreases the sense of hierarchy and power differential between students and faculty. We follow bell hooks (1994) approach, "In my class I do not expect students to take any risk I would not take, to share in any way I would not share" (p. 21).

The free write instructions invite students to write continuously for five minutes writing whatever comes to mind without stopping until the page is filled or time runs out. Participants are advised not to pay attention to spelling or grammar. Instructors establish an expectation of confidentiality about the content of all writing and the privacy of every writer by letting students know all writing and comments stay in the room. With practice, students learn to respect themselves and each other as authors and narrators with important stories to tell and unique perspectives to share. In-class expressive writing is purposefully limited to five minutes. The brief time frame is not as intimidating as a longer time request may be. In addition, when the time is longer or left open, the author may inadvertently go into too much detail, becoming overwhelmed, or feel too exposed. Five minutes provides a reasonable amount of time to write a meaningful story but not too much that a writer might inadvertently overshare or become dysregulated.

After the brief free writing, students and instructors move into small groups to share their stories and receive feedback. The guidelines call for feedback to be affirming, focused on the strengths of the writing without criticism, grammatical corrections, questions, or free association to one's own story. Participants are instructed to listen attentively and respond to each other respectfully just as they would like others to receive their writing. Following a strength-based approach, after a participant shares their story, feedback emphasizes what was strong about the writing and what stayed with you about the story. Attentive listening is required to identify strengths in each story shared. Recognizing what works well in the writing, rather than the usual emphasis on what the author could improve, invites students to reflect positively on their value as storytellers and their identity as emerging writers. The positive feedback encourages students to write more freely and to have more confidence in their ability as writers. Open expression and receptivity to feedback are the important mutative factors. One student remarked, "I started being very nervous about writing. A lot of it is personal. Bit-by-bit I grew more comfortable with it, and it definitely helped me feel more connected to my peers and instructors and build a sense of community." Being in community, creating connection, and having a sense of belonging are key contributors to persistence and success in school. Sharing stories and feedback with authenticity, attunement, and appreciation is a powerfully transformative experience for many students, as evidenced by this comment from a student: "Our stories matter and sharing them helps reduce stigma. It is so beneficial to hear from others and be an active listener as you can come to know more about yourself." Another student observed:

> I liked writing the best because it was very beneficial to me to reflect and realize I am more strong and have more of these qualities than I think I do. Writing made me feel better about myself. I also liked hearing other people's stories. That was the best thing being in class with everyone else. It just felt like a good way to connect and understand everyone.

Similarly, a student stated, "Listening to my peers share meaningful stories in small groups allowed me to gain insight and understand new ideas." Students relate to what they hear in each other's stories and learn two invaluable lessons: First, they learn that they are not alone in their struggles and growing pains; second, through an affirming and strength-based group process, affiliation grows stronger both through realization of similarity and recognition and respect for differences.

## 11.8 Include All

We understand our role and responsibility as strength-based, multicultural educators to reshape the relational space of the classroom to welcome, receive, and value each student in their uniqueness. As instructors, we meet before and after each class to discuss how to make adjustments within the relational container of the classroom so that there is a place provided for everyone to participate, be heard, be seen, and be respected. As one student stated,

> At first it was kind of awkward introducing ourselves to the class. But as the class went by, I got to become friends with some people out of the class this showed me that it doesn't hurt to join in even when you're shy.

Experience and data have shown that the CMCL model works well with multicultural populations (Chandler et al., 2020). The program was specifically designed to work in high-stress, under resourced communities to address social disparities in stress exposure, to accommodate different cultural preferences for pathways to well-being, and to fill the large existing gaps in culturally relevant and resonant resources in college mental health systems of care (Helling & Chandler, 2019). As White college educators of a certain age and generation, we recognized that we could not represent the diverse identities that our students, initially comprised of athletes in the revenue-producing sports of football and basketball, would bring into the classroom. While recruiting, training, and including instructors of color, we are aware that Black faculty and mental health clinicians are chronically underrepresented on predominantly White US campuses and in elite college athletic departments (Kroshus et al., 2023; Helling & Chandler, 2019). Notwithstanding these significant concerns and limitations, we are also mindful of the critical lack of program models designed to meet the needs of college students and athletes of color (The Steve Fund & JED Foundation, 2017). With the pedagogical approach based on peer-focused group interaction through their stories, students connect to each other. As instructors, we can leverage the diversity in our classrooms as one of the strengths of the program by creating a learning environment in which the diverse voices are spotlighted, while the authority and expertise of the faculty are decentralized. Analysis of quantitative data shows unusual model sensitivity and effectiveness with higher stress participants, including athletes of color and first-generation students (Chandler et al., 2020; Helling & Chandler, 2019).

Our students frequently attribute positive change associated with the course experience to peer interaction than with facilitation factors associated with faculty performance. Group-as-a-whole dynamics and peer-to-peer connections provide the culturally resonant mirroring that makes the classroom experience comfortable for Black participants in the absence of a facilitator of their sociocultural identity. The following exchange between students in a breakout group is representative:

WRITER: "I am from somewhere I yet to understand, places I shall not go, loved ones I barely know. I am from a frighten [*sic*] place. A place where memories were hard and tough."

PEER FEEDBACK: "I know that place, I don't know exactly where [you come from] but I know that place."

PEER FEEDBACK: "That's so relatable. I feel you my brother."

Another student described how emerging group norms of engagement, openness, and mutuality, including with instructors, transformed his sense of possibility for learning, connection, and emotional sharing. He wrote,

> In high school I never went to class so I thought I would come here and never go to class. I was surprised that everyone opened up so fast. In the projects where I come from if you tried to express yourself you would get punched, but I finally was able to get things off my chest that I never had before. And not only were my teammates sharing, the teachers were sharing too and that helped everyone to get closer and feel more comfortable.

As facilitators, positioning ourselves as a guide on the side instead of a sage on the stage created space for student voices, student experiences, and student cultural identities to take a central position in the classroom. The student-centered classroom provides the culturally resonant mirroring essential for sustained engagement and learning.

Our research indicates that CMCL helps level the sociocultural playing field and circumvent uncritical replication of prevailing inequities in social capital and social power in the college athletic and student health systems. Students and athletes with higher childhood stress loads show greater improvements in resilience after participating in the CMCL course than their lower stress peers (Chandler et al., 2020). These are important considerations given the elevated stress burdens carried by multicultural students on predominantly White campuses, the lack of culturally relevant psychological wellness resources, and cultural preferences for nonprofessional support resources. The overrepresentation of Black athletes in college sports and the chronic underrepresentation of higher education professionals of color among faculty, administrators, and college mental health staff add to the need for curricular programs that normalize stress, de-pathologize symptoms, and teach life skills so all can succeed.

## 11.9 Recommendations for Strength-Based Prevention

The Changing Minds, Changing Lives resilience program incorporates teaching, research, and policy elements that can be integrated into prevention programs at higher education institutions and in the workplace to buffer stress and improve wellness. The empowerment formula of providing information, opportunities, resources, and relationships offers a ready template for designing program objectives that will meet basic psychological needs and facilitate thriving. The best way to start is to ask the straightforward question, "What is working well?" Once an inventory of assets and a clear sense of your strategic program objectives have been established, strength-based leadership will empower stakeholders to move toward their goals.

Strength-based leadership focuses on sharing assets and commonly held goals to improve morale, facilitate engagement, and enhance performance by:

- Use of surveys or focus groups to identify stakeholder strengths. Working from strengths builds a culture of positivity, mutual support, and respect.

- Create opportunities for students to learn about their strengths and collaborate on developing a plan to put their strengths into action. Collaboration fosters mutual appreciation and connection.
- Invite stories of past experiences that demonstrate managing stress, being resilient and knowing a leader. Student stories bring the expertise of the stakeholders into the room and decenter authority.
- Plan time for structured dialogue and positive feedback that sets judgment aside. Authentic sharing of experiences and receiving affirming, appreciative responses build connection and belonging.
- Develop culturally relevant and accessible resources. Culturally attuned resources foster inclusion, respect differences, and create community solidarity.

The strength-based classroom is an opportunity structure designed to facilitate expression of resilience capacities. Opportunity structures are defined as elements placed in the environment which elicit expression of latent capacity (Ungar, 2018). Think about a climbing structure in a public park, a design element deliberately placed in an environment to afford children an opportunity to exert themselves by climbing. The placement of the structure creates the opportunity for the children to express themselves bodily and to explore their physical power. Offering a strength-based course places that facilitative classroom in the campus environment to afford students the opportunity to stretch and develop their resilience muscles, growing their own well-being. Strength-based leadership and opportunity structures combine well to shape action that promotes wellness behavior.

The tools and techniques of well-designed, interactive, strength-based programs can be successfully employed in campus-level prevention efforts. Significant organizational development to secure support from key decision-makers, along with investment in operational capacity building and training in strength-based teaching, is indispensable to implementation at scale. Bringing resilience work out of the clinic and into the classroom can open doors for broad-based cohort and community-level prevention resulting in a culture change based on wellness.

## References

Bronfenbrenner, U. (1974). Developmental research, public policy and the ecology of childhood. *Child Development*, *45*(1), 1–5.

Chandler, G. (1999). A creative writing intervention to enhance self-esteem and self-efficacy in adolescents. *Journal of Child and Adolescent Psychiatric Nursing*, *12*(2), 70–78. doi.org/10.1111/j.1744-6171.1999.tb00047.x

Chandler, G. (2021). *Positive practices: From stress to strength, build your resilience one neuron at a time*. 2trees, LLC

Chandler G. E., Kalmakis, K. A., Chiodo L., Helling J. (2020) The efficacy of a resilience intervention among diverse, at-risk, college athletes: A mixed-methods study. *Journal of the American Psychiatric Nurses Association. 26*(3), 269–281. doi.org/10.1177/1078390319886923

Chandler, G., Kalmakis, K., Chiodo, L., & Helling, J. (2020). Changing minds, changing lives: A resilience intervention with student athletes. *Journal of American Psychiatric Nurses Association, 26*(3), 269–281. doi.org/10.1177/1078390319886923

Duckworth, A. L., & Seligman, M. P. (2017). The science and practice of self-control. *Perspectives on Psychological Science, 12*(5), 715–718. doi.org/10.1177/1745691617690880

Felitti, V. J., Anda, R. F., Nordenberg, D., Williamson, D. F., Spitz, A. M., Edwards, V., & Marks, J. S. (1998). Relationship of childhood abuse and household dysfunction to many of the leading causes of death in adults: The adverse childhood experiences (ACE) study. *American Journal of Preventive Medicine, 14*(4), 245–258. doi.org/10.1016/S0749-3797(98)00017-8

Grigsby, J., & Stevens, D. (2002) Memory, neurodynamics and human relationships. *Psychiatry, 65*(1), 13–34. doi.org/10.1521/psyc.65.1.13.19762

Hartley, M. (2011). Examining the relationships between resilience, mental health, and academic persistence in undergraduate college students. *Journal of American College Health, 59*(7), 596–604. doi.org/10.1080/07448481.2010.515632

Helling, J., & Chandler, G. (2019). Meeting the psychological growth and health needs of Black college students and athletes: Culture, resonance and resilience. *Journal of College Student Psychotherapy, 35*(2), 152–180. doi.org/10.1080/87568225.2019.1660291

Hooks, B. (1994). *Teaching to transgress.* Routledge.

Houston, J. B., First, J., Spialek, M. L., Sorenson, M. E., Mills-Sandoval, T., Lockett, M., & Pfefferbaum, B. (2017). Randomized controlled trial of the Resilience and Coping Intervention (RCI) with undergraduate university students. *Journal of American College Health, 65*, 1–9. doi.org/10.1080/07448481.2016.1227826

Hunter, A., & Chandler, G. (1999). Adolescent resilience. *Image: Journal of Nursing Scholarship, 31*(3), 243–247. doi.org/10.1111/j.1547-5069.1999.tb00488.x

Kabat-Zinn, J. (1994). *Wherever you go there you are.* Hyperion.

Kalmakis, K., & Chandler, G. (2014). Adverse childhood experiences: Towards a clear conceptual meaning, *Journal of Advanced Nursing, 70*(7), 1489–1501. doi.org/10.111/jan.12329

Kalmakis, K. & Chandler, G (2015). Health consequences of adverse childhood experiences: Systematic review. *Journal of American Association of Nurse Practitioners. 27*(8), 458–465. doi.org/10.1002-2327-6924.12215

Kroshus, E., Coakley, S., Conway, D., et al. (2023). Addressing mental health needs of NCAA student-athletes of colour: Foundational concepts from the NCAA Summit on Diverse Student-Athlete Mental Health and Well-Being. *British Journal of Sports Medicine, 57*, 137–145. doi.org/10.1136/bjsports-2022-105891

Kuh, G. (2008). *High impact educational practices: What are they, who has access and why they matter.* Association of American Colleges and Universities.

Luther, S. S., & Cicchetti, D. (2000). The construct of resilience: Implications for interventions and social policies. *Development and Psychopathology, 12*(4), 857–885. doi.org/10.1017/s0954579400004156

Mahoney, J. W., Gucciardi, D. F., Ntoumanis, N., & Mallet, C. J. (2014). Mental toughness in sport: Motivational antecedents and associations with performance and psychological health. *Journal of Sport & Exercise Psychology*, *36*, 281–292. doi .org/10.1123/jsep.2013-0260

McNaughton-Cassill, M. E., Lopez, S., Knight, C., Perrotte, J., Mireles, N., Cassill, C. K., Silva, S., & Cassill, A. (2021). Social support, coping, life satisfaction, and academic success among college Students. *Psi Chi Journal of Psychological Research*, *26*(2), 150–156. doi.org/10.24839/2325-7342.JN26.2.150

Mrazek, A. J., Ihm, E. D., Molden, D. C., Mrazek, M. D., Zedelius, C. M., & Schooler, J. W. (2018). Expanding minds: Growth mindsets of self-regulation and the influences on effort and perseverance. *Journal of Experimental Social Psychology*, *79*, 164–180. doi.org/10.1016/j.jesp.2018.07.003

Mumford, G. (2015). *The mindful athlete*. Parallax Press.

Nechvatal, J. M., & Lyons, D. M. (2013). Coping changes the brain. *Frontiers in Behavioral Neuroscience*, *7*(13), 1–8. doi.org/10.3389/fnbeh.2013.00013

Pennebaker, J. (1997). *Opening up*. The Guilford Press.

Rogers, H. (2016). *The mindful twenty-something*. New Harbinger Publications, Inc.

Rutter, M. (2012). Resilience as a dynamic concept. *Development and Psychopathology*, *24*, 335–344. doi.org/10.1017/S0954579412000028

Ryan, R., & Deci, E. (2000). Self-determination theory and the facilitation of intrinsic motivation, social development and well-being. *American Psychologist*, *55*(1), 68–78. doi.org/10.1037//0003-066x.55.1.68

Schneider, P. (2003). *Writing alone and with others*. Oxford University Press.

The Steve Fund and JED Foundation. (2017). *Equity in mental health framework: Recommendations for colleges and universities to support the emotional well-being and mental health of students of color*. www.equityinmentalhealth.org/wp-content/uploads/2017/11/Equity-in-Mental-Health-Framework-v17.pdf

Taber-Thomas, B., & Koraly, P.-E. (2015). Emerging adulthood brain development. In J. J. Arnett (Ed.), *The Oxford handbook of emerging adulthood*. Oxford: Oxford Library of Psychology. Academic accessed on 6 Sept. 2023: www.doi.org/10.1093/oxfordhb/9780199795574.013.15

Ungar, M. (2018). *Change your world*. Sutherland House.

Wade, R., Cronholm, P., Fein, J., Forke, C. M., Davis, M., Harkins-Schwarz, M., Pachter, L., & Bair-Merritt, M. (2016). Household and community-level adverse childhood experiences and adult health outcomes in a diverse urban population. *Child Abuse & Neglect*, *52*, 135–145. doi.org/10.1016/j.chiabu.2015.11.021

PART FOUR

# ACROSS THE LIFESPAN: ADULTS AND FAMILIES

# 12 Empowering Mothers and Promoting Resilience in Children Exposed to Intimate Partner Violence

Sandra A. Graham-Bermann

I'm no longer accepting the things I cannot change … I'm changing the things I cannot accept.

—Angela Davis, Ph.D., Professor, University of California Santa Cruz

## 12.1 How Serious Is This Problem for Mothers and Their Children?

### 12.1.1 Prevalence

The National Centers for Disease Control and Prevention defines intimate partner violence (IPV) as physical violence, sexual violence, psychological aggression, and/or stalking in the relationships with a current or former intimate partner (Basile et al., 2011). Physical violence can be measured as mild, moderate, or severe and includes the use of physical force to hurt or attempt to hurt a partner. Sexual violence indicates unwanted contact, ranging from unwanted touching to acts of penetration. Stalking occurs when there is repeated unwanted attention or contact that causes fear of safety for the survivor. This can include stalking via media, as well as contact with those close to the survivor. Psychological aggression takes the form of communication with the intent to control or terrorize a partner and cause emotional and mental harm.

The chronic nature of IPV is reflected in an early study on the prevalence of types of IPV experienced by a diverse group of 221 women who reported that acts of physical violence occurred an average of 15 times in the last year and psychological maltreatment 66 times (Graham-Bermann et al., 2007). Lifetime rates indicate that 1 in 4 women and 1 in 10 men experience any form of IPV across their lifespan, and 1 in 5 women and 1 in 7 men experience severe IPV (Basile et al., 2011). Thus, these figures represent a public health crisis of enormous proportions. The cost to individuals, to families, and to society is vast. In 2003, the National Centers for Disease

Control and Prevention estimated the annual economic cost of IPV to be $5.8 billion, as a result of lost wages, medical services, and costs to the criminal justice system.

While the statistics suggest broad exposure to violence in the relationships of both men and women, the effects and motives for using violence are not the same. Recent studies have sought to contextualize the IPV experiences of men and women. For example, a study of male and female victims of IPV in New Zealand showed women were three times more likely to be injured than men, more likely to experience severe IPV and sexual assault during IPV, and more likely to fear their violent partner (Fanslow et al., 2022). Other studies indicate that women are more likely than men to fight back when IPV is severe and when children are present (Bair-Merritt et al., 2010; Swan & Snow, 2006). However, women's fighting back often results in no effect or escalates the violence (Downs et al., 2007; Fanslow et al., 2015). Thus, in order to understand the effects of IPV and what can be done to assist survivors, we focus on women who are mothers and their children.

### 12.1.2 Prevalence of Children's Exposure

It is estimated that each year more than 15 million children and adolescents live in families with IPV (McDonald et al., 2006). This translates into more than 1 in 15 children being exposed to IPV at home. Initially, there was debate about how much and to which kind of IPV children were exposed and aware. However, several studies indicate that children are eyewitness to IPV in their homes about 80–90% of the time, when it occurs (Fusco & Fantuzzo, 2009; Graham-Bermann et al., 2007). The most common form of IPV witnessed by children is psychological maltreatment (89%) and physical violence (82%), with sexual assaults witnessed least (Graham-Bermann et al., 2007). Children are also made aware of IPV through physical evidence of injury and bruising, witnessing police or ambulance intervention, or simply hearing the assaults being discussed by their parents.

National polyvictimization data show an approximately 56% overlap of IPV with lifetime child maltreatment (Hamby et al., 2010) and a 51% overlap with any other form of child victimization (Finkelhor et al., 2011). Further, Hamby and colleagues found maltreatment of children was most often committed by the IPV perpetrator. Children who witnessed IPV and were abused had greater trauma symptoms than either form of maltreatment alone (Kulkarni et al., 2011). These effects were found to be moderated by child gender, such that boys exposed to IPV were more likely than girls to be the target of parental aggression (Jouriles & LeCompte, 1991).

## 12.2 How Does IPV Effect Children? What Are We Trying to Reduce or Prevent?

### 12.2.1 Anxiety and Aggression

In order to understand the effects of IPV, I first started with focus groups where children talked about being afraid and feeling unprotected. I created a study of fears and worries to ascertain exactly what they were anxious about and compared their responses to a similar group of children who were not exposed to IPV. Thus, a measure of Family Fears and Worries (FFW) was developed and tested (Graham-Bermann, 1996). By asking children to report on the extent to which they were concerned about the behavior of specific family members, I discovered that children in families with IPV were significantly more worried about the harmful behavior of fathers and the vulnerability of mothers, brothers, and sisters than were children in nonviolent families.

Further, while the FFW was significantly associated with internalizing problems, as was expected, it was also related to high levels of aggression (Graham-Bermann, 1996). It was concluded that children who were aggressive and acting out were the most afraid and worried about specific behaviors and specific people in their lives. These findings suggest a context for better understanding children's reactions with focused attention on what they were actually afraid of and worried about. An analysis of fifty years of research on children exposed to IPV consistently indicates high rates of externalizing behavioral problems – that is, aggression, bullying, and delinquency (Holmes et al., 2022). This information is particularly useful when designing an intervention program that directly addresses these issues, as many mothers report difficulty managing their child's aggression.

### 12.2.2 Traumatic Stress

After conducting focus groups and in my therapeutic work, mothers reported that sometimes their children had trouble sleeping, forgetting about what happened, and seemed edgy and highly emotionally reactive – symptoms that fit diagnostic criteria for PTSD in adults. An early study of traumatic stress symptoms in a sample of school-age children exposed to IPV showed 13% met the criteria for a diagnosis of PTSD, with 52% displaying reexperiencing symptoms, 19% symptoms of avoidance, and 42% traumatic arousal symptoms (Graham-Bermann & Levendosky, 1998). The next question was whether symptoms of traumatic stress could be accurately evaluated for younger children. A study of preschoolers in families with IPV revealed that 38% of children who were exposed to traumatic events in addition to IPV had the highest rates of trauma symptoms and behavioral adjustment problems, relative to those who had not experienced additional traumatic events (Graham-Bermann et al., 2012). A third study, this time with Head Start preschool children with experiences of family violence and PTSD, showed a dose–response relationship with eight physical health problems (Graham-Bermann & Seng, 2005) indicating a direct relationship between the amount of exposure to violence and trauma and their number of physical health problems. Those exposed to violence had greatly increased risk of having asthma (1.48 odds ratio), allergies (3.9), ADHD (15.9), gastrointestinal problems (41.7), and headaches (24.0). Exposure to IPV is deemed a traumatic experience for children with far-reaching consequences both in the short term and over time.

The effects of trauma experienced as a result of IPV were also seen in children's lower ability (Graham-Bermann et al., 2010) and in their processing of emotions. Attention bias to threat, as seen in emotional faces, was studied with children exposed to IPV using reaction times with a probe detection task (Swartz et al., 2011). The dot probe test is designed to assess how fast children respond to a threatening image. It measures impaired attention processes. Children diagnosed with PTSD were compared to those without the diagnosis, and children with PTSD evidenced bias in responding to angry faces but not to neutral or happy faces. Given their learned experience with sudden and often unexpected violence, it makes sense that they focus on angry faces and even perceive them to be threatening. The trauma symptom of hypervigilance has been documented in children traumatized by IPV (Galano et al., 2020) and may serve as a defense mechanism to protect them for being caught unawares.

### 12.2.3 Cognitive Functioning

Beyond psychopathology, some mothers were concerned that their children were adopting unhealthy gender roles, with reports of some even condoning the violence against their mother or mimicking the violent behavior modeled by their fathers. I wanted to determine if IPV affects how children conceive of the roles of men and women in the family and the acceptability of violence as a solution to interpersonal problems. Such cognitions provide a road map for what is possible in social interaction and the considerations of family life in the future. However, new measures were needed to evaluate these constructs. In order to ascertain school-age children's cognitions concerning IPV, the Attitudes About Family Violence (AAFV) measure was created to assess their ideas about the acceptability of violence in the family and its relationship to adjustment (Graham-Bermann et al., 2007). Howell and colleagues tested a preschool version of the measure with similar items developmentally altered and found children holding the most maladaptive beliefs showed the greatest aggression (Howell et al., 2012).

In order to understand what children consider to be appropriate roles of men and women in the family, I also created the Family Stereotypes Card Sort (Graham-Bermann & Brescoll, 2000). Evaluation with a school-age sample showed significant associations among stereotypes and exposure to IPV within boys, younger children, and non-White children. These groups were more likely to hold extreme beliefs about the acceptability of male power and violence privilege. However, we know that children differ in the extent to which they exhibit IPV effects.

### 12.2.4 Profiles of Adjustment

I wanted to go beyond documenting dysfunction in order to seek out contributions to children's functioning and to include strengths as outcomes in that analysis. The first studies to differentiate the effects of IPV on children were conducted by Hughes and Luke in 1998. Using cluster analysis to distinguish typologies of adjustment from measures of psychopathology and self-esteem, they found the majority of children (approximately 60%) doing moderately well with mild symptoms and average-to-high self-esteem. The rest were suffering varying levels of psychological distress. In 2000, Grych and colleagues published a cluster analytic study with the same constructs with children exposed to IPV and reported five similar patterns (Grych et al., 2000). Profiles were multiple externalizing problems (aggression), multiple internalizing problems (anxiety, depression), externalizing alone, mild distress, and no problems.

In order to ascertain elements of strength and resilience and thus identify both deficits and potential protective factors, I added measures of social competence and self-competence to the assessment of behavioral adjustment in children exposed to IPV (Graham-Bermann et al., 2009). Results showed clusters of those who were struggling (45%), with severe problems (24%), with depression (11%), and deemed resilient (20%), who scored not only low in psychopathology but also high in social and self-competence. Most recently, Cameranesi and colleagues added biological measures of chronic health conditions, medication prescriptions, doctors' visits, and hospitalization in addition to psychopathology, taking a biopsychosocial approach to profiles of adjustment (Cameranesi et al., 2022). Their latent class analysis revealed four profiles, including multiple mild problems, multiple severe problems, resilient, and a fourth profile of externalizing problems characteristic of boys and severe physical health problems characteristic of girls. Thus, it is clear that not all children are affected in the same way. Of great interest was the consistent finding throughout these studies that a considerable group of children did not show deleterious effects, at least at the time of evaluation – they appeared to be resilient.

### 12.2.5 What Have We Learned about Positive Adjustment?

Resilience is a process, whereby those who are exposed to significant adversity show positive adaptation (Luthar et al., 2000). As discussed earlier, studies have identified children who do not show adverse consequences to IPV, at least at the time of evaluation. They appear to be competent in social relationships, have high self-esteem, function adequately, and consider themselves to be liked by others. A sample of preschool-aged children exposed to IPV was evaluated to identify which risk factors and which protective factors were associated with resilient functioning (Howell et al., 2010). Here, being older, having a mother with better parenting skills, fewer mental health problems, and less violence exposure predicted children's stronger emotional regulation and social skills. Conversely, young children, those exposed to more IPV and more severe IPV, were at greater risk for negative outcomes. In other studies, boys and girls are found equally likely to be resilient and, in general, there are few studies with outcome differences in terms of race or ethnicity (Sternberg et al., 2006).

## 12.3 How Can We Assist Children? What Actions Should We Take?

Overall, the ability to regulate one's emotions, get along well with other people, and to be able to adjust following exposure to potentially traumatic events are all hallmarks of successful adaptation considered to be necessary for optimal development. Thus, targets for intervention with children include reducing internalizing problems, such as anxiety and symptoms of depression, helping them to cope when distressed, discovering their attitudes and beliefs about violence, and exploring family and gender stereotypes. The high rates of children's internalizing and externalizing problems point to the need for activities that augment emotion regulation, enhance the ability to identify feelings, and build capacity to understand and practice how to handle conflict. Children's anxiety is centered on their fears and worries that can be reduced with safety planning (Miller et al., 2012). Essential programs also promote factors that are associated with resilience. By utilizing evidence-based therapeutic activities, we can augment children's self-esteem and sense of competence while reducing the negative effects of IPV.

## 12.4 What Are the Effects of IPV on Mothers? What Can Be Offered to Aid Their Healing?

Perhaps the most important moderator of children's adjustment is the functionality of their mother. Women who have been abused commonly suffer consequences in most areas of their lives, from disruptions in work and education to physical and mental health problems, economic loss, and challenges in relationships with family and friends.

### 12.4.1 Death and Injury

According to the CDC, more than half of female homicides are committed by a male intimate partner (Petrosky et al., 2017). Approximately 1,300 women die of IPV each year in the United States. Physical injury is a common outcome of IPV, with CDC reporting 35% of female survivors sustaining injury. When a diverse group of 221 survivors was asked to report on the worst violence that occurred in the last year, 70% indicated that they sustained an injury and 12% reported injury to their child (Graham-Bermann et al., 2007). Of these mothers, 31% reported mild injury that required no intervention (bruises, swelling), 33% had moderate injury (cuts, sprains, bite marks), and 20% had severe injuries requiring immediate medical attention (broken bones, stabbings, concussions).

Valera (2020) notes that most women experience severe violence to their head and upper torso. While traumatic brain injury (TBI) has primarily been studied with athletes, Valera and Kucyi (2017) estimate that 1.6 million abused women suffer TBI each year, with rates greatly increased during the COVID-19 pandemic (Valera, 2020). While long-term TBI effects are less studied in this population, short-term effects include disruption in cognitive functioning, psychological problems, and deterioration in brain health – symptoms that can be confused with other diagnoses.

### 12.4.2 Mental Health, Anxiety, Depression, and Traumatic Stress

Meta-analyses of mental health studies show consistent associations among depression, anxiety, traumatic stress, PTSD, and IPV (Lagdon et al., 2014). Symptoms of depression and depressive disorder are common in women who experience IPV. A meta-analysis of 37 studies revealed a twofold to threefold increased risk for major depressive disorder and one and one half- to twofold increased risk for postpartum depression among abused, compared to nonabused women (Beydoun et al., 2012).

Approximately half of the women living with IPV are traumatized by their experiences and have PTSD (Graham-Bermann & Miller, 2013). Most have moderate to high levels of anxiety and depression, making it difficult to navigate their circumstances, make plans, and find help (Oram et al., 2022). In biological terms, exposure to frequent traumatic events can overload the body's neuroendocrine response to stress, making it more difficult to recover each successive time, thereby hampering the ability to process and manage emotions (Goldberg et al., 2023).

CDCP also reports a heightened risk of physical health problems ranging from death to various degrees of injury that result from assaults, such as concussions, diseases, heart attacks, and strokes. They are also at risk for future victimization that only exacerbates existing problems.

### 12.4.3 Parenting under Stress

Beyond physical and mental health problems, women who experience IPV are challenged in parenting and caretaking, in part because they are parenting children with serious adjustment disorders, while also trying to remain stable and recover from the violence themselves. A number of studies show that the negative effects of IPV on parenting are related to women's mental health, specifically depression and traumatic stress (Levendosky & Graham-Bermann, 2001; Levendosky et al., 2003). Women with fewer mental health problems were found to be more effective parents, despite their chaotic environment. These women were more supportive and responsive to their children's needs and gave their children more attention than other mothers in similar circumstances. In fact, Levendosky and colleagues recently reviewed the literature and concluded that a comprehensive model of effects shows that most child outcomes are mediated through mothers' parenting and the child's emotion regulation (Bogat et al., 2023). There is no doubt that mothers who have experienced IPV are parenting under duress.

## 12.5 What Are the Problems We Need to Address in Preventive Intervention Programs for Women Who Have Experienced IPV?

Given the results of research studies with women who have experienced IPV, it is clear that their needs are many. They may be injured, isolated, anxious, or traumatized by IPV, in need of information, access to resources and services, a safety plan, and struggle to move forward. If there are physical injuries, women need referrals to affordable and appropriate medical care. Their continued safety is also paramount. In order to prepare women for the possibility of future victimization, safety planning is an essential element in any program for women who have experienced IPV. Providing social support is also important as, in order to exert and maintain control, perpetrators often isolate their partner from her family and friends. Building social support and restoring connections with others are paramount to emotional healing.

The format of the program also promotes healing. Meeting in groups helps women to heal the isolation that comes from living in a relationship characterized by IPV. Further, the women know firsthand what others in their group are going through, thus reducing stigma and enhancing trust. They are the experts in IPV. In order to reduce the effects of trauma, it is important to provide a supportive place for women to discuss their experiences and share feelings, fears, and worries about their past circumstances. Trauma symptoms of avoidance and the potential for reexperiencing the trauma when discussing it are reduced in the context of such conversations with others. When there is no pressure or expectation that women will reveal disturbing elements of their experiences, as may sometimes be the case in individual therapies, women may be more comfortable when disclosure is optional. Support also comes from sharing information about local resources and strategies for coping with others.

Parenting stress is a very real concern for mothers who have experienced IPV. When mothers use effective techniques to manage their child's behavior, the children's adjustment improves, thereby reducing their own stress (Graham-Bermann, Howell et al., 2011). But many women have not been able to parent effectively, in part due to the parenting they received in their family of origin (Levendosky & Graham-Bermann, 1998). Thus, it helps empower women by offering the opportunity to discuss parenting concerns and challenges in managing their child's behavior. Group leaders can work with and assist women by providing information and encouragement in using new behavior management techniques. Beyond reducing problems, preventive intervention programs should also seek to enhance protective factors that have been identified in research studies. Here, mothers can work to reduce their child's anxiety by developing skills in talking with their child about upsetting events, including IPV. Another example is emphasizing and using positive parenting practices that mothers can consider as further avenues for change.

## 12.6 Designing the Kids' Club and Moms' Empowerment Programs

The Kids' Club (KC) and Moms' Empowerment Program (MEP) were developed and pilot tested with groups of women and children living in shelters who identified issues of concern (Graham-Bermann, 1989/1992, 1989/1994). Relevant outcomes were then examined in empirical studies, sometimes requiring the creation of new measures. The 10-session programs employ evidence-based practices and have a group format, found to be developmentally appropriate for children and clinically important for the women. Group process and proven techniques derived from individual clinical practice are hallmarks of both programs.

The programs can take place in a range of settings including community settings, shelters, and clinical service agencies. Group leaders have been community service providers, students, as well as trained professionals. The programs are primary prevention such that they seek to prevent negative outcomes. They are also secondary prevention programs in that they seek to reduce the negative impact of IPV before it creates permanent damage.

## 12.7 The Kids' Club (KC) Program

The KC program is grounded in the knowledge that children exposed to IPV may be distressed and anxious, may have learned harmful patterns of behavior, and may have developed attitudes and beliefs about violence that put them at risk for less optimal development. The KC program develops coping skills and fosters resilience with activities and lessons that address emotions, emotion regulation, fears and worries, how to manage anger, safety planning, and other problem-solving skills.

The CDC funded an evaluation to ascertain whether participation in the KC reduced children's internalizing and externalizing behavior problems and reduced their negative attitudes and beliefs about violence (Graham-Bermann et al., 2007). Three conditions were compared in this randomized control trial – children in the KC child-only group (CO), those whose mothers also participated in the MEP (CM group), and a comparison group of mothers and children with treatment as usual (CG group). Pre-, post-, and eight-month follow-up assessments were conducted for 221 mother/child dyads. Analyses using HLM provided evidence of significant change from baseline, with CM children showing the greatest improvement in both externalizing problems and attitudes about violence relative to CO and CG groups. From baseline to follow-up, 79% fewer children were in the clinical range on externalizing problems and 77% fewer children in the CM group were in the clinical range on internalizing problems.

## 12.8 Preschool Kids' Club (PKC) Program

A second semi-randomized control trial was conducted with a diverse group of 120 children, four to six years of age, and their mothers who had experienced IPV (Graham-Bermann et al., 2015). Given the wish to intervene earlier in the life of the child, we sought to discover whether the program was equally effective when working with younger children and their mothers. The PKC compared CM and CG groups focusing on change in internalizing problems, post-intervention and at eight-month follow-up. The PKC also differed in being offered twice a week over five weeks with an average attendance of six sessions.

Intent-to-treat analyses (everyone initially in the study) showed significantly reduced internalization problems for CM girls, relative to CG girls, but not for boys in either group. Per protocol analyses (comparing those who participated in the program to those who did not), a reduced number of internalization problems were shown for both CM boys and girls. While the findings were not as strong as those found for older children, reliable change was greater for CM versus CG preschool children at follow-up with 23% no longer in the clinical range (CG = 8%), 22% changed to the normal range (CG = 5%). We also examined what led to change in internalizing symptoms for children and found that those who spontaneously disclosed the fighting in their family during group discussions had less anxiety than those who did not disclose (Graham-Bermann et al., 2011). It should be noted here that at no time is a child required to discuss traumatic events. Attention problems were also evaluated. While no change of inattention or hyperactivity symptoms were found immediately post-intervention, significantly greater change was found one year later for PKC children exposed to high levels of IPV, relative to CG children, and those exposed to less IPV (Clark et al., 2021).

## 12.9 The Moms' Empowerment Program (MEP)

The MEP was created to provide a supportive group where women who had experienced IPV could meet together to discuss important issues, share information, and receive resource materials from trained leaders. The focus on parenting was implemented as a primary concern of the mothers in the focus groups, and given the belief that by helping the mother to address her parenting concerns, we could also help the child. Still, their own experiences of IPV were shared and discussed. Recall that most of these are women dealing with children with behavioral adjustment problems, few resources, immense parenting stress, as well as struggling with their own mental health issues. Program sessions address fears and worries about children, voluntarily sharing and naming IPV experiences, safety planning, managing and changing children's behavior, support for talking with children about IPV, finding community resources, and stress management techniques for themselves and for their child. Thus, the program was designed to empower women by addressing their issues, enhancing their coping, and reducing their traumatic stress.

The CDC-funded randomized control trial compared MEP groups from baseline to post-intervention and again from post-intervention to eight-month follow-up. The CM group showed the greatest improvement in depression and positive parenting skills, relative to women in the CO or CG groups (Graham-Bermann & Miller-Graff, 2015). Further, mothers in the CG group showed deterioration in their parenting over time. At baseline, 81% of the women in the study were diagnosed with PTSD. Women in the CM group had the greatest reduction in traumatic stress symptoms over time, relative to women in the CO or CG groups who did not participate in the program. Further, the reliable change index showed 85% of mothers in the CM group no longer had PTSD at the eight-month follow-up (Graham-Bermann & Miller-Graff, 2013). These findings rival those of other studies using trauma-focused interventions with reliable change rates ranging from 63 to 72% (Bradley et al., 2005).

The implications of these findings go beyond value to the women in the program, as the change in mothers' mental health, more specifically in post-traumatic stress symptomology, was found to mediate the relationship between children's intervention participation and change in child internalizing symptoms (Graham-Bermann et al., 2011). In these ways, help to the mother also helps the child and, transactionally, children with fewer adjustment problems reduce parenting stress.

Outcomes of the MEP evaluation of the mothers of preschoolers (PKC) showed improvement in trauma symptoms over follow-up (eight months after the end of the program) but not in the short term (immediately after the program) (Graham-Bermann et al., 2018). However, we identified a curvilinear relationship between the number of sessions attended and reduced trauma symptoms. Reductions were seen only after the seventh session of the program, with older mothers evidencing greater change. Again, the mothers attended twice each week, but attendance was low (on average six sessions), indicating that efforts to assist younger children and their mothers might do well to offer benefits that enhance program participation. Such benefits can include providing money for transportation and parking and providing meals before sessions. Additional findings from this study include less use of physical punishment for MEP mothers of preschool-age children relative to CG mothers (Grogan-Kaylor et al., 2019), greater use of positive parenting techniques (Howell et al., 2015), and less exposure to IPV at both post-intervention and follow-up, relative to CG mothers (Miller et al., 2014).

An eight-year follow-up of the PKC and MEP evaluation was conducted to ascertain whether any of the changes found for mothers and preschoolers would hold over a longer term, from when the children were 4 to 6 years old to when they were 12 to 14 years old. The most important finding was that those in the MEP were exposed to significantly less violence over eight years than those who did not participate in the program eight years ago (Stein et al., 2022). Mothers who attended more MEP sessions showed fewer symptoms of traumatic stress at the eight-year follow-up (Galano et al., 2021). Further, changes in child internalizing problems that were identified in the PKC study were maintained eight years later, into early adolescence, but only for those who received an effective dose of the program – in this case, attending at least eight sessions (Galano et al., 2020).

## 12.10 Creating Cultural Adaptations for Prevention Practice

Each of these programs – the KC children, the PKC for preschoolers, and the MEP for their mothers – have proven to be popular, in that they have been adopted for use in 38 states and several countries. In order to do this work and to learn while adapting the KC program and MEP for different cultures and communities, I have worked closely with leaders and stakeholders in Alaska, Canada, Texas, and Sweden. Each of these collaborations required obtaining an understanding of the cultural context in which IPV takes place, learning about the resources available in each community and listening to community leaders who shared information about cultural issues that need to be considered when adapting the programs for their setting. In each setting, we discussed and made plans together to integrate diversity issues into the program. It should be noted that it can take many months and sometimes years to form successful collaborations and respectful partnerships. Some examples are shared later in this chapter.

## 12.11 Empowering Communities through Research Collaborations

### 12.11.1 Alaska

After I received a request by the State of Alaska's Council on Domestic Violence and Sexual Assault (CDVSA) to adapt the programs for use with Alaskan women and children, I researched issues related to IPV in Alaska. Recent figures show approximately half of adult Alaskan women experience IPV in their lifetime, with numbers rising each year (Alaska Department of Public Safety, 2020). Agencies such as CDVSA do make a difference, but I discovered that helping resources are not equally available in all areas, with some remote and rural areas even being cut off from law enforcement due to lack of connecting roads. The population of Alaska consists of 64.5% people who are identified as White, 6.6% Asian, and 3.6% African American or Black residents. Native Alaskans make up 15.7% of the population and are represented by more than 125 recognized tribes. Indigenous people in the Tlingit and Haida tribes reside primarily in southeast coastal Alaska, where the programs were to be offered, with the hope that they would be distributed to other areas.

After trips to Juneau over a three-year period and meetings with the CDVSA team and local leaders, I came to have a broader understanding of the issues facing Alaskan women and children and their community strengths. We discussed the cultural values that could be represented within each program. It became clear that the KC program and MEP already embodied many elements of Native approaches to intervention, such as healing as a way to achieve homeostasis or balance, including elements of mental, physical, emotional, and spiritual well-being, understanding historical contexts, and using storytelling with local symbols. Both the KC program and MEP already meet in a talking circle (another cultural practice that represents equality), and we discussed the possibility of smudging at the start of meetings. Having food at meetings and providing enough time to talk and catch up were similar values. Both programs already incorporate hands-on activities, so ways of incorporating meaningful crafts were also discussed.

This cultural adaptation work necessitated updating the children's workbooks and rethinking assessment materials. For example, together we chose measures to evaluate children's behavior that reflect both strengths and challenges. We agreed to adopt a lethality assessment of violence exposure rather than longer measures and to drop the usual assessment of mental health, such as measuring depression symptoms, due to state shelter rules against monitoring emotional stability. Shelters providing services to all Alaskan women and children who had experienced IPV were identified, with service providers meeting in Juneau for several days of discussion and a workshop on implementing the program in their setting. In the end, we had a highly diverse sample of women who are identified as White (47.5%), Alaska Native (36.1%), mixed race (3.3%), Latina (3.3%), Native American (1.6%), and Asian/Pacific Islander (1.6%) (Burrage, Gagnon, & Graham-Bermann, 2021). Their children were identified primarily as Alaska Native (41%), with White (36.1%), mixed race (14.1%), Native American (1.6%), Asian/Pacific Islander (1.6%), Latino/a (1.6%), and other ethnicities (3.3%). The data are being analyzed and will be published with CDVSA staff as co-authors (Burrage et al., 2021).

### 12.11.2 Canadian First Nations and Aboriginal Families

Next, the Canadian government funded a grant to adapt the programs for use solely with Indigenous and First Nations people. I joined researchers from universities in two provinces in Canada for a number of meetings with tribal leaders, who were integrally connected with the shelters and community service centers for Native Americans. Those meetings took many turns and phases where the research team introduced us and described the project. Given the long history of abuse by the government toward their population, we knew it was not going to be an easy collaboration. While I brought gifts from Michigan and honored the tribal leaders in the initial meeting, it would have been better, in retrospect, to begin the first meeting by simply asking for their thoughts, plans, input, and taking more time to get acquainted. However, over time we were able to develop a good relationship of respect and trust. We found ways to include many more tribal leaders in different phases of the program, in the role of paid advisors, as storytellers in the KC program, and in discussing historical trauma with women in the MEP. The meetings would begin with a smudging ceremony led by a community elder, and the adapted programs would belong to the tribes. That project was interrupted due to COVID-19, with plans to continue this coming year.

### 12.11.3 Spanish Language Adaptation

Because many agencies and groups inquired about a Spanish language version of the MEP, the Latina MEP (LMEP) was developed in consultation with community leaders in Texas, Ohio, and Michigan. Graduate students and I traveled to Texas to work with the director of a community center for Latina women who was also a faculty member at the University of Texas at Brownsville at the time. It was ideal to collaborate with someone intimately familiar with issues in her community and to have access to the right population. Fewer adaptations were made to the programs, but other elements were discussed and brought into the training sessions for group leaders, such as ways to address the sometimes conflicting values of the role of women in Latinx families, issues of immigration, threats of deportation, language barriers to getting help, finding Latinx-friendly community resources, and isolation.

Students provided the program and conducted interviews in Toldeo, Ohio, and Pontiac, Michigan. The research team also worked with service providers in Texas who also conducted some interviews with the mothers and children as part of the program evaluation. However, as we discovered later, not all of the questions were being asked. Interviews were much shorter as a result. In the end, missing data prohibited analyzing the children's data for outcomes. We discovered this quandary in doing applied research where the salience of protecting the community took precedence over the needs of the research project. Still, we were able to test the efficacy of the Spanish language version of the program. A total of 93 low-income, mostly immigrant Latinas were included in this community trial (Galano et al., 2017; Stein et al., 2021). The MEP was effective in reducing women's symptoms of traumatic stress and depression compared to those who did not participate in the program. Comparison mothers had the option to participate after the 10-week intervals. The training materials have been translated into Spanish, which broadens the reach of the programs to many more communities.

### 12.11.4 Sweden: Barnsclubben (Kids Club)

Collaboration with colleagues in Sweden began with one social worker in the town of Kristinehamn who requested program materials and then wrote a small grant to have in-person training for her agency. She invited her mentor from Örebro University and so began the evaluation project of a Swedish version of the program (Cater & Grip, 2014). Some of the reactions of the Swedish service providers to program materials were eye-opening. First, by law, they were obligated to include males who were victims of IPV in their programs, although none participated in the program evaluation.

The issue of managing child behavior was the subject of much discussion. Given the many problems that most children suffer when exposed to IPV, parenting under stress is a serious and frustrating issue for the mothers and, thus, is addressed in the MEP. The program is not prescriptive in advising parents to use any particular form of discipline but does offer suggested methods approved by the AMA and pediatrics associations for helping children to resolve conflicts and to better manage their behavior. These include "time out" or taking the child aside to discuss the problem, then giving choices, rather than any form of corporal punishment. The use of physical punishment is a hot topic when discipline is debated in MEP groups in the United States. The group leaders said that it would be not acceptable in Sweden to humiliate a child by separating that child from the group. Physical punishment of the child, even spanking, would never be allowed. They cited the United Nations Convention on the Rights of the Child that champions the child's right to be respected and not physically assaulted (interestingly, only two countries have not ratified that UN Convention – the United States and Somalia!). Most other elements of the program were similar. The group leaders particularly enjoyed the program, although those whose work was primarily based on individual therapy found it harder to adapt to the group format. The evaluation combined the KC program and MEP with other community services with positive results (Cater & Grip, 2014). Subsequently, all program materials were translated into Swedish.

## 12.12 Summary of Key Recommendations for Prevention Practice

Effective preventive intervention programs should:

- rely on a solid base of evidence for their effectiveness,
- have a supportive atmosphere,
- employ activities that build and allow for the practice of skills,
- be culturally relevant,
- include evaluations,
- rely on trained providers,
- use training manuals to ensure that the programs are provided consistently,
- provide support and consultation for staff.

A final note – It is critically important to recognize the need for organizational support and the opportunity for consultation for those who are service providers working with women and children exposed to IPV. This essential work can be difficult, rewarding, challenging, and exhausting at times, such that long-term provider success will require the ability to monitor one's own symptoms of distress and to understand and implement useful avenues for self-care. As Mother Teresa has said, "To keep the lamp burning, we have to keep putting oil in it."

## Additional Resources

Graham-Bermann, S. A. (Ed.). (2018). *Cultural considerations in intervention with women and children exposed to intimate partner violence.* Nova Science Publishers, Inc.

Graham-Bermann, S. A., & Edleson, J. L. (Eds.). (2001). *Domestic violence in the lives of children: The future of research, intervention, and social policy.* American Psychological Association Books.

Graham-Bermann, S. A., & Levendosky, A. A. (Eds.). (2011). *How intimate partner violence affects children: Developmental research, case studies, and evidence-based treatment.* American Psychological Association.

Johnson, L., & Stylianou, A. M. (2020). Coordinated community responses to domestic violence: A systematic review of the literature. *Trauma, Violence, & Abuse, 23*(2), 506–522. https://journals.sagepub.com/doi/10.1177/1524838020957984

Preventing Intimate Partner Violence. *CDC's fact sheet that includes definitions, consequences, and strategies for preventing intimate partner violence.* www.cdc.gov/violenceprevention/pdf/ipv/IPVfactsheet_2020_508.pdf

## References

Alaska Department of Public Safety. (2020). *Alaska victimization survey.* State of Alaska Department of Public Safety. https://dps.alaska.gov/AST/PIO/PressReleases/CDVSA-Releases-2020-Alaska-Victimization-Survey-Results

Bair-Merritt, M. H., Shea Crowne, S., Thompson, D. A., Sibinga, E., Trent, M., & Campbell, J. (2010). Why do women use intimate partner violence? A systematic review of women's motivations. *Trauma, Violence & Abuse, 11*(4), 178–189. doi.org/10.1177/1524838010379003

Basile, K. C., Black, M. C., Breiding, M. J., Smith, S. G., Walters, M. L., Merrick, M. T., Chen, J., & Stevens, M. R. (2011). *National intimate partner and sexual violence survey (NISVS): 2010 summary report.* Atlanta, GA: National Center for Injury Prevention and Control, Centers for Disease Control and Prevention. www.cdc.gov/violenceprevention/pdf/nisvs_report2010-a.pdf

Beydoun, H. A., Beydoun, M. A., Kaufman, J. S., Lo, B., & Zonderman, A. B. (2012). Intimate partner violence against adult women and its association with major depressive disorder, depressive symptoms and postpartum depression: A systematic review and meta-analysis. *Social Science & Medicine, 75*(6), 959–975. doi.org/10.1016/j.socscimed.2012.04.025

Bogat, G. A., Levendosky, A. A., & Cochran, K. (2023). Developmental consequences of intimate partner violence on children. *Annual Review of Clinical Psychology, 19*, 303–329. doi.org/10.1146/annurev-clinpsy-072720-013634

Bradley, R., Greene, J., Russ, E., Dutra, L., & Westen, D. (2005). A multidimensional meta-analysis of psychotherapy for PTSD. *The American Journal of Psychiatry, 162*(2), 214–227. doi.org/10.1176/appi.ajp.162.2.214

Burrage, R., Gagnon, M. B., & Graham-Bermann, S. A. (2021). Trauma history and social support among women American Indian/Alaska Native and non-native survivors of intimate partner violence. *Journal of Interpersonal Violence, 36*(5–6). doi.org/10.1177/0886260518772103

Cameranesi, M., Shooshtari, S., & Piotrowski, C. C. (2022). Investigating adjustment profiles in children exposed to intimate partner violence using a biopsychosocial resilience framework: A Canadian population-based study. *Child Abuse & Neglect, 125* (March), 105453. doi.org/10.1016/j.chiabu.2021.105453

Cater, Å., & Grip, K. (2014). Kids Club in Sweden: Results from a feasibility study of a method to support children who have experienced violence against their mother. In B. Anders & O. Lindberg (Eds.), *Working papers and reports, social work*, 4. Örebro University.

Clark, H. M., Grogan-Kaylor, A. C., Galano, M. M., Stein, S. F., & Graham-Bermann, S. A. (2021). Treating attention problems in children exposed to intimate partner violence: Evaluating the Preschool Kids' Club. *Children and Youth Services Review, 128*. doi.org/10.1016/j.childyouth.2021.106138

Downs, W. R., Rindels, B., & Atkinson, C. (2007).Women's use of physical and non-physical self-defense strategies during incidents of partner violence. *Violence Against Women, 13*(1), 28–45. doi.org/10.1177/1077801206294807

Fanslow, J., Gulliver, P., Dixon, R., & Ayallo, I. (2015). Hitting back: Women's use of physical violence against violent male partners, in the context of a violent episode. *Journal of Interpersonal Violence, 30*(17), 2963–2979. doi.org/10.1177/0886260514555010

Fanslow, J. L., Malihi, Z., Hashemi, L., Gulliver, P., & McIntosh, T. (2022). Prevalence of interpersonal violence against women and men in New Zealand: Results of a cross-sectional study. *Australian and New Zealand Journal of Public Health, 46*(2), 117–126.

Finkelhor, D., Turner, H., Hamby, S. L., & Ormrod, R. (2011). *Polyvictimization: Children's exposure to multiple types of violence, crime, and abuse*. OJJDP Juvenile Justice Bulletin, NCJ235504, 1–12. US Government Printing Office.

Fusco, R. A., & Fantuzzo, J. W. (2009). Domestic violence crimes and children: A population-based investigation of direct sensory exposure and the nature of involvement. *Child Youth Services Review, 31*(2), 249–256. doi.org/10.1016/j.childyouth.2008.07.017

Galano, M. M., Grogan-Kaylor, A. C., Stein, S. F., Clark, H. M., & Graham-Bermann, S. A. (2017). Posttraumatic stress disorder in Latina women: Examining the efficacy of the Moms' Empowerment Program. *Psychological Trauma: Theory, Research, Practice, and Policy, 9*(3), 344–351. doi.org/10.1037/tra0000

Galano, M. M., Grogan-Kaylor, A. C., Stein, S. F., Clark, H., & Graham-Bermann, S. A. (2020). Dyadic profiles of traumatic stress symptoms in mothers and children experiencing intimate partner violence. *Child Psychiatry and Human Development, 52*, 943–955. doi.org/10.1007/s10578-020-00973-y

Galano, M. M., Stein, S. F., Clark, H. M., Grogan-Kaylor, A. C., & Graham-Bermann, S. A. (2022). Eight-year trajectories of behavior problems and resilience in children exposed to early-life intimate partner violence: The overlapping and distinct effects of individual and family factors. *Development and Psychopathology*, 1–13. doi.org/10.1017/S0954579422000104

Galano, M. M., Stein, S. F., Grogan-Kaylor, A. C., Clark, H. M., & Graham-Bermann, S. A. (2021). Investigating the effects of the Moms' Empowerment Program on eight-year traumatic stress symptom trajectories in women with histories of IPV. *American Journal of Orthopsychiatry, 91*(6), 776–788. doi.org/10.1037/ort0000577

Goldberg, X., Espelt, C., Nadal, R., Alon, Y., Palao, D., Bar-Haim, Y., & Armario, A. (2023). Blunted neurobiological reactivity and attentional bias to threat underlie stress-related disorders in women survivors of intimate partner violence. *Psychological Medicine*, 1–12. doi.org/10.1017/S0033291723000910

Graham-Bermann, S. A. (1989/1992). *The Kids' Club: A preventive intervention program for children exposed to domestic violence*. Graham-Bermann Programs, LLC.

Graham-Bermann, S. A. (1989/1994). *The Moms' Empowerment Program: A training manual*. Graham-Bermann Programs, LLC.

Graham-Bermann, S. A. (1996). Family worries: The assessment of interpersonal anxiety in children from violent and nonviolent families. *Journal of Clinical Child Psychology*, *25*(3), 280–287. doi.org/10.1207/s15374424jccp2503_4

Graham-Bermann, S. A., & Brescoll, V. (2000). Gender, power, and violence: Assessing the family stereotypes of the children of batterers. *Journal of Family Psychology*, *14*(4), 600–612. doi.org/10.1037/0893-3200.14.4.600

Graham-Bermann, S. A., Burrage, R., & Carey, E. (2018, July). *The Kids' Club enhances social support for Alaskan children exposed to intimate partner violence. In chairperson, community-based intervention for families experiencing intimate partner violence: Exposure, posttraumatic stress, and resilience*. International family violence and child victimization research. International Family Violence and Child Victimization Research Conference, Portsmouth, NH.

Graham-Bermann, S. A., Castor, L., Miller, L. E., & Howell, K. H. (2012). The impact of additional traumatic events to trauma symptoms and PTSD in children exposed to intimate partner violence (IPV). *Journal of Traumatic Stress*, *25*(4), 393–400. doi .org/10.1002/jts.21724

Graham-Bermann, S. A., Gruber, G., Howell, K. H., & Girz, L. (2009). Factors discriminating among profiles of resilience and psychopathology in children exposed to intimate partner violence (IPV). *Child Abuse & Neglect*, *33*(9), 648–660. doi .org/10.1016/j.chiabu.2009.01.002

Graham-Bermann, S. A., Howell, K. H., Lilly, M. M., & Devoe, E. (2011). Mediators and moderators of change in adjustment following intervention for children exposed to intimate partner violence (IPV). *Journal of Interpersonal Violence*, *26*(9), 1815–1833. doi.org/10.1177/0886260510372931

Graham-Bermann, S. A., Howell, K. H., Miller, L. E., Kwek, J., & Lilly, M. (2010). Traumatic events and maternal education as predictors of verbal ability for preschool children exposed to intimate partner violence (IPV). *Journal of Family Violence*, *25*(4), 383–392. doi.org/10.1007/s10896-009-9299-3

Graham-Bermann, S. A., Kulkarni, M., & Kanukollu, S. (2011). Is disclosure therapeutic for children following exposure to traumatic violence? *Journal of Interpersonal Violence*, *26*(5), 1056–1076. doi.org/10.1177/0886260510365855

Graham-Bermann, S. A., & Levendosky, A. A. (1998). Traumatic stress symptoms of children of battered women. *Journal of Interpersonal Violence*, *13*(1), 111–128. doi .org/10.1177/088626098013001007

Graham-Bermann, S. A., Lynch, S., Banyard, V., Devoe, E., & Halabu, H. (2007). Community based intervention for children exposed to intimate partner violence: An efficacy trial. *Journal of Consulting and Clinical Psychology*, *75*(2), 199–209. doi .org/10.1037/0022-006X.75.2.199

Graham-Bermann, S. A., & Miller, L. E. (2013). Intervention to reduce traumatic stress following intimate partner violence: An efficacy trial of the Moms' Empowerment Program (MEP). *Psychodynamic Psychiatry*, *41*(2), 327–348. doi.org/10.1521/pdps.2013.41.2.329

Graham-Bermann, S. A., & Miller-Graff, L. E. (2015). Community-based intervention for women exposed to intimate partner violence: A randomized control trial. *Journal of Family Psychology*, *29*(4), 537–547. doi.org/10.1037/fam0000091

Graham-Bermann, S. A., Miller-Graff, L. E., Howell, K. H., & Grogan-Kaylor, A. (2015). An efficacy trial of an intervention program for young children exposed to intimate partner violence. *Child Psychiatry & Human Development*, *46*(6), 928–939. doi.org/10.1007/s10578-015-0532-4

Graham-Bermann, S. A., & Seng, J. S. (2005). Violence exposure and traumatic stress symptoms as additional predictors of health problems in high-risk children. *Journal of Pediatrics*, *146*(3), 349–354. doi.org/10.1016/j.jpeds.2004.10.065

Grogan-Kaylor, A. C., Galano, M., Howell, K. H., Miller-Graff, L. E., & Graham-Bermann, S. A. (2019). Reductions in parental use of corporal punishment on preschoolers in the Moms' Empowerment Program. *Journal of Interpersonal Violence*, *34*(8), 1563–1582. doi.org/10.1177/0886260516651627

Grych, J. H., Jouriles, E. N., Swank, P. R., McDonald, R., & Norwood, W. D. (2000). Patterns of adjustment among children of battered women. *Journal of Consulting and Clinical Psychology*, *68*(1), 84–94. doi.org/10.1037/0022-006X.68.1.84

Hamby, S., Finkelhor, D., Turner, H., & Ormrod, R. (2010). The overlap of witnessing partner violence with child maltreatment and other victimizations in a nationally representative survey of youth. *Child Abuse & Neglect*, *34*(10), 734–741. doi.org/10.1016/j.chiabu.2010.03.001

Holmes, M. R., Berg, K. A., Bender, A. E., Evans, K. E., O'Donnell, K., & Miller, E. K. (2022). Nearly 50 years of child exposure to intimate partner violence empirical research: Evidence mapping, overarching themes, and future directions. *Journal of Family Violence*, 1–13. doi.org/10.1007/s10896-021-00349-3

Howell, K. H., Graham-Bermann, S. A., Czyz, E., & Lilly, M. (2010). Assessing resilience in preschool-age children exposed to intimate partner violence. *Violence and Victims*, *25*(2), 150–164. doi.org/10.1891/0886-6708.25.2.150

Howell, K. H., Miller, L. E., & Graham-Bermann, S. A. (2012). Evaluating preschool children's attitudes and beliefs about intimate partner violence. *Violence and Victims*, *27*(6), 941–956. doi.org/10.1891/0886-6708.27.6.941

Howell, K. H., Miller, L. E., Barnes, S. E., & Graham-Bermann, S. A. (2015). Promoting resilience in children exposed to intimate partner violence through a developmentally informed intervention: A case study. *Clinical Case Studies*, *14*(1), 31–46. doi.org/10.1177/1534650114535841

Howell, K. H., Miller, L. E., Lilly, M. M., Burlaka, V., Grogan-Kaylor, A. C., & Graham-Bermann, S. A. (2015). Strengthening positive parenting through intervention evaluating the Moms' Empowerment Program for women experiencing intimate partner violence. *Journal of Interpersonal Violence*, *30*(2), 232–252. doi.org/10.1177/0886260514533155

Hughes, H. M., & Luke, D. A. (1998). Heterogeneity in adjustment among children of battered women. In G. W. Holden, R. Geffner, & E. N. Jouriles (Eds.), *Children exposed to family violence* (pp. 185–222). American Psychological Association Books.

Jouriles, E. N., & LeCompte, S. H. (1991). Husbands' aggression toward wives and mothers' and fathers' aggression toward children: Moderating effects of child gender. *Journal of Consulting and Clinical Psychology*, *59*(1), 190–192. doi.org/10.1037/0022-006X.59.1.190

Kulkarni, M., Graham-Bermann, S. A., Rauch, S. A. M., & Seng, J. (2011). Witnessing versus experiencing direct violence in childhood as correlated with adulthood PTSD. *Journal of Interpersonal Violence*, *26*(6), 1264–1281. doi.org/10.1177/0886260510368159.

Lagdon, S., Armour, C., & Stringer, M. (2014). Adult experience of mental health outcomes as a result of intimate partner violence victimisation: A systematic review. *European Journal of Psychotraumatology*, *5*(1), 24794. doi.org/10.3402/ejpt.v5.24794

Levendosky, A. A., & Graham-Bermann, S. A. (1998). The moderating effects of parenting stress on children's adjustment in woman-abusing families. *Journal of Interpersonal Violence*, *13*(3), 383–397. doi.org/10.1177/088626098013003005

Levendosky, A. A. & Graham-Bermann, S. A. (2001). Parenting in battered women: The effects of domestic violence on women and children. *Journal of Family Violence*, *16*(2), 171–192. doi.org/10.1023/A:1011111003373

Levendosky, A. A., Huth-Bocks, A. C., Shapiro, D. L., & Semel, M. A. (2003). The impact of domestic violence on the maternal-child relationship and preschool-age children's functioning. *Journal of Family Psychology*, *17*(3), 275–287. doi.org/10.1037/0893-3200.17.3.275

Luthar, S. S., Cicchetti, D., & Becker, B. (2000). The construct of resilience: A critical evaluation and guidelines for future work. *Child Development*, *71*(3), 543–562. doi.org/10.1111/1467-8624.00164

McDonald, R., Jouriles, E. N., Ramisetty-Mikler, S., Caetano, R., & Green, C. E. (2006). Estimating the number of American children living in partner-violent families. *Journal of Family Psychology*, *20*(1), 137–142, doi.org/10.1037/0893-3200.20.1.137

Miller, L. E., Howell, K. H., & Graham-Bermann, S. A. (2014). The effect of an evidence-based intervention on women's exposure to intimate partner violence (IPV). *American Journal of Orthopsychiatry*, *84*(4), 321–328. doi.org/10.1037/h0099840

Miller, L. E., Howell, K. H., Hunter, E. C, & Graham-Bermann, S. A. (2012). Enhancing safety planning for young children exposed to intimate partner violence. *Child Care in Practice*, *18*(1), 67–82. doi.org/10.1080/13575279.2011.621885

Oram, S., Fisher, H. L., Minnis, H., Seedat, S., Walby, S., Hegarty, K., Rouf, K., Angénieux, C., Callard, F., Chandra, P. S., Fazel, S., Garcia-Moreno, C., Henderson, M., Howarth, E., MacMillan, H. L., Murray, L. K., Othman, S., Robotham, D., Rondon, M.B., … Howard, L. M. (2022). The Lancet Psychiatry Commission on intimate partner violence and mental health: Advancing mental health services, research, and policy. *The Lancet Psychiatry*, *9*(6), 487–524. doi.org/10.1016/S2215-0366(22)00008-6

Petrosky, E., Blair, J. M., Betz, C. J., Fowler, K. A., Jack, S. P., & Lyons, B. H. (July 21, 2017). Racial and ethnic differences in homicides of adult women and the role of intimate partner violence – United States, 2003–2014. *Morbidity and Mortality Weekly Report*, *66*(28), 741–746. doi.org/10.15585/mmwr.mm6628a1External

Stein, S. F., Galano, M. M., Grogan-Kaylor, A. C., Clark, H. M., Ribaudo, J. M., & Graham-Bermann, S. A. (2022). Predictors of intimate partner violence victimization by multiple partners over 8 years. *Journal of Traumatic Stress*, *35*(1), 222–234. doi.org/10.1002/jts.2272

Stein, S. F., Grogan-Kaylor, A. C., Galano, M. M., Clark, H. M., & Graham-Bermann, S. A. (2021). Contributions to depressed affect in Latina women: Examining the effectiveness of the Moms' Empowerment Program. *Journal of Interpersonal Violence*, *36*(5–6), 2298–2323. doi.org/10.1177/0886260518760005.

Sternberg, K. J., Baradaran, L. P., Abbott, C. B., Lamb, M. E., & Guterman, E. (2006). Type of violence, age, and gender differences in the effects of family violence on children's behavior problems: A meta-analysis. *Developmental Review*, *26*(1), 89–112.

Swan, S. C., & Snow, D. L. (2006). The development of a theory of women's use of violence in intimate relationships. *Violence Against Women*, *12*(11), 1026–1045. doi.org/10.1177/1077801206293330

Swartz, J. R., Graham-Bermann, S. A., Mogg, K., Bradley, B. P., & Monk, C. S. (2011). Attention bias to emotional faces in young children exposed to intimate partner violence. *Journal of Child & Adolescent Trauma*, *4*(2), 109–122. doi.org/10.1080/19361521.2011.573525

Valera, E. M. (2020). When pandemics clash: Gendered violence-related traumatic brain injuries in women since COVID-19. *E Clinical Medicine*, *2*, 100423. doi.org/10.1016/j.eclinm.2020.100423

Valera, E., & Kucyi, A. (2017). Brain injury in women experiencing intimate partner violence: Neural mechanistic evidence of an "invisible" trauma. *Brain Imaging and Behavior*, *11*(6), 1664–1677. doi.org/10.1007/s11682-016-9643-1

# 13 Culturally Sensitive Health Promotion and Health Care to Prevent Chronic Diseases in Black Communities

Carolyn M. Tucker, Guillermo Wippold, Julia Roncoroni, and Kirsten G. Klein

Anything worth doing ain't easy.

—Roy Nathaniel Tucker,
[Expression in a motivational talk with disadvantaged youth]

Chronic disease is defined by the World Health Organization (WHO) as a disease that typically has a long duration, a slow progression, and that is not communicable. Because many chronic diseases have similar risk factors, it is not unusual for individuals to have multiple, co-occurring chronic diseases. For example, adult obesity that is an epidemic disease in the United States (Mitchell et al., 2011), commonly co-occurs with type 2 diabetes (Geiss et al., 2010), hypertension and coronary heart disease (Eckel & Krauss, 1998), and several cancers (Renehan et al., 2008). This is alarming because it is known that the rate of obesity is higher among Black adults (49.6%) compared to Hispanic adults (44.8%), and non-Hispanic White adults (42.2%) (Hales et al., 2020), and that the rate of obesity is higher among Black women (56.6%) than Hispanic women (50.0%), non-Hispanic White women (42%) (Hales et al., 2020), and men of all races/ethnicities. Compared to Hispanics and non-Hispanic Whites, Black adults also have the highest rates of the following obesity, co-occurring chronic diseases: hypertension (Aggarwal et al., 2021), type 2 diabetes (CDC, 2022), and several cancers such as colorectal cancer, prostate cancer, and breast cancer. Although it is well known that regular health-care use can help prevent and reduce the negative impact of multiple chronic diseases, many Black adult patients with such diseases underutilize available primary health care (Stepanikova & Oates, 2017).

Culturally sensitive health care is key to promoting health and preventing disease among Black adults. Research conducted with Black Americans has identified perceived cultural insensitivity of health-care providers as a major barrier to health-care use among these individuals (Tucker, Moradi et al., 2014). Additionally, culturally insensitive health-care systems have been identified as major contributors to poor health outcomes among racial/ethnic minorities. Patient-centered, culturally sensitive health care has therefore been identified as a best-practice approach for improving health outcomes and for reducing health disparities. This type of care involves providers and staff (a) being aware of their biases (e.g., racial and income-related biases) and realizing that patients also have biases (e.g., provider preferences based on race) that may impact health-care use; (b) empowering patients to be respected partners who have interpersonal control in the clinical encounter; (c) engaging in behaviors that enable their patients to feel comfortable, respected, and trusting in patient–provider interactions; and (d) fostering a physical and social environment in the clinical setting that enables patients to feel a sense of belonging (e.g., have minority-focused magazines in waiting areas and culturally diverse front desk staff) (Tucker et al., 2011). The importance of patient-centered culturally sensitive health care is highlighted by a study involving 229 patients (48% African American; 52% White), which found that provider cultural sensitivity predicted treatment adherence among the African American patients (Tucker, Marsiske et al., 2011).

Given the serious consequences of chronic diseases and their high rates among Black communities, prevention of chronic diseases among these communities is critically important. Such prevention of chronic diseases can occur through culturally sensitive health promotion programs that are (a) designed to promote modifiable healthy lifestyle behaviors, (b) anchored in a community-based participatory research (CBPR) approach, and (c) holistic (i.e., target mental, physical, social, and spiritual health-related outcomes). The importance of targeting modifiable lifestyle behaviors is evidenced by campaigns spearheaded by the Centers for Disease Control and Prevention (CDC) that links chronic diseases and risk behaviors, which are modifiable (CDC, 2013). Though, it is recognized that health promotion campaigns among Black Americans are limited in impact. Campaigns that do not align with the values, perspectives, and preferences of these individuals produce limited health-related results. The CBPR approach requires involvement of community members as equitable partners in every aspect of the prevention program. Because of the involvement of the target community in the entire research process, health promotion campaigns anchored in CBPR naturally align with the values, perspectives, and preferences of the target community and are considered viable strategies to reduce health disparities and prevent chronic health conditions. Holistic refers to giving attention to the whole person, including the mental, social, and spiritual aspects of that person. This approach to health promotion aligns with qualitative research conducted with Black Americans indicating that these individuals have a conceptualization of health that encompasses multiple domains (i.e., physical, psychological, spiritual, and social) (Griffith et al., 2018; Hankerson & Bailer, 2015;

Namageyo-Funa et al., 2015). In this chapter, we describe two grant-funded, evidence-informed, culturally sensitive health promotion programs for Black adults. The first is called the Health-Smart Holistic Health (HSHH) Program for Black seniors ages 55 and older (Tucker et al., in press). This is a holistic health promotion program rooted in CBPR. The second is called the Health-Smart for Weight Loss (HSWL) Program (Tucker et al., submitted for publication). This health promotion program is also a holistic health promotion program rooted in CBPR that sought to promote weight loss and weight loss maintenance among Black women with obesity.

## 13.1 The Health-Smart Holistic Health Program for Black Seniors

Black older adults are disproportionately impacted by structural barriers, such as poverty and discrimination, which contribute to adverse health conditions (Chatters et al., 2020; Graham, 2020). Given the documented limitations of "one-size-fits-all" approaches (i.e., approaches that are not tailored for individuals and often produce limited results), it is important to develop culturally relevant interventions that promote health and prevent disease among Black older adults that take into account the aforementioned structural barriers (Minvielle, 2017; Wippold et al., 2021). The Health-Smart Holistic Health Program for Black Seniors (called here the HSHH Program) is such a program. The HSHH Program has been repeated with different seniors each year from 2019 to the present year (i.e., 2022). It is designed to address social isolation, food insecurity, and financial insecurity that negatively impact the health and health-related quality of life of older adult residents in Jacksonville, Florida's Health Zone 1 (Year 1: $n$ = 600, Year 2: $n$ = 500, Year 3: $n$ = 300, and Year 4: $n$ =150). Health Zone 1 in Jacksonville has the highest rates of poverty, chronic disease, and heart disease among the six health zones in this city. Health Zone 1 also has the highest percentage of racial/ethnic minority residents (81.2%) and the highest percentage of Black residents (85%) of all of the six Jacksonville health zones.

## 13.2 Theoretical Background and Intervention Description

The HSHH Program was based on the Health Self-Empowerment Theory (HSET; Tucker et al., 2009, 2018) and the Minority Health and Health Disparities (NIMHD) Research Framework (National Institute on Minority Health and Health Disparities, 2021). HSET highlights the importance of five modifiable cognitive behavioral variables that influence health-promoting behaviors among underserved individuals. These variables are (a) health motivation, (b) health self-praise, (c) coping style (problem-solving, spiritual, religious, and/or emotion-focused coping), (d) health responsibility and knowledge, and (e) health self-efficacy. There is ample evidence that HSET predicts health-related behaviors among underserved individuals (Tucker, Butler, Kaye et al., 2014; Tucker, Butler, Loyuk et al., 2009; Tucker, Wippold et al., 2014; Wippold et al., 2019). Given their low perceived or actual power over their health, low-income Black older adults may be empowered and more able to engage in healthy lifestyle behaviors by focusing on such personal, psychological, and spiritual/religious variables. Support for this view has come from research showing that the Health-Smart Behavior Program™, which is also rooted in HSET, has been effective in promoting weight loss among low-income Black older adults (Tucker et al., 2016, 2017).

The NIMHD Research Framework (National Institute on Minority Health and Health Disparities, 2021) highlights the complex and multifaceted nature of health disparities impacting Black older adults and other minorities by drawing attention to determinants of health under several domains of influence (i.e., biological, behavioral, physical/built environment, sociocultural environment, and health-care system) and different levels of influence (i.e., individual, interpersonal, community, and societal), while emphasizing a lifespan perspective (National Institute on Minority Health and Health Disparities, 2021). The HSHH Program targeted determinants at the individual (e.g., loneliness), interpersonal (e.g., social isolation), and community (e.g., food security) levels of influence, all of which typically increase the risk for poor health outcomes among low-income Black older adults (Chatters et al., 2020; Schulz et al., 2020).

Drawing on HSET and the NIMHD Research Framework, the major components of the HSHH Program are (a) the Health-Smart Behavior Program™ (commonly called Health-Smart) – which promotes health-smart behaviors (i.e., healthy eating, physical activity, and depression and stress management) and has been adapted to increase food security and social connection among older adults; (b) a food pantry program implemented at churches in Health Zone 1; (c) a cellphone-based Social Connection and Food Security (SCFS) App that was developed for this program in order to promote social connection; and (d) a job training and placement, financial literacy, and asset security program for family members who contribute to participating older adults' financial situation either directly or indirectly (e.g., through providing them with free transportation). This latter program was implemented by the Jacksonville Urban League.

This iteration of Health-Smart that was adapted for the HSHH Program was implemented by trained Black community members who served as Health Empowerment Coaches (HECs). HECs led a goal-setting session, group discussion sessions, and group physical activities. During the goal-setting session, HECs individually met with participants to facilitate these participants' setting of a SMART (i.e., specific, measurable, attainable, realistic, and time-bound) physical activity goal and healthy eating goal. HECs also led nine weekly two-hour group discussion sessions with the program participants. In these group sessions, participants discussed the content in the Health-Smart Behavior Resource Guide for Adults that is a culturally relevant resource guide created by the research team that includes information on healthy eating and drinking, physical activity, stress and depression management behaviors, and strategies for overcoming barriers to these behaviors. HECs also encouraged participants to engage in moderate-to-intense physical activity as they were able, with a target of 150 minutes per week. Toward the end of the intervention program, participants attended Health Smart Expert Panels. These panels consisted of invited health experts (e.g., medical doctors, dietitians, nurses, mental health professionals, physical fitness experts), as well as community members that have made positive lifestyle changes. The participants in the HSHH Program asked panel members anonymous health-related questions.

As previously described, participants in the HSHH Program were provided access to food pantries that were implemented at 10 churches in Jacksonville's Health Zone 1. These pantries provided free, healthy foods and were financially supported by grant funds awarded to the principal investigator (PI) for the HSHH Program. The pantries were used 2,737 times in the first program year, and about this same usage has occurred annually to date. Finally, family members who contributed to the participating older adults' financial situation were offered a job training and placement, financial literacy, and asset security program. However, only approximately 10% of the family members of the program participants enrolled in this latter program because of several reasons, including difficulty reaching these family members, low literacy levels, and problematic background records.

Although participants received opportunities for social connection as participants in Health-Smart, the SCFS App was also developed to increase these opportunities. In the first of the two-hour group sessions, the HECs taught the program participants how to use this app. The SCFS app allowed Health-Smart Program participants to chat with each other and allowed all community members to seek consultation regarding their physical and mental health, with possible referrals to health services in their community.

During Year 2, the HSHH Program was paused for six months because of COVID-19. In consultation with participants and relevant stakeholders, the PI and research team determined that a technology-enhanced version of the program should be developed and implemented. This decision was made given emerging research on the disproportionate impact of the pandemic on low-income Black older adults' health and social connection (Cohen & Tavares, 2020; Vasquez Reyes, 2020). The adaptation of the HSHH Program to a technology-enhanced version of the program occurred in conjunction with community stakeholders. This adaptation included a drive-through pantry program and delivery of Health-Smart via Zoom version. To support older adults who struggled with use of technology, a Zoom and conference call training and support component was added to group discussions. Additionally, technical support was provided by the HECs and research assistants.

For the purpose of the online implementation of Health-Smart, materials were digitized and uploaded to the internet. The research team also developed a website to deliver the physical activity component. The website included (a) links to Zoom-based fitness programs, like Zumba®, that fostered social connection among participants and (b) a platform that participants could use to interact with one another and participate in fitness-based games. Student research assistants organized and attended Zoom-delivered fitness programs. The SCFS app's use continued given its compliance with COVID-19-related social distancing recommendations.

## 13.3 Social Justice/Diversity Emphasis

The HSHH Program is based on principles of socially just leadership, which focuses on supporting groups most affected by health disparities, such as Black older adults, in achieving health justice (Tucker et al., 2017). Because it is based on these principles, the program included the following best practices: (a) involvement of diverse, multidisciplinary, and representative leadership teams; (b) establishment of an egalitarian leadership structure; (c) promotion of equal power, participation, and influence; (d) identification of mutually beneficial activities and goals; (e) promotion of facilitative attitudes and values and implementation of structures for sustained goal attainment; and (f) empowerment of members of groups experiencing health disparities.

This program was a collaborative multidisciplinary effort among (a) two University of Florida health centers, where participant program evaluation data were collected (i.e., weight, blood pressure, and responses to questionnaires that assessed stress, depression, healthy eating, and physical activity), (b) 20 churches serving a Black congregation; (c) University of Florida faculty and students who were part of the research team, (d) community member researchers called community scientists, (e) community member leaders who were members of the research team, and (f) local stakeholders such as Feeding North Florida Food Distribution Center. Other important partners included health promotion groups such as the Jacksonville Area Health Education Center that offered free healthy eating classes to participants who completed Health-Smart, and the Jacksonville Institute of Food and Agricultural Sciences Extension Office that offered similar services and vegetable gardening education. Multidisciplinary teams have been praised for their potential to promote health equity and reduce health disparities (Haq, 2017).

The team of academic and community member interventionists and researchers collaborated to design and implement the HSHH Program. This collaboration in design and implementation ensured that the intervention aligned with the values, preferences, and perspectives of the low-income Black older adult program participants. This included the coaches who implemented the Health-Smart component of the program and participant enrollers/data collectors (community scientists) from the target community, all of whom participated in research meetings. Transparent procedures were used to elect program leaders in a way that promoted representation and participation; as an example, HECs were nominated by the participating churches that grew from 10 churches to 20 in Year 1 of the program to 20 churches in Year 2 of the program. All community members who participated in planning, implementing, and evaluating the program were trained as needed and compensated fairly for their time.

Community members were also crucial in deciding on the goals of the program. These goals were determined in collaboration with church leaders and in response to a needs assessment in Health Zone 1. Additionally, the community member researchers/interventionists were asked whether they had the capacity and/or desire to continue the intervention program during the pandemic. Their input was that the program should be continued during the pandemic.

Notably, the HSHH Program was designed to be sustainable. The trust and bidirectional learning between the academic and community member research team members informed and supported the implementation and sustainability of the program. As another example, in 2021, a survey of transportation needs was conducted. A transportation alliance that was comprised of eight community members not a part of our research team but living in Health Zone 1 and one community research team member worked with the Jacksonville Transportation Authority (JTA) executives and city leaders to obtain survey-based bus transportation policy changes. To evaluate the program, mixed methods were used that relied on community input. Results were interpreted with the help of the community at town halls.

### 13.3.1 Practical Recommendations for Individuals Interested in Implementing the HSHH Program

Following are several practical recommendations for individuals interested in implementing a program similar to the HSHH Program in their community or another community (i.e., the target community):

1. Reflect on whether or not one is willing to work hard to build the trust of target community – work that includes having meetings after 5:00 p.m. with members of the target community and waiting months before collecting

data for publication. Find reasons to feel passionate about the program as community members can tell if outsiders of their community genuinely care about community members.

2. Review the most recent health needs assessment for the target community to be sure that the program of interest addresses one or more of the priority concerns identified in that assessment.
3. Meet with members/leaders in the community who are interested in health/wellbeing of their community (e.g., church leaders) for the purpose of obtaining their feedback on the program idea and soliciting input on the most important health priorities in their community. It is important that this feedback and input help guide program intervention planning.
4. Work to develop equitable partnerships with the aforementioned community members/leaders. Such partnerships ideally should be consistent with the CBPR approach, which requires that partners be involved in all aspects of research planning, implementation, and evaluation and that the target community receives benefits and resources (e.g., materials, equipment, part of the grant funding, and payment of community members more than a living wage for their program participation).
5. Provide leadership roles and titles for community member research partners just as is provided for the university/academic partners – titles such as program manager, associate program manager, community scientists.
6. Make sure that the university/academic team of researchers are culturally diverse and include members of the race/ethnicity and age of the target community. This increases the likelihood that the team will be accepted as partners in the target community.
7. Establish a community advisory board with the assistance of the community member partners. This board should ideally be selected because of the strengths (e.g., is a member of an organization that serves individuals being targeted in the intervention program) and resources (has access to funding to support implementation of the intervention program) that they bring to the board.
8. Include community members as leaders in trainings designed to promote cultural sensitivity among all intervention program team members.
9. Meet with members of the local institutional review boards (IRBs) to develop practical strategies for enabling community members to become IRB-approved community scientists (i.e., individuals approved to enroll and collect data from study participants).
10. Use a "talk less and listen more" policy from university/academic team members in meetings with community leaders and community member research partners.
11. Hold town hall meetings to share research findings and challenges with members of the target community.

12. Provide training and consultation to community member research partners and community leaders that will enable sustainability of the intervention program if it is shown to produce some positive health outcomes.
13. Include community research partners as co-authors of publications about the intervention program that they help implement and/or evaluate.

There are also some important recommendations for evaluating programs similar to the HSHH Program when it is implemented by individuals in their community or another community. Following are these evaluation recommendations:

1. Educate community leaders and research partners involved with the research about the importance of program evaluation and research designs to evidence the beneficial effects of the intervention program.
2. Obtain evaluation data from those who implement the intervention and those who support the intervention, as well as from the participants in the intervention. All of these evaluation data will help determine the broad impact of the intervention and how the intervention can be improved.
3. Obtain qualitative evaluation data (e.g., focus group data) and quantitative evaluation strategies (e.g., questionnaire data and biometric data such as blood pressure).
4. Use focus groups and interviews that seek to determine program weaknesses and needed program changes to overcome these weaknesses as well as to improve program delivery and impact.
5. Collect process evaluation data such as dropout, the percentage of invited participants who decided not to participate in the intervention program, and the reasons for dropping out and not participating. This information can help determine ways to make intervention programs more accessible and acceptable to all in a target community.

## 13.4 Health-Smart for Weight Loss (HSWL) Program

Black women have the highest prevalence of obesity in the United States. Despite the high rate of obesity among Black women, there is a significant need for effective weight loss and weight loss maintenance strategies for them. The HSWL Program was designed to address this need and was two-phased. The first phase tested the impact of a culturally sensitive, evidence-based program (i.e., the Health-Smart Behavior Program™ [Health-Smart]) for reducing weight among Black women with obesity that was conducted in 20 primary care clinics and implemented over the course of 6 months by trained community health workers (CHWs). The second phase tested the comparative effectiveness of two 12-month clinic-based, physician-implemented weight-loss maintenance programs at these same 20 primary care clinics. Immediately following participation in the 6-month Health-Smart, all clinics and participating patients and physicians within each clinic were randomized to one of two 12-month, physician-implemented weight loss maintenance programs. Those two weight loss maintenance programs were the (1) patient-centered, culturally sensitive weight loss maintenance program (PCCS-WLM) and (2) standard behavioral weight loss maintenance program (SB-WLM), which had a major focus on motivational interviewing (Tucker et al., 2022).

## 13.5 Theoretical Background and Intervention Description

### 13.5.1 Phase 1: Health-Smart

All participating women completed a six-month version of Health-Smart to promote initial weight loss. This program was described in the preceding HSHH Program section of our chapter. Unlike previous iterations of Health-Smart, this version of Health-Smart was implemented by trained community health workers (CHWs). Following their participation in this program, all clinics, and therefore the participants and physicians within each clinic, were randomized to one of the two weight loss maintenance programs – the PCCS-WLM and the SB-WLM programs.

### 13.5.2 Phase 2: PCCS-WLM and SB-WLM Interventions

The PCCS-WLM Intervention was based on the Patient-Centered, Culturally Sensitive Health Care (PC-CSHC) Model (Tucker et al., 2011). The PC-CSHC Model asserts that (a) patient-perceived provider cultural sensitivity promotes patients' trust in their provider, satisfaction with provider's care, and perceived interpersonal control; (b) the latter two variables impact treatment adherence (e.g., dietary adherence) via physical stress; and (c) physical stress, satisfaction with provider's care, and perceived interpersonal control also directly promote treatment adherence. A test of this model indicated that it is a good fit for Black patients and non-Hispanic White American patients; however, the link between perceived provider cultural sensitivity and satisfaction with provider's care was stronger among the Black patients; furthermore, among the Black patients only, perceived interpersonal control had a significant positive impact on dietary adherence, and physical stress had a significant negative effect on treatment adherence (Tucker et al., 2011). In another test of the first part of this model, it was found that the relationship between provider cultural sensitivity and health-care satisfaction was mediated by trust in one's provider and patient-perceived provider impartiality (fairness) – a core aspect of health-care justice (Tucker, Moradi et al., 2014).

One implication of these findings is that training medical professionals in cultural sensitivity is key to promoting health among underserved individuals (Tucker et al., 2011).

Additionally, prior to developing the abovementioned training for the physicians who implemented the interventions in our HSWL Program, the PI and her team conducted focus groups with Black women who were not participants in the present study who have obesity or were overweight (Tucker et al., 2021) to determine the desired and undesired weight-focused behaviors of providers in clinical encounters with Black women who have obesity. Based on the results of these focus groups and the PC-CSHC Model, the HSWL Program began with online training of physicians about the major content of the Health-Smart Program followed by in-person training on how to (a) talk with their Black women patients about their weight, weight loss goals, barriers to their weight-loss goals, and strategies for overcoming their goal barriers; (b) deliver this talk in culturally sensitive ways (i.e., in ways that enable Black women patients to feel comfortable with, trusting of, and respected by the physicians talking with them); (c) assist their patients with engaging in self-identified strategies for achieving and sustaining their self-selected health-smart goals for weight loss and overall health; (d) promote patients' use of the health-smart behaviors learned in Health-Smart; (e) display behaviors and attitudes in physician–patient interactions with Black women patients that are provider cultural sensitivity indicators in published literature, but customized for use when counseling Black women patients with obesity; and (f) display behaviors and attitudes that Black women have identified as important when discussing obesity and weight loss. It was posited that this PCCS-WLM physician-implemented intervention would yield better results (i.e., more participants experiencing weight loss maintenance) than the physician-implemented SB-WLM intervention due to the intervention's alignment with the preferences and values of Black women with obesity.

The SB-WLM was based on a commonly used approach to weight loss maintenance – a behavioral motivational interviewing emphasized approach. This program was designed to enable physicians to (a) conduct motivational interviews with their patients about their weight loss goals and behavioral strategies to achieve these goals; (b) know empirically supported behavioral change principles that have been used to help patients maintain weight loss in previous interventions; (c) communicate how to use these empirically supported behavioral change principles to have patients initiate or maintain their self-selected health-smart goals related to weight loss and/or weight loss maintenance; and (d) conduct motivational interviews to communicate empathy and understanding to patients who are struggling to maintain their weight loss and/or accomplish a health-smart behavior goal.

## 13.6 Social Justice/Diversity Emphasis

Similar to the HSHH Program, the HSWL Program was developed to promote a positive and sustainable health-related impact on the lives of Black women with obesity. Specifically, this impact was achieved by the (1) involvement of patients, community member focus group members, and clinic directors as study partners (i.e., a CBPR approach); (2) tailoring of the physician training to the cultural preferences and values of the target group; (3) engagement of CHWs and physicians as interventionists within longstanding primary care clinics; and (4) involvement of clinic staff (e.g., medical assistants and office managers) in integrating CHWs into the clinic so that they could implement Health-Smart in designated clinic areas during clinic hours and in the evenings when the clinics were closed. The HSWL Program was also based in HSET.

The interventions leveraged the expertise of Black women with obesity or who were overweight, in addition to other professionals (e.g., a study advisory board consisting of physicians, an insurance company representative, and community members) as stakeholders to help develop, implement, and evaluate the intervention. This approach drew on the tenets of CBPR and centered the voices of participants, which resulted in an intervention designed by and for Black women with obesity. Such an approach aligns the intervention with the preferences, values, and perspectives of these women – an approach that holds promise in promoting health equity (Wippold, Frary, Abshire et al., 2021). Recently, national funding organizations such as the Patient-Centered Outcomes Research Institute and the National Institutes of Health have advocated for the involvement of members of the target community and those with diverse perspectives (e.g., researchers and professionals from other fields).

Notably, the HSWL Program sought to improve health among a "hard-to-reach" group. The National Institutes of Health Revitalization Act of 1993 mandated for the proportional representation of racial/ethnic minorities in health-related research. Despite this mandate, Black adults continue to be underrepresented in such research (Chen et al., 2014; Vickers & Fouad, 2014). This underrepresentation is extremely problematic given that Black adults experience a disproportionate amount of health disparities and have little representation in health-related research to reduce these disparities.

Finally, the engagement of CHWs and physicians as implementers of the Health-Smart Program and the PCCS-WLM Intervention lends support for the sustainability of these health promotion efforts. This is because many health promotion efforts successfully implemented by academic researchers alone typically cease to continue when the project terminates. Health promotion efforts implemented by CHWs, physicians, and other nonacademic partners, along with academic research partners, can continue to promote health among the target community long after the cessation of the program.

### 13.6.1 Practical Recommendations for Individuals Interested in Implementing the HSWL Program

Following are several practical recommendations for individuals interested in implementing a program similar to the HSWL Program in their community primary care clinics or in primary care clinics in other communities (i.e., the target primary care clinics):

1. Include the administrators and directors of the target primary care clinics as coinvestigators in the proposed program as these individuals have much influence on the needed participation of all clinic staff and providers in the program. It is critically important to have the aforementioned administrators and directors actively involved in the initial meetings to plan the intervention program.
2. Arrange for strong monetary and other incentives (e.g., free continuing education units) for physicians as well as the support staff (e.g., medical technicians) to participate in the intervention program.
3. In program planning, identify structural barriers to patients' participation in the intervention program such as transportation and lack of babysitters and develop strategies for overcoming these barriers.
4. Include a physical fitness professional or exercise physiologist who can design physical activities that are safe for older individuals and individuals with physical limitations such as arthritis.
5. Use recruitment flyers that have pictures of individuals who look like someone who could be a member of the target community. If the target group is a group for whom English is often not their first language, make sure that the words on the flyer are in both the first language of the group and in English.
6. Avoid training physicians to implement weight loss interventions in the evenings after a long day of seeing patients, as it is challenging to fully engage these physicians in this training even when they desire the training and perceive it as important.
7. Make sure that the directors of the participating clinics inform all clinic staff about the intervention program, the roles of the community health workers (CHWs) in the program, and the need to welcome the CHWs and integrate them as members of the clinic staff.
8. Conduct focus groups with the participating physicians and clinical staff early in the intervention program to identify ways to improve the intervention as it was being implemented.

9. Hire enough research coordinators such that each can oversee program implementation at a maximum of four clinics, as programs like the HSWL Program are time-intensive and complex.
10. It is important that the administrator and directors of the clinic be involved in establishing a plan for sustaining the program as devoting time for physicians to implement weight loss maintenance interventions requires a commitment of money to pay for this time – money that can only be approved by the administrators of the primary care clinics participating in the intervention program.
11. Involve primary care clinic directors and administrators as well as community research partners in grant writing training so that they can write grants to obtain funding to help sustain their intervention program.

There are also some important recommendations for evaluating a program similar to the HSWL Program when it is implemented in community primary care clinics by individuals in their community or another community. Following are these evaluation recommendations:

1. Evaluation of the perceived impact of the intervention program and needed changes in the program ideally should occur at all program levels, including the administrator, director, physician, clinic staff, CHW staff, and patient participant level. It is important for these impact data to be obtained periodically throughout the program, rather than just at the end of the program, so that any needed program adjustments can be made early in the process of implementing the program.
2. Evaluation of the program on participating patients' health outcomes needs to be assessed not only by weight/BMI and blood pressure changes but also by changes in cholesterol, triglycerides, and blood glucose levels.
3. Given the mind–body–spirit health connection, it is important to include measures of program impact in all three of these health domains.
4. It is important that program evaluation questionnaires used with Black adults and other people of color include such target groups in the standardization group for each questionnaire.
5. Use focus groups and structured interviews (i.e., qualitative assessment methods) to obtain program evaluation data. These assessment methods are culturally sensitive in many ways including because they do not require good reading and writing skills.
6. Produce video testimonials from patient participants in which these patients discuss the impact of the intervention program as such videos are powerful patient participant and physician participant recruitment tools.
7. Allow adequate time for multilevel evaluations of the intervention program and its impact when designing the program timeline. It is typical to plan for these evaluations to occur in one month, though in reality they require two to three months.

8. Involve representatives from among the patients and clinic staff at the participating primary care clinics as well as the administrator(s) of these clinics and the community and academic research team members in making meaning of all the program evaluation and program impact data obtained.
9. Include the aforementioned representatives in a town hall meeting where study findings and related evaluation data are presented.
10. Include training in program implementation impact and overall program evaluation in the plan for sustaining the intervention program at the participating clinics.

## 13.7 Conclusion

There is much evidence regarding the high prevalence of chronic diseases and the underutilization of health care in Black communities in general and in low-income Black communities in particular. The outcome of this reality for many Black adults is morbidity and premature death. Thus, prevention of chronic diseases in Black communities must be a national priority as evidenced by needed system-level health care, health promotion, economic, educational, and environmental changes. Given that these changes will not come in the lifetime of many living Black adults, it is extremely important that academic researchers form equitable partnerships with community members and health-focused funders to conduct intervention research focused on developing and testing multilevel intervention programs to prevent and/or reduce chronic diseases. It is important that such intervention research is culturally sensitive and individual and community empowerment-oriented.

In sum, prevention of chronic diseases among Black adults involves empowering members of Black communities to take charge of their health under whatever conditions that exist in their lives and promoting nonracist and culturally sensitive health-related policies and systems that facilitate this empowerment. Examples of such empowerment that can occur immediately are training community members to be researchers, training academic researchers to be culturally sensitive, training all researchers to conduct CBPR, and including community members as coinvestigators and collaborators on research grants. Such empowerment actions are not easy, but anything worth doing "ain't" easy.

## Acknowledgments

The HSHH Program was funded by the Humana Foundation (PI: Tucker; AWD05408; AWD07906; AWD09725).

The HSWL Program was funded by the Patient-Centered Outcomes Research Institute (PI: Tucker; PCORI/AD-1609-36187).

## Recommended Resources

Agency for Healthcare Research and Quality. (2021). *National healthcare disparities report, 2021*. Rockville, MD. www.ahrq.gov/research/findings/nhqrdr/nhqdr21/index.html

American Association of Retired Persons. (2020). *The pandemic effect: A social isolation report*. https://connect2affect.org/wp-content/uploads/2020/10/The-Pandemic-Effect-A-Social-Isolation-Report-AARP-Foundation.pdf

Centers for Disease Control and Prevention. (2013). CDC health disparities and inequalities report – United States. *Morbidity and Mortality Weekly Report, 62*(3). www.cdc.gov/mmwr/pdf/other/su6203.pdf

National Institute on Minority Health and Health Disparities. (2017). *NIMHD research framework*. https://nimhd.nih.gov/researchFramework.

Patient-Centered Outcomes Research Institute. (2022, March 4). *Do Black women with obesity lose weight and keep the weight off when offered culturally sensitive treatment programs?* Patient-Centered Outcomes Research Institute. www.pcori.org/research-results/2017/do-black-women-obesity-lose-weight-and-keep-weight-when-offered-culturally-sensitive-treatment-programs

Tucker, C. M., Roncoroni, J., & Buki, L. P. (2019). Counseling psychologists and behavioural health: Promoting mental and physical health outcomes. *The Counseling Psychologist, 47*(7), 970–998. https://psycnet.apa.org/doi/10.1177/0011000019896784

Tucker, C. M., Williams, J. L., Roncoroni, J., & Heesacker, M. (2017). A socially just leadership approach to community-partnered research for reducing health disparities. *The Counseling Psychologist, 45*(6), 781–809. https://psycnet.apa.org/doi/10.1177/0011000017722213

US Preventive Services Task Force. (2018). Behavioral weight loss interventions to prevent obesity-related morbidity and mortality in adults: US Preventive Services Task Force recommendation statement. *Journal of the American Medical Association, 320*(11):1163–1171. doi.org/10.1001/jama.2018.13022

## Community Partners

Florida Community Health Workers Coalition. www.flchwcoalition.org/

The Florida Community Health Worker Coalition, Inc. is a statewide partnership dedicated to the support and promotion of the CHW profession through collaboration, training, advocacy, and leadership development.

Jacksonville Institute of Food and Agricultural Extension Office. https://sfyl.ifas.ufl.edu/duval/

The Jacksonville Institute of Food and Agricultural Extension Office's mission is to continually enhance the quality of life for a unified Jacksonville through strengthening decision-making, knowledge application, economic security, environmental care, and leadership skills for all citizens.

Jacksonville Transportation Authority. www.jtafla.com/

The Jacksonville Transportation Authority, an independent state agency serving Duval County, has multimodal responsibilities. JTA designs and constructs bridges and highways and provides varied mass transit services. These include express and regular bus service, community shuttles for a neighborhood ride, a downtown Skyway monorail, the St. Johns River Ferry, the Gameday Xpress for various sporting events at TIAA Bank Field, paratransit for the disabled and elderly, and Ride Request on-demand services.

Northeast Florida Area Health Education Center. www.northfloridaahec.org/about/
The Northeast Florida Area Health Education Center's mission is to enhance access to quality health care, particularly primary and preventive care, by improving the supply and distribution of healthcare professionals via strategic partnerships with academic programs, communities, and professional organizations.

## References

Aggarwal, R., Chiu, N., Wadhera, R. K., Moran, A. E., Raber, I., Shen, C., Yeh, R. W., & Kazi, D. S. (2021). Racial/ethnic disparities in hypertension prevalence, awareness, treatment, and control in the United States, 2013 to 2018. *Hypertension*, 78(6), 1719–1726. doi.org/10.1161/hypertensionaha.121.17570

Chatters, L. M., Taylor, H. O., & Taylor, R. J. (2020). Older Black Americans during COVID-19: Race and age double jeopardy. *Health Education & Behavior*, *47*(6), 855–860. doi.org/10.1177/1090198120965513

Chen, M. S., Lara, P. N., Dang, J. H. T., Paterniti, D. A., & Kelly, K. (2014). Twenty years post-NIH Revitalization Act: Enhancing minority participation in clinical trials (EMPaCT): Laying the groundwork for improving minority clinical trial accrual. *Cancer*, *120*(S7), 1091–1096. doi.org/10.1002/cncr.28575

Cohen, M. A., & Tavares, J. (2020). Who are the most at-risk older adults in the COVID-19 era? It's not just those in nursing homes. *Journal of Aging & Social Policy*, *32*(4–5), 380–386. doi.org/10.1080/08959420.2020.1764310

Eckel, R. H., & Krauss, R. M. (1998). American Heart Association call to action: Obesity as a major risk factor for coronary heart disease. *Circulation*, 97(21), 2099–2100. doi.org/10.1161/01.cir.97.21.2099

Geiss, L. S., James, C., Gregg, E. W., Albright, A., Williamson, D. F., & Cowie, C. C. (2010). Diabetes risk reduction behaviors among U.S. adults with prediabetes. *American Journal of Preventive Medicine*, 38(4), 403–409. doi.org/10.1016/j.amepre.2009.12.029

Graham, J. (2020, September 3). *Why Black aging matters, too*. Kaiser Health News. https://khn.org/news/why-black-aging-matters-too/

Griffith D. M., Cornish E. K., Bergner E. M., Bruce M. A., & Beech B. M. (2018). "Health is the ability to manage yourself without help": How older African American men define health and successful aging. *Journals of Gerontology: Series B*, *73*(2), 240–247. doi.org/10.1093/geronb/gbx075

Hales, C. M., Carroll, M. D., Fryar, C. D., & Ogden, C. L. (2020). Prevalence of obesity and severe obesity among adults: United States, 2017–2018. *NCHS Data Brief*, 360, 1–8. https://stacks.cdc.gov/view/cdc/85451/cdc_85451_DS1.pdf

Hankerson S. H., Suite D., & Bailey R. K. (2015). Treatment disparities among African American men with depression: Implications for clinical practice. *Journal of Health Care for the Poor and Underserved*, *26*(1), 21–34. doi.org/10.1353%2Fhpu.2015.0012

Haq, C. (2017). The path to health equity through multidisciplinary collaboration. *Journal of Patient-Centered Research and Reviews*, *4*(4), 208–210. doi.org/10.17294%2F2330-0698.1615

Mitchell, N. S., Catenacci, V. A., Wyatt, H. R., & Hill, J. O. (2011). Obesity: Overview of an epidemic. *Psychiatric Clinics of North America*, 34(4), 717–732. doi.org/10.1016/j.psc.2011.08.005

Minvielle, E. (2017). Toward customized care comment on "(re) making the procrustean bed? Standardization and customization as competing logics in healthcare." *International Journal of Health Policy and Management*, *7*(3), 272–274. doi.org/10.15171/ijhpm.2017.84

Namageyo-Funa, A., Muilenburg, J., & Wilson, M. (2015). The role of religion and spirituality in coping with type 2 diabetes: A qualitative study among Black men. *Journal of Religion and Health*, *54*(1), 242–252. doi.org/10.1007/s10943-013-9812-0

National Institute on Minority Health and Health Disparities. (2021, April 15). *National Institute on Minority Health and Health Disparities research framework.* www.nimhd.nih.gov/about/overview/research-framework/nimhd-framework.html

Renehan, A. G., Tyson, M., Egger, M., Heller, R. F., & Zwahlen, M. (2008). Body-mass index and incidence of cancer: A systematic review and meta-analysis of prospective observational studies. *The Lancet*, 371(9612), 569–578. doi.org/10.1016/s0140-6736(08)60269-x

Schulz, A. J., Mehdipanah, R., Chatters, L. M., Reyes, A. G., Neblett, E. W., & Israel, B. A. (2020). Moving health education and behavior upstream: Lessons From COVID-19 for addressing structural drivers of health inequities. *Health Education & Behavior*, *47*(4), 519–524. doi.org/10.1177/1090198120929985

Stepanikova, I., & Oates, G. R. (2017). Perceived discrimination and privilege in health care: The role of socioeconomic status and race. *American Journal of Preventive Medicine*, 52(1), S86–S94. doi.org/10.1016/j.amepre.2016.09.024

Tucker, C. M., Anton, S., Marsiske, M., Wippold, G., Bilello, L., Henry, M., Shah, N., Gautam, S., Klein, K., Mathews, A., Webb, F., & Desmond, F. (2022). *A cluster randomized trial to test a culturally sensitive versus a standard behavioral intervention to promote weight loss maintenance among Black women primary care patients.* (Submitted for publication).

Tucker, C. M., Butler, A., Kaye, L. B., Nolan, S. E. M., Flenar, D. J., Marsiske, M., Bragg, M., Hoover, E., & Daly, K. (2014). Impact of a culturally sensitive health self-empowerment workshop series on health behaviors/lifestyles, BMI, and blood pressure of culturally diverse overweight/obese adults. *American Journal of Lifestyle Medicine*, *8*(2), 122–132. doi.org/10.1177/1559827613503117

Tucker, C. M., Butler, A. M., Loyuk, I. S., Desmond, F. F., & Surrency, S. L. (2009). Predictors of a health-promoting lifestyle and behaviors among low-income African American mothers and White mothers of chronically ill children. *Journal of the National Medical Association*, 101(2), 103–110. doi.org/10.1016/S0027-9684(15)30821-X

Tucker, C. M., Marsiske, M., Rice, K. G., Jones, J. D., & Herman, K. C. (2011). Patient-centered culturally sensitive health care: Model testing and refinement. *Health Psychology*, *30*(3), 342–350. doi.org/10.1037/a0022967

Tucker, C. M., Roncoroni, J., Klein, K. G., Derias, T. O., Ateyah, W., Williams, J., Nmezi, N. A., Shah, N. R., Bilello, L. A., & Anton, S. (2021). Views of Black women patients with obesity on desired and undesired weight-focused clinical encounters. *Clinical Obesity*, *11*(5), e12468. doi.org/10.1111/cob.12468

Tucker, C. M., Roncoroni, J., Wippold, G. M., Marsiske, M., Flenar, D. J., & Hultgren, K. (2018). Health self-empowerment theory: Predicting health behaviors and BMI in culturally diverse adults. *Family & Community Health*, *41*(3), 168–177. doi.org/10.1097/FCH.0000000000000195

Tucker, C. M., Smith, T. M., Wippold, G. M., Whitehead, N. E., Morrissette, T. A., Williams, J. L., Ukonu, N. A., Arthur, T. M., Sealy, Y. M., & Crosier, B. S. (2016). Impact of a university-community partnership approach to improving health behaviors and outcomes among overweight/obese Hispanic adults. *American Journal of Lifestyle Medicine*, *11*(6), 479–488. doi.org/10.1177/1559827615623773

Tucker, C. M., Wippold, G. M., Roncoroni, J., Henry, M. A., Klein, K. G., Garrepy, M., Ateyah, W., Burwell, A., Walker, H., Clements, L. M., Kelly Pryor, B. N., & Fullwood, D. (2022). Impact of the health-smart holistic health program: A CBPR approach to improve health and prevent adverse outcomes for Black older adults. *Journal of Prevention and Health Promotion*, *3*(4), 589–607. doi.org/10.1177/26320770221099586

Tucker, C. M., Wippold, G. M., Smith, T. M., Desmond, F. F., Arthur, T. M., Butler, A. M., Pauly, R. R., & Surrency, S. L. (2014). Association of health self-empowerment with health-promoting behaviors among chronically Ill African American and non-Hispanic White adolescents. *Journal of Health Care for the Poor and Underserved*, *25*(4), 2019–2031. doi.org/10.1353/hpu.2014.0168

Tucker, C. M., Wippold, G. M., Williams, J. L., Arthur, T. M., Desmond, F. F., & Robinson, K. C. (2017). A CBPR study to test the impact of a church-based health empowerment program on health behaviors and health outcomes of Black adult churchgoers. *Journal of Racial and Ethnic Health Disparities*, *4*(1), 1–9. doi .org/10.1007/s40615-015-0203-y

Vasquez Reyes, M. (2020). The disproportional impact of COVID-19 on African Americans. *Health and Human Rights*, *22*(2), 299–307.

Vickers, S. M., & Fouad, M. N. (2014). An overview of EMPaCT and fundamental issues affecting minority participation in cancer clinical trials: Enhancing minority participation in clinical trials (EMPaCT): Laying the groundwork for improving minority clinical trial accrual. *Cancer*, *120*, 1087–1090. doi.org/10.1002%2Fcncr.28569

Wippold, G. M., Frary, S. G., Abshire, D., Wilson, D. K., (2022). Improving recruitment, retention, and cultural saliency of health promotion efforts targeting African American men: A scoping review. *Annals of Behavioral Medicine*, *56*(6), 605–619. doi.org/10.1093/abm/kaab079

Wippold, G. M., Tucker, C. M., Roncoroni, J., & Henry, M. A. (2021). Impact of stress and loneliness on health-related quality of life among low-income senior African Americans. *Journal of Racial and Ethnic Health Disparities*, *8*(4), 1089–1097. doi .org/10.1007/s40615-020-00865-w

Wippold, G. M., Tucker, C. M., Smith, T. M., Whitehead, N. E., Kang, S., Guastello, A. D., Morrissette, T. A., Arthur, T. M., & Desmond, F. F. (2019). An examination of health-promoting behaviors among Hispanic adults using an activation and empowerment approach. *Progress in Community Health Partnerships: Research, Education, and Action*, *13*(1), 9–17. doi.org/10.1353/cpr.2019.0004

# 14 PIER: A Clinical/Epidemiologic System for Prevention of Psychosis

Donna Downing, Rebecca Jaynes, Alexander Kopelowicz, Sarah Lynch, William R. McFarlane, Liisa Sloat, Barbara Stuart, and Barbara C. Walsh

## 14.1 Theoretical and Scientific Background

The Psychosis Identification and Early Referral (PIER) program was developed in 2000 to undertake early detection, intervention, and prevention of psychosis throughout an entire urban catchment area by providing treatment during the prodromal, or clinical high risk (CHR), period. The intent was to reduce the incidence of psychotic disorders and schizophrenia specifically for a defined population, while also rigorously testing the efficacy of family-aided assertive community treatment (FACT) as a preventive treatment (McFarlane et al., 1992). The PIER program (a) developed a community-wide referral network, (b) mounted a major public education campaign, and (c) operated a special multidisciplinary team to treat young people identified as at the highest risk of initial onset of psychosis. The focus was on a defined catchment area, Greater Portland, Maine, with a population of about 340,000 (McFarlane et al., 2010). This chapter will describe the model's theoretical, epidemiological, and clinical background; the model itself; evidence for its efficacy; and the complicating factors often experienced in promulgating and disseminating it across large epidemiologic catchment areas.

## 14.2 Indicated Prevention in Medical Disorders

The theoretical and strategic foundation of the PIER model is that of indicated prevention: identifying and intervening after the onset of a disease state but before the onset of acute and severe symptoms. As in most cancers, onset for schizophrenia has the same progression. Stage 1 is the premorbid period, usually prior to adolescence, during which subtle neurologic and cognitive impairments can be identified, but not psychotic symptoms and, to date, not sufficiently predictive of psychosis. Stage 2 is the target for indicated prevention, as it is for the PIER model: gradual onset in adolescence or early adulthood of subtle and intermittent psychotic symptoms and cognitive impairments notable to the individual and often to concerned and observant others. Stage 3 is the onset of full psychosis with loss of insight, usually manifested by frank hallucinations and fixed delusional ideation, which tend to provoke behavioral disturbance and interference with even the most basic human capacities. Stage 3 is that which is required for the diagnosis of schizophrenia. Stage 4 involves psychotic relapses and severe, often lifelong disability at the emotional, cognitive, intellectual, and functional levels. The design of the approach builds on the remarkable successes of indicated prevention in cardiac disease and many cancers, even when cure and primary prevention have remained elusive (Luepker et al., 1994). The major difference between the psychotic and cardiac or oncological disorders is the age of onset: psychosis strikes and disables young people at the very beginning of their independent, reproductive, and productive lives, while cancer and heart disease strike at the end of life, accounting for a substantial proportion of mortality but not lifelong illness and disability.

The other major theoretical foundation of the PIER model is summarized by the biosocial hypothesis that *major psychiatric disorders are the result of the continuous interaction of specific biological factors with specific psychosocial factors* (McFarlane, 2002). Particularly with respect to schizophrenia, these biological factors include genetic abnormalities; cerebral cortical deficits; and neurochemical, neuroendocrine, and anatomic abnormalities. The effect of these changes becomes evident as neurocognitive losses and sensory abnormalities early in the prodromal period and later as hallmark early psychotic symptoms (Woodberry et al., 2013). The psychosocial factors include the multitude of stressors during adolescence and young adulthood. These include increasing academic demands, social pressures, and romantic disappointments.

In this framework, the interactions involve cognitive impairment leading to academic difficulty that in turn elicits criticism and rejection from parents and teachers, which then leads to increased anxiety, provoking adrenergic and dopaminergic activation, and further deterioration in cognitive functioning. The tragedy is that the psychoses elicit in the social environment the very phenomena that have been most directly associated with clinical and functional deterioration: social isolation; stigma, social rejection, criticism, hostility; and, occasionally, outright physical or sexual abuse. Thus, the earliest signs of an emerging psychosis arise during adolescence because of neurodegenerative processes, psychosocial stress, and hormonal changes. The current approach rests on the assumption that these processes can be altered and even reversed by earlier treatment.

The major qualifier to a comprehensive theoretical foundation is that at the biological, psychological, and psychosocial levels, young people at risk for psychosis are inherently and markedly heterogeneous. For instance, as for ultimate diagnosis, a substantial proportion are actually experiencing the onset of a severe mood disorder, not schizophrenia, although psychosis is a marker for worse severity and a poor prognosis. In addition, several other syndromes manifest as psychosis, including obsessive–compulsive disorder, posttraumatic stress disorder, schizotypal and borderline personality disorders, autism spectrum disorders, substance abuse, acute drug toxicity, and a few rare medical disorders. These diagnoses are manifestations of a variety of underlying and evolving biological abnormalities, which makes pharmacological intervention quite complicated. Indeed, the current international consensus is that antipsychotic drugs should not be offered routinely as an initial preventive treatment. Consider also the developmental stages encompassed within the age range of highest risk: 10–35. Some of those presenting with early psychotic symptoms are prepubertal, while others will be approaching middle age. The most common ages are 14–20, but that range still involves major differences in psychosocial and brain development. Presenting symptoms, course, and age of onset vary by sex. Males tend to be identified earlier during onset secondary to behavioral changes. Females tend to have a later onset, but often go undetected because they cover their symptoms and adapt until cognitive losses become evident to parents and teachers.

Family emotional environments vary widely from extremely critical, rejecting, and even abusive parents or siblings to remarkably understanding, affectionate, and committed immediate family members (McFarlane & Cook, 2007). Fortunately for preventive intervention, the latter form is by far the most common. Some families have only a single parent, while others will present with a large, concerned, and available network. The community environment will vary depending on many factors, especially cultural norms and economic status. Some ethnic cultures strongly stigmatize any form of psychotic illness, making intervention and even identification difficult. A consistent finding is that as poverty increases in a community, the likelihood of very early intervention decreases, consistent with disparities in health in medical disorders generally (McFarlane et al., 2015).

The young person's and the family's religion will usually determine how symptoms are interpreted, sometimes dramatically at odds with current scientific understandings. Confusion about sexual orientation is a stressor, both psychologically and socially (Haas & Drescher, 2014). Youth and their family members vary from one extreme to the other on awareness, insight, and acceptance of risk and preventive intervention. Lack of acceptance may eliminate the possibility of prevention and increases risk for suicide. In summary, while the biosocial perspective improves identification and treatment of prodromal symptoms, the clinician must consider a substantial number of other factors – the "specifics" of brain biology and the social environment – to understand and effectively intervene in an individual in the throes of onset of an initial psychosis (McFarlane et al., 2015).

## 14.3 Public Health Effects and Burden of Disease of Psychotic Disorders

The psychoses are often ignored when considering public health, but they have major effects on the total burden of disease. Among all medical disorders, schizophrenia is one of the most disabling and costly (Rupp & Keith, 1993). It is the most severe mental disorder, creating continuous disability for a lifetime in most cases. Nearly 1% (between 0.27% and 0.83%) of the population suffers directly from this disorder, even though the incidence is low at about 0.2 per 1,000 per year (Eaton, 1999). In market economies, schizophrenia is the fifth leading cause of disability and premature mortality among all medical disorders. It is a devastating disorder for families and communities, whose members often assume major caretaking burdens because of the profound functional deficits that this disorder imposes. Psychotic forms of major depression and bipolar disorder add to the prevalence of psychotic disorder to a total of 2.5–3% of population (Kessler et al., 2005). Twenty-five percent of all hospital admissions and disability payments in the United States are accounted for by patients with severe mental illness, most of them for schizophrenia or other psychotic disorders. It is a major drain on the economy; recent estimates put direct and indirect costs to the nation for schizophrenia alone at more than $62 billion per year (Wu, 2005; Murphy et al., 2021). Recent meta-analyses have found that schizophrenia exacts a 25-year reduction in life expectancy (Parks et al., 2006; Hjorthøj et al., 2017).

## 14.4 Historical Background: Previous Studies and Trials

Long a desired goal, but increasingly a focus of research on clinical practice, prevention of psychosis has emerged as one of the most promising and impactful areas of investigational interest and effort in psychiatry. Spurred by long-term studies that have associated worse outcomes with longer duration of untreated psychosis, research has focused on improving the accuracy of prediction based on clinical and neurocognitive measures and on refining treatments for the earliest symptoms of the psychoses. Several groups, especially in Europe and Australia, have developed treatment programs explicitly designed to intervene early in the first episode (Fusar-Poli et al., 2017). Recently, they have gone on to intervene in the period between onset of attenuated psychotic symptoms and the onset of frank psychosis (i.e., in the prodromal or CHR phase; Fusar-Poli et al., 2013). Given the substantial burdens to the individual, family, community, and economy that these disorders impose when they cause lifelong disability, the initiative to attempt prevention was obvious, even though daunting in its complexity.

The cohort to be identified and treated preventively is already experiencing the onset of psychotic symptoms and is often impaired cognitively and functionally. The extent of illness is subthreshold to the level needed to meet current criteria for a schizophrenic or psychotic mood disorder. Therefore, intervention at this stage is indicated prevention. Further, the question of whether intervention delays or prevents illness onset is left to longer term research. Even delaying onset is seen as valuable, because achieving developmental milestones and cognitive maturation appears to be a defense against the neurologic consequences of long-term psychotic disorders (Woodberry et al., 2013). From a lay perspective, most persons during the prodromal phase are not seen as mentally ill.

These efforts have borne success, with some ambiguity as to the most effective preventive interventions. Initial meta-analyses of early randomized controlled trials suggested that receiving *any* trial intervention (e.g., family psychoeducation, cognitive-behavioral therapy, omega-3 fatty acids, antipsychotic medications) reduced transition to psychosis by 50% at 12 months (van der Gaag et al., 2013). A more recent umbrella review of 42 meta-analyses published between 2013 and 2019 concluded that no robust evidence yet exists to favor any indicated intervention over another for preventing the onset of psychosis (Catalan et al., 2021).

Regarding family intervention, in a randomized controlled trial, FACT led to a significantly lower rate of conversion to psychosis in a sample of people with schizotypal personality disorder, a diagnostic group at high risk for psychosis (Nordentoft et al., 2006). In a study of single-family psychoeducation (family-focused treatment (FFT)), CHR participants randomized to FFT were less likely to convert to psychosis than those assigned to a comparator condition that included three educational sessions (1/55 or 1.8% vs. 5/47 or 10.6%; adjusted odds ratio = 4.7; Miklowitz et al., 2014). The efficacy of psychoeducational multifamily groups (PMFGs) in relapse prevention has been documented in established and first-episode psychotic disorders (Dyck et al., 2000; Fjell et al., 2007; McFarlane, Link et al., 1995; McFarlane, Lukens et al., 1995; Melle et al., 2006; Petersen et al., 2005). PMFGs led to lower rates of relapse and higher rates of engagement, occupational functioning, and retention in treatment (McFarlane et al., 1999; McFarlane et al., 1996; Nordentoft et al., 2006).

## 14.5 PIER Model

### 14.5.1 Overview

The goal of early intervention is to identify and treat young people at risk before they experience a full psychosis. A key and essential component of the PIER approach is a community outreach and education program targeting potential referral sources to (a) increase knowledge of early warning signs for psychotic disorders, (b) increase appropriate referrals of youth at risk, (c) create and educate a system of professional and community member early identifiers, and (d) decrease barriers to early identification. Once identified and referred for preventive treatment, the at-risk person is offered FACT. The

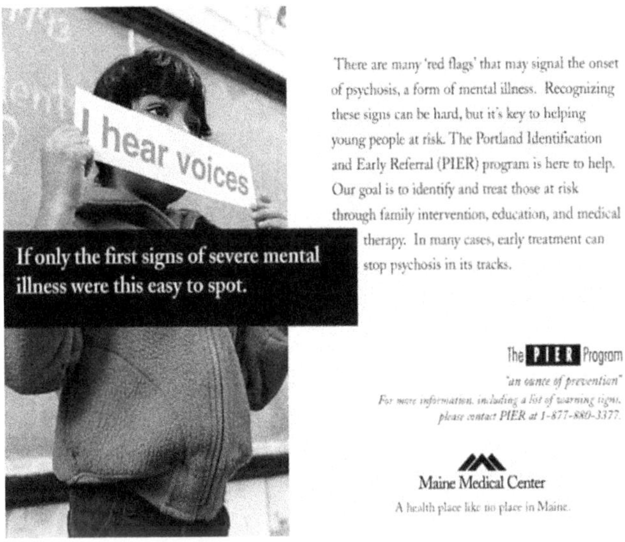
I hear voices
If only the first signs of severe mental illness were this easy to spot.
There are many 'red flags' that may signal the onset of psychosis, a form of mental illness. Recognizing these signs can be hard, but it's key to helping young people at risk. The Portland Identification and Early Referral (PIER) program is here to help. Our goal is to identify and treat those at risk through family intervention, education, and medical therapy. In many cases, early treatment can stop psychosis in its tracks.
The PIER Program
"an ounce of prevention"
For more information, including a list of warning signs, please contact PIER at 1-877-880-3377.
Maine Medical Center
A health place like no place in Maine.

Figure 14.1 Example of an early intervention for psychosis ad campaign (courtesy of PIER Training Institute)

FACT model includes a multidisciplinary team comprised of a psychiatrist or nurse practitioner, nurse, occupational therapist, licensed clinical counselors (MSW, MFT, CPC, PsyD, or PhD), and an educational/employment specialist (ES). The FACT team provides proactive outreach and in vivo treatment that is family-based and client-centered. Each family is assigned a primary clinician and is offered case management, PMFG, supported employment and education, occupational therapy (OT), cognitive-behavioral therapy for psychosis, and psychiatric treatment. PMFG attendance is an expectation of all treatment families, while the intensity of other treatment interventions is dependent on the client's level of functioning and symptom acuity.

### **14.5.2** Community Outreach

When the PIER program community outreach education model was first established in 2000, no American examples were available to use as a model for its community outreach for mental health services, although there was growing international evidence to support the approach(Falloon, 1992; Yung et al., 1996; Joa et al., 2008; Krstev et al., 2004). Although community education and outreach are traditional public health approaches (Luepker et al., 1994; World Health Organization, 2004), until recently no published data existed on their use or outcomes for the prevention of, or early intervention in, major mental illness in the United States. Developments such as the success of the PIER model (Figure 14.1), along with recent studies, have consistently demonstrated that community members and health-care professionals can effectively identify and refer those who are manifesting the early signs of a psychotic disorder (Lynch et al., 2016).

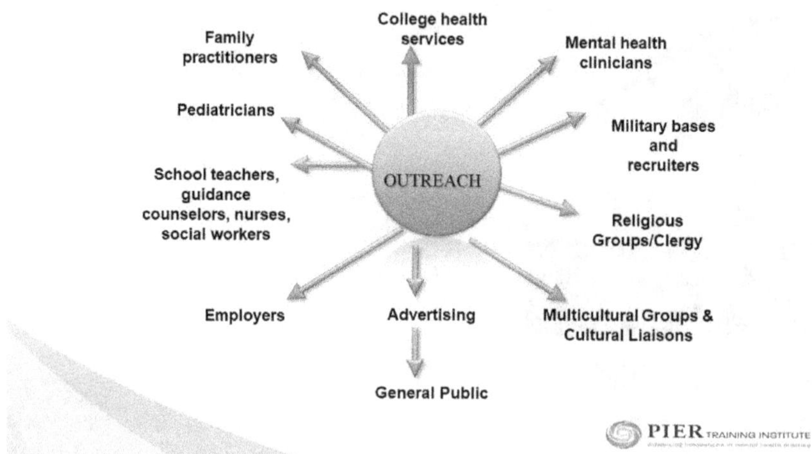


Figure 14.2 Community outreach plan example

## 14.6 Implementing Community Education

Early identification of psychosis depends on the accurate recognition of the earliest warning signs in a young person between the age of 12 and 25 years occurring in themselves or by someone in that person's occupational or social network. It is in the implementation of the PIER model outreach processes that the theory behind the comprehensive model turns to practice, as unique geographic, cultural, socioeconomic, and political opportunities and barriers come into play. When each city, town, or state owns a stake in the outcome of not just the early intervention program, but more generally in the well-being of young people in their community, implementation is more likely to be successful (Figure 14.2).

## 14.7 PIER Model Community Outreach Education

The PIER model community outreach and education plan includes a multi-tiered plan that can maximize earliest possible intervention. The PIER model community education methods include the following:

- developing a plan for community education, including defining the area to be served, estimating opportunities and likely challenges, defining staff roles and leadership, and identifying professional sectors, agencies, and public constituencies to be contacted and provided with education;
- establishing an external steering council and advisory committee to broaden stakeholdership in the outreach effort and to aid in developing awareness and contacts throughout the relevant professional and public sectors in a target community;
- mapping the specific sectors to be contacted and educated, including for young people between 12 and 25 years, a network that primarily includes

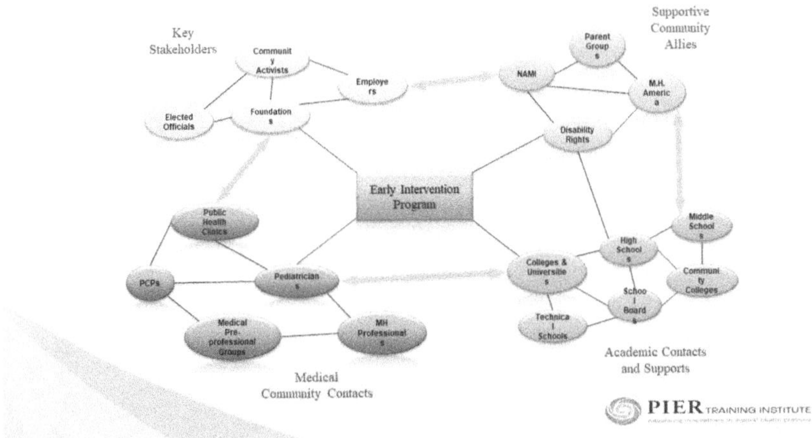


Figure 14.3 Community mapping tool (courtesy of PIER Training Institute)

educational professionals, health-care providers, friends and family members, mental health clinicians, social and human service providers, community agencies, law enforcement, military officers, judicial agencies, and multicultural groups (see Figure 14.3);

- developing or obtaining existing and tested educational materials for those respective sectors and professional groups;
- organizing a systematic and ongoing program of outreach and community education;
- educating professional and public audiences;
- training community professionals to explain symptoms and encourage using treatment options for those experiencing onset;
- establishing a system of rapid referral for assessment and treatment;
- over time, following up on previous educational events and efforts to maintain community knowledge and motivation to refer; and
- providing initial and repeat evaluations of the community education effort to identify successes, remaining challenges, and the fidelity of the outreach efforts to model criteria (Ruff et al., 2012).

For teams committed to prevention, a six-hour, initial, individualized outreach training is followed by up to two years of ongoing supervision, fidelity review of materials, and program certification requirements in outreach/community education. The training and supervision are designed to promote increased independence over time, individually address the barriers, and build upon the natural relationships and inherent opportunities specific to their community. Specifically, the PIER model promotes long-term engagement with program participants and families to become speakers and contributors to outreach campaigns, which in turn allows for earlier identification.

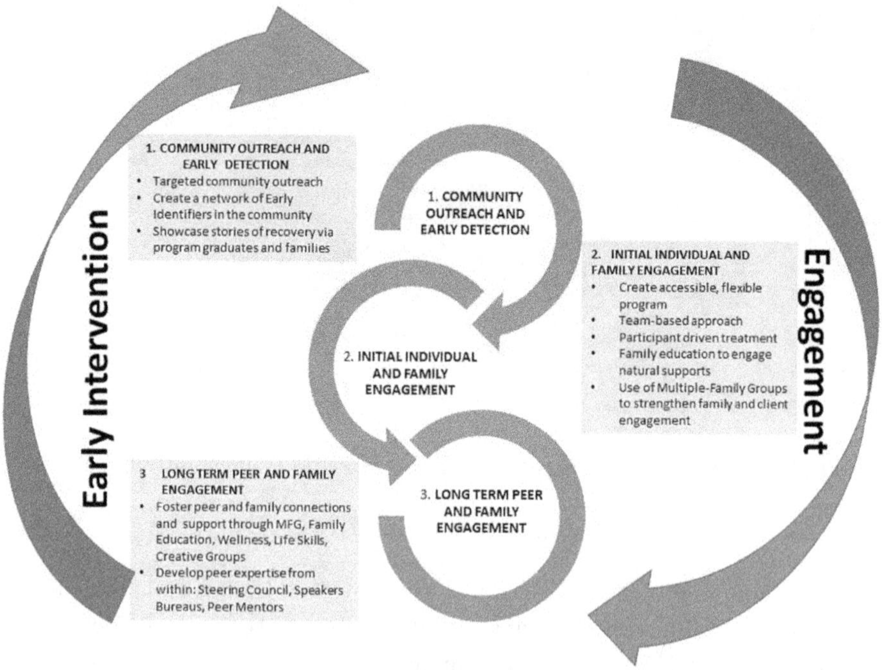


Figure 14.4 Engaging families and individuals in care

The PIER program community outreach education model has been successfully replicated in multiple agencies, counties, and statewide mental health systems with documented success in significantly improving access to care for mental health systems that had been described as "initially inaccessible" systems of care (Joly, 2012). In a 2013 study, PIER reported that all of their six geographically, socioeconomically, and culturally diverse sites yielded appropriate referrals for youth at risk for psychosis (Lynch et al., 2016). The model illustrated in Figure 14.4 conceptualizes how the PIER model integrates long-term family engagement and peer-to-peer connections with outreach education to create a self-sustaining model of community engagement and education.

This self-sustaining model of outreach education and long-term engagement through peer-to-peer connections facilitates community education that, over time, requires less effort to maintain, so long as the program is well evaluated and maintains fidelity over time (Ruff et al., 2012).

## 14.8 Assessment of Risk

Even though psychosis is a universal illness observed all around the world in various countries and cultures, and despite all the recent advances in early psychosis research, we still do not have a standard laboratory test to mark its presence (McGlashan et al., 2010). Psychosis presents differently in all individuals and does not impact everyone in the same way. Diagnosing the recent onset phase of psychosis and the CHR phase of psychosis is dependent on symptoms that can be observed by others or reported by the individual themselves. Assessing an individual for these conditions requires a high level of sensitivity to existing symptoms, the fact that symptoms can be nonspecific and change over time, and the normal course of development of young people. In addition to possessing a specific understanding of the course of psychotic disorders, professionals must possess proficiency in performing psychiatric assessments. They must recognize that stigma is widely endorsed and impacts thinking and behavior toward individuals with mental illness (Judd & Park, 1996) The prejudicial effects of this type of stereotyped thinking contribute to the fact that fewer than half of the nearly 50 million Americans estimated to live with a serious mental illness seek proper treatment (NIMH, 2017).

Assessment of early psychosis is an ongoing process and allows for the possibility that the diagnosis may change over time. Individuals requesting this evaluation are experiencing some level of distress from their experiences, and even if they do not meet the criteria for the at-risk or early-onset phase, they need support and, more often than not, treatment for a nonpsychotic disorder. Establishing an open discussion regarding the future course of action is important for the person being assessed.

The evaluation serves as the primary means for understanding a person's experiences and leads to a diagnosis and treatment plan, a crucial component of early identification and intervention work. Poor evaluation interviews and/or misinterpretation of a person's presentation can be detrimental to their future well-being and subsequent treatment (U.K. Essays, 2013). It is imperative to establish an atmosphere that is relaxed and nonjudgmental and allows the development of a trusting relationship to ensure the success of this evaluation. The Structured Interview of Psychosis-Risk Syndromes (SIPS; McGlashan et al., 2010) is one of the most commonly used instruments throughout the world for diagnosing and evaluating individuals with a CHR syndrome (Granö et al., 2014; McGlashan, 2010). The SIPS is a semi-structured interview used for diagnosing either a CHR syndrome for psychosis or cases of first-episode psychosis (FEP) (McGlashan, 2010). It contains a severity rating scale (SOPS), a well-anchored Global Assessment of Functioning (GAF; Hall, 1995), the DSM-IV schizotypal personality disorder checklist, a brief grid capturing the family history of psychosis, and the Criteria of Psychosis-Risk Syndromes (COPS), Presence of Psychosis Scale (POPS), and DSM-5 Attenuated Psychosis Syndrome criterion sets. The assessment is valid for individuals between the ages of 10 and 45 who have a minimum IQ scale of 70 and who are experiencing symptoms that are either distressing or interfering with their functioning.

The primary aims of the assessment are to identify a past or current fully psychotic episode, to date the onset of the first psychotic episode if it is present, to identify one or more of the at-risk syndromes of psychosis, and to rate the current severity of symptoms. While an individual cannot be fully psychotic and meet the at-risk criteria at the same time, they can meet criteria for more than one of the at-risk syndromes at the same time: the brief intermittent psychosis risk syndrome, the attenuated positive symptom psychosis risk syndrome, and the genetic risk and deterioration psychosis risk syndrome. The three CHR syndromes are designed to predict the onset of psychosis as a broad construct, not only schizophrenic psychosis but also psychosis in affective, posttraumatic stress, and obsessive–compulsive disorders.

It is important to conduct a prescreening assessment to minimize the stress associated with the evaluation of psychosis. The purpose of the prescreening is to establish the basic eligibility criteria needed to conduct a valid assessment and to establish that the SIPS is warranted for the individual. Once the decision is made to conduct the assessment, it is important to introduce the assessment in a way that also reduces the stress associated with having a psychiatric assessment. It is important to stress the fact that the SIPS is a semi-structured risk assessment in which everyone is asked the same questions, so the individual might relate to some of the questions but not to others. It is also important to state that there are no right or wrong answers, because we all have different experiences. Additionally, it needs to be stressed that just having the interview does not mean that others think the person is already having a psychotic episode; doing so helps normalize the experience of the interview, allows the individual to endorse their experiences, and opens the door for future therapeutic interventions.

The final step in the assessment process is notifying the individual, and their family if appropriate, of the outcome of the assessment. If the problem identified does not involve risk, they are referred elsewhere for further evaluation or treatment. If a risk is present, they must be informed of this fact, emphasizing that risk means probability, not an inevitability. It is crucial to describe the treatment recommendations in detail and to set a tone that is optimistic and emphasizes hope for recovery. Ensuring this state-of-the-art assessment process facilitates effective early identification and intervention in early psychosis.

## 14.9 Family Intervention

### 14.9.1 Engaging the Family in Treatment throughout the Program and Beyond

Engaging families early during onset of psychosis is critical because young people are most likely living with family members and reliant on them to access treatment. Family involvement leads to earlier identification and better outcomes. Family members can play an indispensable role in providing history, helpful insights, and ongoing support to their loved one. Family members caring for a loved one experiencing a first psychosis report a high level of distress and longer term impact on their own well-being, as the episode can be traumatic for the entire family. Families coping with how to help a young person with untreated psychosis may experience fear, isolation, and distress.

Family interventions that focus on providing information, improving communication, decreasing stress, problem-solving, and providing a shared understanding of psychosis reduce hospitalizations and relapse rates (Lucksted et al., 2012; McFarlane, 2010). Communication difficulties, hostility, and criticism have been linked to increased relapse, risk for conversion to psychosis, and lower social and role functioning (Thompson et al., 2019). Conversely, positive family involvement leads to decreased symptoms and improved social functioning at the earliest onset of symptoms (McFarlane et al., 2015). Family intervention is particularly important when affected individuals perceive their family functioning to be unsupportive, maladaptive, or strained (Thompson et al., 2019). Research suggests that early intervention benefits not only individuals but family dynamics (Hinojosa-Marqués et al., 2022; Miklowitz et al., 2014).

The PMFG model addresses the family system as a critical resource and partner. The PMFG is an effective and efficient way to deliver treatment because it builds community, helps people hear things from others who have lived with similar experiences, promotes different learning styles, and holds people accountable for small steps toward their goals. The community that is built in PMFG treatment can lead to family engagement beyond the program. The PIER program has a family advisory council and speakers' bureau of families who formerly participated in the program and share their stories on a regular basis with new families considering treatment. PIER also offers a weekly parent-to-parent virtual group with a combination of parent alumni, current parents, and prospective parents. Parents can access support and find community with other families even before entering the program. As programs become more established, this network of families becomes critical to the success of community outreach, program recruitment, and engagement.

### 14.9.2 Family Psychoeducation Treatment Model

The PMFG model addresses the family's need for information, clinical guidance, and ongoing support during the recovery of their loved one (McFarlane, 2002). The model is based on a partnership between the client, family (broadly defined as the client's trusted supports), and treatment team. Most families are new to psychosis and benefit from education and partnership with providers to dispel misinformation and to better understand how to help their loved

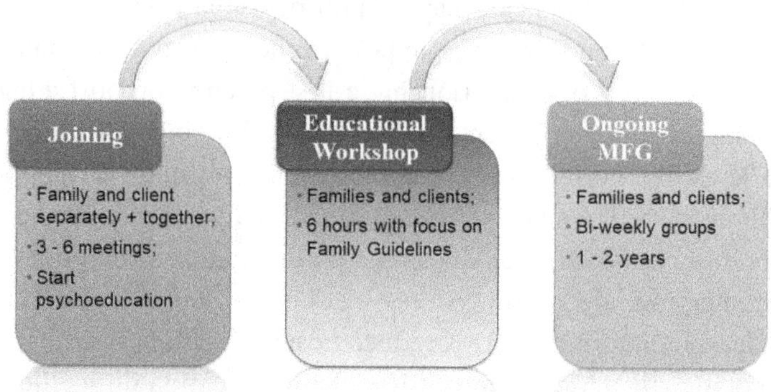


Figure 14.5 Stages of psychoeducation multifamily group

one. Single- or multiple-family intervention is offered with flexibility to accommodate family schedules, understand barriers, and address needs. The PMFG addresses isolation, stigma, family stress, and burden with empathy, education, skill-building, and community. The following three phases of PMFG offer a combination of single-family joining, educational workshops, and ongoing groups by developmental stage (Figure 14.5).

### 14.9.3 Joining

The first stage of the family psychoeducation model is "joining" with the family (Minuchin, 1974). In the PMFG model, group facilitators initially meet with the participating families for at least three single-family sessions. The purpose of these sessions is to learn about each family member's experiences, reactions, support networks, and past involvement with mental health services. This conversation allows families space to explore how they are coping and address barriers to treatment. Joining allows family members to build trust and comfort with the group facilitators.

### 14.9.4 Educational Workshops

Comprehensive monthly educational workshops enable families and community members alike to learn about psychosis as a spectrum of changes in thinking, perceptions, and mental processing. The educational workshop offers information about the window of opportunity for early intervention and an explanatory model of early psychosis including biological, psychological, social, and systemic influences. The workshop is led by the multidisciplinary team members, including peer and family program alumni. Families are invited to see psychosis on a continuum from normal human experiences to experiences

1. Go slow *recovery can take longer than you want it to*
2. Keep it cool *try to avoid over-loading, information processing can be hard during this time, especially if under stress*
3. Give each other space *alone time can be self-care, try not to hover*
4. Observe limits *clear rules can help everyone*
5. Ignore what you can't change *let some things slide, just not violence*
6. Keep it simple *say what you need to as simply, clearly, and positively as possible*

6. Carry on business as usual *re-establish family routines, stay in touch with family and friends*
7. Consider medication use *medication can help symptoms, work with your doctor to see what might work for you*
8. Consider not using drugs and alcohol *they can worsen symptoms*
9. Attend to early warning signs *know what your triggers are*
10. Lower expectations temporarily *see incremental progress*
11. Solve problems step by step

Figure 14.6 Family guidelines

that are more severe, distressing, and impact functioning. Peer support specialists and program alumni share personal stories and invite attendees to join in experiential role play that builds empathy and understanding. There is an emphasis on the research that supports early intervention and a message of hope. Families are presented with guidelines for recovery, which are geared toward the whole family and reinforced regularly in groups (Figure 14.6).

### 14.9.5 Ongoing Multifamily Groups

After the joining and the workshop, the first two groups provide a structured, safe environment for families to get to know one another and find commonalities. Since PMFG is a rolling group (which was adapted for early psychosis), families in later stages of recovery take the lead in sharing their stories including onset of symptoms, changes over time, and what helps them feel hopeful. The ongoing problem-solving model begins with socializing and then a check-in with each member of the group about what is going well and what could be better. The facilitators select a problem to work through using open conversation, weighing safety factors, risks for relapse, recent changes in functioning, and challenges with family guidelines. At the same time, the facilitators ensure rotation of problems so that they are specific to the individual, and balance exists between family members and participants. Members tend to relate to one another's challenges and learn from being in the role of helper. Facilitators model open, transparent communication as they lead the group in generating solutions and forming a specific action plan. Over time, PMFG becomes a central "hub" for the PIER program, reinforcing the important concept of making natural connections outside of traditional treatment settings. Groups celebrate the small successes and see growth over time. Group members validate and empathize with others during the predictable ups and downs of recovery.

Given that social networks are already diminished in the early stages of psychosis, PMFGs are key to building these connections and offering a space to practice social reciprocity during a critical developmental stage for the participant and the family.

### 14.10 Occupational Therapy and Employment Specialist Services in the PIER Model

As a coordinated, integrated, and person-centered program, the PIER model includes supported education and employment (SEE) services for CHR and FEP clients. These services can prevent or reverse functional and cognitive decline, minimize isolation, improve socialization, and help individuals get back on track with developmental tasks, especially school and work (Bond et al., 2015).

In the PIER model, these services are typically provided by OT practitioners and ESs, who bring specialized skills to SEE. They collaborate with the client, family, team members, school personnel, employers, and community providers to facilitate functional improvement and promote recovery. Initial evaluations provide important information about (a) functional, sensory, and cognitive abilities; (b) self-perceptions of functioning; (c) school and work interests and experiences; (d) future goals; and (e) psychosocial aspects of the individual's life. Assessment results are shared with the client, family, team, and community members in functional terms, leading to a comprehensive treatment plan. Even though SEE services are offered at the client's pace, conversations about returning to school or work ideally begin as soon as the individual enters the program.

The client–clinician relationship is important, but not more so than the relationship developed between the client and other team members. In the PIER model, the ES, OT, and case manager (CM) establish rapport early with the participant and family by using specific strategies, such as being introduced at the initial intake session or within the first two appointments, as well as frequent participation in clinical sessions to foster connections with services. The likelihood of engagement and full participation is highest when the individual and family participate in a *joining* session with team members in preparation for multifamily group psychoeducation.

Early intervention service programs that emphasize school and work participation for FEP clients have early engagement and high rates of school and work involvement (Humensky et al., 2017). There is compelling evidence that when supported employment is offered to FEP youth to assist with school and work challenges, in addition to treatment as usual (TAU), outcomes can be significantly better than TAU alone (Baksheev et al., 2012; Killackey et al.,

2019). Supported employment services increased participants' employment rates in one review to 56% compared to 23% for controls (Bond et al., 2015; Rosenheck et al., 2017).

## 14.11 Supported Education

Supported education includes individual skill development as well as collaboration with schools (Substance Abuse and Mental Health Services Administration, 2011; see Resources). CHR and FEP symptoms reflect underlying cognitive impairments, which interfere with functioning and make new learning challenging. Some students stop attending school or fall far behind in their studies due to increased anxiety, symptoms of psychosis, and learning challenges, which increases stress for the student and family. The client may or may not have difficulties with routine tasks and activities of daily living (ADLs), but often has trouble concentrating, associating new information with learned information, making decisions, and prioritizing steps in a task. These latter abilities are all necessary for successful school performance.

The individual's functional and cognitive abilities are assessed by the OT and ES in real-life one-on-one sessions, as well as with formal, standardized assessments. This information is then shared with the intention of designing a client-centered educational plan based on the individual's cognitive and functional abilities and learning needs. Guidance is offered to clients and family members for self-advocacy, including information about local and state educational laws. Often, the OT and/or ES become educational advocates for a student by attending 504 or Individual Educational Plan (IEP) meetings. They can offer information to school staff about the biology of psychosis and how it impacts learning. Once everyone involved with the individual's education understands how altered brain functioning interferes with learning, appropriate accommodations can be developed. When school supports and accommodations are in place, the client typically feels less stressed and can better manage symptoms, the school environment, and new learning.

Some assessment tools used by occupational therapists are (a) the Adolescent/Adult Sensory Profile (AASP; Brown & Dunn, 2002), a self-questionnaire that gathers important information about an individual's sensory preferences; (b) the Assessment of Motor and Process Skills (AMPS; Fisher & Jones, 2010), an observation tool of the performance of everyday tasks in natural settings that is client-centered and administered by someone trained and certified in the tool; (c) the Test of Everyday Attention (TEA; Robertson et al., 1994), a psychology assessment tool that provides information about the eight areas of attention; (d) the Canadian Occupational Performance Measure (COPM; Carswell et al., 2004), an OT tool that quickly reviews an individual's performance areas and assists in goal-setting by asking the individual to rate their satisfaction with the task and perception of their performance; and (e) self-evaluation checklists for general performance, school performance, and work performance. These checklists are useful in beginning dialogues about perceived challenges and goals for improved functioning, socialization, and management of symptoms, and many of them can be found in *The Navigate Complete SEE Manual* (http://navigateconsultants.org/2020manuals/see_2020.pdf). In addition, this manual offers useful checklists that the ES, CM, or OT can use to gain a better understanding of the individual's challenges with cognition and functional performance areas, such as ADLs, sleep hygiene, avocational interests, socialization, school, and work.

## 14.12 Supported Employment

Supported employment is a vocational service that assists individuals with finding and keeping a job that pays a competitive wage, capitalizes on personal strengths and interests, and provides the necessary support to be successful in the workplace (Wehman & Moon, 1988). This support can reduce stress, which can lead to reduced anxiety and improved functioning. Examples of specific supported employment services include, but are not limited to identifying career goals, working on prevocational skills, finding a job, keeping a job, connecting to resources, updating or creating a résumé, on-site job coaching, preparing for an interview, and improving interview skills. Employment with appropriate supports can be beneficial for the CHR or FEP individual who wants to work. Work can be therapeutic in that it builds self-esteem and confidence, provides a pathway to independence and self-reliance, improves social skills and relationships, develops coping skills, broadens interests in all life areas, and provides a sense of contributing to society.

Ensuring a good job match often depends on the skills of an ES and OT, and most importantly, the individual's work interests. There are multiple online and paper/pencil assessments the ES can administer to the client, such as (a) a comprehensive assessment of work history, volunteer work, and education; (b) an assessment of environmental preferences; and (c) an inventory of strengths and barriers. Through discussion, the ES conducts a complete inventory of the individual's career and education to get a full picture of current and future school and work goals.

The support of team, family, and community members can be key to the success of the job search, placement, and continuation in the job. The ES might network with local employers to develop jobs and/or develop accommodations for existing positions, including coaching the individual to share their learning style with the employer if they do not want to disclose mental health symptoms, providing education about disclosing to employers, helping prepare them for work, and providing job coaching (on-site or outside of work) through the State Department of Vocational Rehabilitation. The OT provides information about cognition, functioning, and work environments in which the individual might be the most successful to assist with finding a good job match. Additionally, multi-family group psychoeducation can be a helpful venue for discussing school and work challenges, since other CHR and FEP youth and their families can identify with those issues and offer suggestions and even job leads.

## 14.13 Clinical Interventions

### 14.13.1 FACT: Team Organization and Functioning

Because the reader may be unfamiliar with specific features of ACT, we will describe them here, dividing the model into its constituent elements for heuristic purposes. As it has been applied in most instances, ACT is a comprehensive, biopsychosocial intervention designed to improve the community functioning of those with severe mental illness, thereby diminishing reliance on inpatient care while improving quality of life. The strategies are derived from the Program for Assertive Community Treatment in Madison, Wisconsin (Stein & Test, 1980). Because ACT has been well studied and described over the last four decades, we are providing only a brief synopsis here (McFarlane et al., 2000; Stein & Test, 1980).

### 14.13.2 Integration of the Patient's Life into the Community

This model is conceived as an alternative to hospitalization by providing the patient with a viable support system in the community. As suggested by the name, ACT calls for an assertive approach with considerable outreach and proactive monitoring in which ACT staff function as direct providers of individualized therapeutic and rehabilitation services, rather than as service brokers.

### 14.13.3 In Vivo Teaching of Coping and Problem-Solving Skills

Patients must not only have adequate access to all material resources but learn how to use them effectively to meet the demands of community life. In addition, problems of daily living and educational or vocational adjustment arise frequently and require an array of problem-solving skills. As much as possible, teaching these skills takes place "in vivo," that is, side-by-side in the natural settings of the patient.

### 14.13.4 Prevention of Onset, Relapse, and Crisis Intervention

Monitoring of social stressors such as life events or transitions and responding immediately and assertively are essential for the prevention of FEP or relapse. Such actions require a proactive stance and an awareness of prodromal signs on the part of the treatment team. Medication management and monitoring is an integral feature of this approach and requires close collaboration with the prescribing psychiatrist, who is a member of the FACT team. The team is available on a 24-hour basis to respond to client emergencies and is reachable by all concerned parties, especially for family members.

### 14.13.5 Graduated Increase in Patient Responsibilities

The ACT approach maintains a continuous rehabilitative stance in looking for opportunities to help the patient move in the direction of their established goals and independence. An assertive but graduated approach is maintained to support patients in their striving toward higher functional levels; however, we also recognize that precipitous and premature advances can contribute to the resurgence of prodromal symptoms and ultimately lead to a full psychosis. Therefore, an increase in support, advance guidance for family and friends, careful preparation, and symptom monitoring accompany any significant increase in functional demands.

### 14.13.6 Support and Education of Community Members

Community members, especially the patient's family and employers, frequently react to patients' behavior in ways not supportive of community tenure. The goal of the FACT team is to aid these key community members by providing them with ongoing support and guidance.

### 14.13.7 Team Approach

FACT is provided by a team composed of staff from the major mental health disciplines, whose members are known to all the team's clients and serve relatively interchangeable functions. It functions within a tightly organized, pragmatic, and hierarchical structure with an emphasis on goal-oriented treatment planning. Daily schedules and staff assignments are based on client needs and staff availability. The team reviews every case daily and does in-depth treatment planning once or twice weekly, focusing on individual cases.

### 14.13.8 Psychiatric Treatment

FACT includes careful assessment by a psychiatrist for psychotic symptoms and possible psychotic disorder, but also for medical and substance abuse disorders that may contribute to, or in some cases, fully explain the incipient psychosis and other severe symptoms. A FACT team nurse continues to monitor the young person during treatment to track side effects of any medications, assess ongoing health and safety status, intervene to avert crises, and work with the psychiatrist to provide hospitalization when necessary. The current standard of care includes providing psychotropic medication in low and carefully monitored doses for mood and anxiety disorders but using antipsychotic drugs only for rapidly increasing psychotic symptoms and potential suicide, also in low doses.

## 14.14 When ACT and Multifamily Groups Are Combined

The original intention in combining PMFGs and ACT was to enhance outcomes by adding the clinical effects of each modality. As we learned, in very high-risk and treatment-resistant populations, there appears to be a limit to the reduction in clinical morbidity that is possible with these methods and pharmacotherapy. However, there are additive effects for the family intervention in the functional domain, especially in employment, relief of family burdens, and improvement in family emotional well-being. What can account for these effects? The following section describes processes that occur, perhaps uniquely, in FACT when multifamily groups are conducted by a team that is also intensively working with the ill member of the family.

The most obvious effect is that all efforts, whether by professionals, family members, friends, or others in the community, can be coordinated. The multifamily group then functions as a clearinghouse for all the various actions that are being taken by and on behalf of the person receiving services. It is crucial to ensure that contradictory directions are not being suggested to the patient by family, clinicians, and rehabilitation professionals. The multifamily group serves as a place to plan out what the family will do in crisis situations and what the team will do as well. The team routinely and regularly shares the immediate and longer term next steps with the family, allowing discussion and melding of intentions and actions into a coherent plan. At the more general level, the regular meetings of the group promote sharing of information of all appropriate types, in all directions among patients, family members, and clinicians, across families and even between groups. Participants speak more openly, honestly, and coherently than in individual therapy or single-family settings. Family members find that the presence of other families is conducive to more open communication. Multifamily group leaders often observe that they learn more from families about the life events that might trigger decompensation during friendly socializing than during more focused interviewing. Members of different families regularly share information about resources and opportunities in their communities, some of which may be unknown to clinicians or rehabilitators. This sharing of information is routine within natural networks and is one of their most valuable functions. Information sharing and coordination makes comprehensive treatment possible, meaning that multiple interventions can occur simultaneously.

## 14.15 Individual Counseling: Cognitive-Behavioral Therapy for Psychosis

PIER integrates cognitive-behavioral therapy for psychosis (CBTp) as the primary modality for individual therapy. CBTp has both a strong foundation in traditional cognitive-behavioral therapy and psychosis-specific strategies to decrease symptoms and improve functioning. Across the spectrum of psychosis, CBTp helps reduce positive symptoms of psychosis, improve mood symptoms, decrease hospitalizations, improve medication adherence, and maintain treatment gains over time; in early psychosis, CBTp has been shown to reduce the incidence of conversion to psychosis (van der Gaag et al., 2013).

### 14.15.1 CBTp – Basic Tenets

CBTp is a change-based psychotherapy that promotes recovery through structured, focused sessions that are personalized to the client's goals and emphasize work outside of sessions (Figure 14.7).

CBTp builds off the basic cognitive-behavioral model that explores the connectedness of thoughts, emotions, and behavior and specifically adds prompts for psychotic thoughts and perceptual changes, as well as physical sensations. From a cognitive perspective, psychosis can be described as an extension of overconfidence in one's beliefs and experiences which often results in a sense of rigidity of thought and/or experience, which frequently involves either

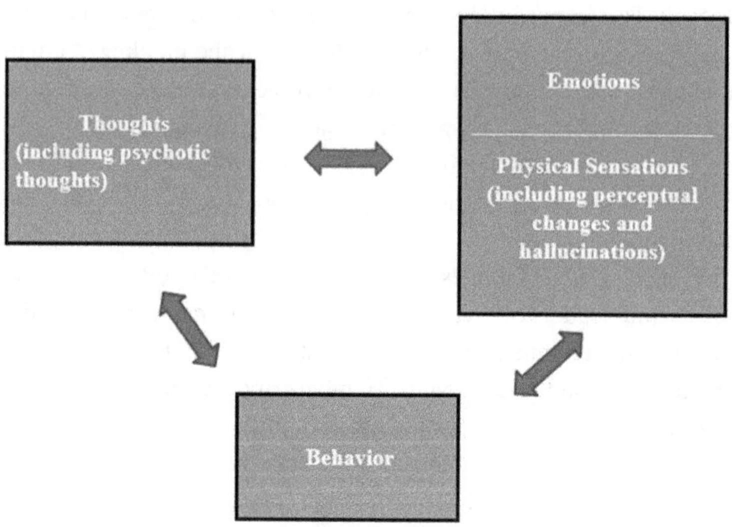


Figure 14.7 Cognitive-behavioral model

misattribution or another cognitive distortion from classic CBT. These factors almost always create some dissonance for the individual, whether within the self (e.g., self-view at odds with functioning or confusion of experience), between self and others (i.e., relationships), or between self and external environment (e.g., work/life impact).

### 14.15.2 Goals of CBTp

Building a sense of trust is a key component in CBTp. The goals of counseling are not to challenge beliefs directly, as that could disrupt trust, but instead to introduce flexibility of perspective. This introduction involves an intentional distancing from experience and thoughts, which allows for improved self-awareness and personal efficacy. When the trusting therapeutic relationship is combined with the working atmosphere of structured sessions and homework, the client and therapist begin to work on moving toward a neutral or curious perspective on symptoms. They also adopt a "living with" approach to symptoms which builds upon symptom-specific coping skills.

### 14.15.3 CBTp Treatment Duration within the PIER Model of Care

In early psychosis, CBTp treatment typically lasts 6–18 months, broken down into the following phases: phase 1: engagement and introduction to CBTp, phase 2: assessment and goal-setting, phase 3: CBTp interventions and coping skill development, phase 4: progress tracking and treatment generalization, and phase 5: relapse prevention.

Within the PIER model, the CBTp treatment phases align with treatment within the full multidisciplinary team and work to strengthen family and natural supports. As treatment progresses, the PIER participant takes increased ownership of skills and session topics to enhance skill acquisition and relapse prevention. Particularly toward phases 4 and 5, the participant and their natural and/or family support often take the lead, and the therapy becomes a touchpoint for the progress that is primarily made outside of sessions. Similarly, CBTp treatment steps and homework often overlap with multifamily group participation.

## 14.16 Empirical Effects of the PIER Model of Prevention

The PIER program was initiated in 2000. Youths and young adults aged 12–35 years were identified by professionals in a wide variety of educational, health, and mental health settings. PIER program staff assessed, confirmed risk of psychosis, and provided treatment for 24 months to eligible and consenting young people ($N = 148$). The monthly rate of first hospital admission for psychosis was the outcome measure for efficacy of identification and intervention. Admission rates before and after the program began accepting referrals were compared, both in the experimental area (Greater Portland) and in aggregated urban areas of Maine (control areas). Autoregressive integrated moving average (ARIMA) models were used to assess the effect. PIER's first six years showed a 26% drop in first psychiatric hospitalizations for psychotic disorders in the Greater Portland catchment area, compared to an 8% rise during the same period in the aggregated urban areas that served as the control. The net result was a 34% decrease from the expected rate (McFarlane et al., 2014). PIER demonstrated that population-wide early identification is feasible, and that preventive intervention can reduce rates of initial hospitalizations for psychosis in a midsized city.

The other published study (McFarlane et al., 2015) with a family intervention as the centerpiece of an indicated prevention treatment described the results of the Early Detection and Intervention for the Prevention of Psychosis Program (EDIPPP). Funded by the Robert Wood Johnson Foundation, this project followed youth aged 12–25 years from 2007 to 2012 using a risk-based allocation study design and regression discontinuity analysis. The sites were Portland, ME; Queens, NY; Ann Arbor MI; Albuquerque, NM; Salem, OR; and Sacramento, CA. Those indicating early, or prodromal, symptoms of psychosis were invited for an orientation to the study and evaluation for pre-psychosis symptoms using the SIPS (McGlashan et al., 2010). Those meeting study criteria were assigned to one of three conditions based on their symptoms: clinically low risk (CLR), clinically high risk (CHR), or early first episode of psychosis (EFEP). The lower risk group served as the control condition, receiving whatever services their families chose in the community, including no treatment services. Three hundred thirty-seven young people (mean age 16.6) were assigned to the FACT group (CHR or EFEP, 250 young people) or comparison group (CLR, 87 young people). Study participants were assessed over 24 months for positive, negative, disorganized, and general symptoms; Structured Clinical Interview for DSM-IV Disorders (SCID-IV) diagnoses; social and role functioning; substance abuse; family functioning; and neurocognitive status. Across the six sites, rates of first hospital admissions for the same age group five to seven years prior to the intervention were compared to three years after initiation of the assigned intervention. Those rates were compared to a large adjacent control catchment area for both periods. Using the PIER/FACT model, the team provided proactive outreach and treatment to the CHR/EFEP cohort, but not to the CLR cohort.

FACT was significantly more effective in decreasing positive and negative symptoms among both the higher risk and early FEP groups, compared to the community care received by the lower risk group, adjusting for the baseline difference in positive symptoms. Rates of conversion to psychosis (6.3% in the higher risk group, compared to 2.3% in the lower risk group) and first negative event did not differ significantly, consistent with the goal of treatment: to have actual negative outcomes in the high-risk groups to equal the low or no-risk control group. The proportion of conversions was lower than expected, compared to prior studies that have averaged 29%. In the group receiving treatment, participation in work or school was 83% at baseline and remained the same 24 months later, while participation among the lower risk group fell from 84% to 79%. First-episode hospitalization rates for at-risk young people were down in all the sites where data were available. For example, the rate in the Portland area fell 24% when the five-to-seven-year period prior to the intervention was compared to three years after its start. During the same period, the hospitalization rate went up in three other cities in Maine by 8%. In summary, early identification and intervention with FACT during the period prior to onset of frank psychosis was found to be effective in six highly representative US cities. The substantial scale of the treatment effects, combined with the diversity of the sample and sites, suggests that wider dissemination and testing is warranted and would be likely to lead to reduction in burden of disease.

## 14.17 Practical Development, Adaptation, and Implementation

The replication of the PIER model from Portland was an inherent aspect of the EDIPPP effectiveness trial (McFarlane et al., 2015). The sites were selected to provide a large sample that was as representative of the US population as possible. That study demonstrated that replication of the program was followed by replication of its outcomes. In that process, a method for training and fidelity monitoring was developed that allowed the team to go on to implement programs across the United States that are continuing at the time of this writing (www.piertraining.com). The guiding principles for that extension emphasized the challenges of expanding the mission of mental health services to include indicated prevention, the necessity for in-depth training in evidence-based clinical treatments, careful adaptation to the community and its varied constituent populations, and ongoing formative evaluation, supervision, and fidelity review to assure that outcomes equal or exceed those in the preceding clinical trials. In practice, replication has also had to surmount the COVID-19 pandemic, extensive turnover in staffing, and continuing budget challenges for the agencies implementing the prevention program for the public entities providing the needed funding.

To date, programs have been established in San Diego and Pomona, Imperial, Los Angeles, Ventura, Santa Clara, and Contra Costa Counties in California; the entire State of Delaware; Weber County, Utah; Southern

Maine; Nashville and surrounding counties in Tennessee; southwestern South Carolina; and, in collaboration with other training groups, the five counties of the San Francisco Bay area and most of Oregon. Most of these programs have been initiated by and integrated into existing large mental health centers and agencies. Almost all have combined their first episode of psychosis and CHR cases into a single PIER program. Because these programs all have defined catchment areas, they now serve over 12% of the American population, with that proportion increasing annually. While the training and supervision have assured fidelity, several adaptations have been developed which have improved the fit of some programs with their respective communities.

For instance, the program in San Diego recruited young people with established but recovered diagnoses of a psychotic disorder to act as peer supports, working closely with the FACT team to carry out parts of the treatment plan, especially in relation to education, social functioning, and recreation. That modification is now included in the California programs and several others. Several programs have engaged family members who have completed the treatment to provide education and guidance to families as they enter. The Weber County, Utah, program added a brief psychosis screening survey to the standard intake process for all patients entering a large community mental health center; identification of young people at risk increased substantially. As a result of the COVID-19 pandemic, many PMFGs have been conducted by videoconferencing, as have the training and supervision for several new sites. The impression of the authors is that both the groups and the training and supervision have achieved nearly the same results in virtual format as when done in person. Most recently, the model has been expanded by integrating cognitive-behavioral therapy for psychosis, cross-linking specific interventions coming from the CBTp with those from the PMFG and supported education/employment and OT. Each of these examples illustrates the necessity to adapt PIER as an evidence-based model to both the specific community and population being served, to the exigencies imposed by major socioeconomic trends, and by the emergence of new scientific knowledge and clinical methods with demonstrated efficacy.

## 14.18 Social Justice, Ethnic, and Racial Diversity Adaptations

The PIER model is patient- and family-centered. One major implication is that the cultural, ethnic, racial, language, and generational status of each individual will determine even the most basic aspects of early identification, let alone acceptance and relevance of preventive treatment. The program must address the needs of the entire local population, including the diversity of that population and the existing disparities in health status and access to treatment to achieve public health goals. There are several ways that the approach has addressed these issues. Perhaps the most effective method occurs before a single at-risk youth is engaged: recruiting staff for the program that represent the diverse microcommunities that the program serves. A common presentation is a young person, the son or daughter of immigrants, who is fluent in English and understands many aspects of American culture but whose parents do not speak English, are resistant to accepting, and may even be frightened by their offspring's new culture. The joining process is greatly facilitated by having a staff member who speaks the language and understands the intergenerational conflict that is so common in immigrant families. The basic tenets of PMFG emphasize a model of cultural humility (openness to learn), as well as cultural competence (expectation to know the beliefs and social behaviors of the cultural groups). As such, using interpreters and cultural facilitators, as well as simply asking questions to learn more about the nuances of the familial and cultural backgrounds, helps program staff that do not match the cultural demographic to continue to lead the group in a culturally informed and inclusive way.

Further, understanding how each culture views psychosis is crucial to the educational process for both patient and family members. In our experience, each member of the family can have radically different concepts regarding psychosis and the actual symptoms being experienced by the at-risk member of the family. It is rare to have any of those concepts match modern scientific knowledge about brain dysfunction or the critical role of psychosocial stress. Thus, the initial conversation with the youth and family involves a delicate exploration of what they think is causing the difficulty, followed by a sensitive explanation of what the program intends to do about it. The education provided as an integral part of family psychoeducation offers a clear and nonjudgmental alternative explanation, coupled again with explicit guidance to alleviate the most significant symptoms and impairments.

Other components of the model address diversity issues and racial inequities. The outreach in communities experiencing discrimination usually reaches organizations and groups that reflect the trusted preferences of that culture. These include religious organizations, minority advocacy associations, elders that serve as community leaders and/or traditional healers, the police, and athletic clubs, as well as schools, agencies, and clinics. Outreach materials are translated or even prepared exclusively for a particular culture. For instance, the PIER trainers of Latino background have prepared introductory videos and brochures reflecting specific language and cultural references about psychosis. The educational materials provided as part of the PMFG are translated and the groups themselves conducted in the language of most of the members by staff who are as fluent as possible. For some cultures, group participation is not acceptable, so the family psychoeducational component is provided on a single-family basis until the family feels comfortable and can use the social support and collective guidance of the PMFG. Family members who have completed the program are recruited to serve as culturally specific guides and supports to parents who are distressed by losing aspects of their culture and/or are confused by or in disagreement with the educational material and the standard family guidelines. Respecting traditional explanations for psychosis while offering scientific alternatives is key to helping youth and family to accept intervention and work collaboratively with the staff, particularly in relation to educational and employment goals.

## 14.19 Recommendations for Evaluation

Research is needed to ensure that early psychosis interventions reach everyone who needs them, especially given the fact that individuals who have experienced discrimination have a higher risk of onset of a psychotic disorder (McFarlane et al., 2015). We expect that over the next decade, more effective treatments with better evidence will emerge and should be adopted within the services that offer prevention for psychotic disorders. In the meantime, the PIER model has been in use and under study for over 20 years with good results, widespread implementation, and a minimum of risk for harm to youth and their families.

## Resources for Greater Detail

Recent books provide much more detail as to the technical aspects of early intervention, including in the prodromal phase. Key articles from the literature are highlighted here to supplement the information for prospective clinical teams as they undertake implementation.

1. www.piertraining.com outlines the methods used for training and clinical supervision for new teams.
2. Hardy, K. V., Ballon, J. S., Noordsy, D. L., & Adelsheim, S. (Eds.). (2019). *Intervening early in psychosis.* American Psychiatric Association Publishing.
3. McGlashan, T. H., Walsh, B., & Woods, S. W. (2010). *The psychosis risk syndrome.* Oxford University Press.
4. McFarlane, W. R. (2002). Multifamily groups in the treatment of severe psychiatric disorders. Guilford Press.
5. Hagen, R., Turkington, D., Berge, T., & Grawe, R. W. (Eds.). (2011). *CBT for psychosis*. Routledge.
6. McFarlane, W. R. et al. (2014). Reduction in incidence of hospitalizations for psychotic episodes through early identification and intervention. *Psychiatric Services*, *65*(10), 1194–1200. doi.org/10.1176/appi.ps.201300336

7. Woodberry, K. A. et al. (2010). Neuropsychological profiles in individuals at clinical high risk for psychosis: Relationship to psychosis and intelligence. *Schizophrenia Research*, *123*(2–3), 188–198. doi.org/10.1016/j.schres.2010.06.021
8. McFarlane, W. R. et al. (2015). Clinical and functional outcomes after 2 years in the early detection and intervention for the prevention of psychosis multisite effectiveness trial. *Schizophrenia Bulletin*, *41*(1), 30–43. doi.org/10.1093/schbul/sbu108
9. The entire issue of Adolescent Psychiatry, *2*(2), provides a broad perspective on early intervention and the theoretical background for the large EDIPPP effectiveness trial. https://benthamscience.com/public/journal/109
10. Fusar-Poli, P. et al. (2013). The psychosis high-risk state: A comprehensive state-of-the-art review. *JAMA Psychiatry*, *70*(1), 107–120. doi.org/10.1001/jamapsychiatry.2013.269
11. The *Navigate Complete SEE Manual* (http://navigateconsultants.org/2020manuals/see_2020.pdf) offers useful tools such as checklists, that the ES, case manager, or OT can use to gain a better understanding of the individual's challenges with cognition and functional performance areas, such as ADLs, sleep hygiene, avocational interests, socialization, school, and work.
12. Online resources for functional assessments can be found at O*NET OnLine (www.onetonline.org) or the Substance Abuse and Mental Health Services Administration (www.samhsa.gov).
13. Substance Abuse and Mental Health Services Administration (2011). *Supported Education: Building Your Program.* HHS Pub. No. SMA-11-4654, Rockville, MD: Center for Mental Health Services, Substance Abuse and Mental Health Services Administration, U.S. Department of Health and Human Services.

## References

Baksheev, G. N., Allott, K., Jackson, H. J., McGorry, P. D., & Killackey, E. (2012). Predictors of vocational recovery among young people with first-episode psychosis: Findings from a randomized controlled trial. *Psychiatric Rehabilitation Journal*, *35*(6), 421–427. doi.org/10.1037/h0094574

Bond, G. R., Drake, R. E., & Luciano, A. (2015). Employment and educational outcomes in early intervention programmes for early psychosis: A systematic review. *Epidemiologia e Psichiatria Sociale*, *24*(5), 446–457. doi.org/10.1017/S2045796014000419

Brown, C., & Dunn, W. (2002). *Adolescent/adult sensory profile: User's manual.* The Psychological Corporation.

Carswell, A., McColl, M. A., Baptiste, M. L., Polatajko, H., & Pollock, N. (2004). The Canadian occupational performance measure: A research and clinical literature review. *Canadian Journal of Occupational Therapy*, *71*(4), 210–222. doi.org/10.1177/000841740407100406.

Catalan, A., Salazar de Pablo, G., Vaquerizo Serrano, J., Mosillo, P., Baldwin, H., Fernandez-Rivas, A., Moreno, C., Arango, C., Correll, C. U., Bonoldi, I., & Fusar-Poli, P. (2021). Annual Research Review: Prevention of psychosis in adolescents – Systematic review and meta-analysis of advances in detection, prognosis and intervention. *Journal of Child Psychology and Psychiatry and Allied Disciplines*, *62*(5), 657–673. doi.org/10.1111/jcpp.13322

Dyck, D. G., Short, R. A., Hendryx, M. S., Norell, D., Myers, M., Patterson, T., McDonell, M. G., Voss, W. D., & McFarlane, W. R. (2000). Management of negative symptoms among patients with schizophrenia attending multiple-family groups. *Psychiatric Services*, *51*(4), 513–519. doi.org/10.1176/appi.ps.51.4.513

Eaton, W. W. (1999). Evidence for universality and uniformity of schizophrenia around the world: Assessment and implications. In W. F. Gattaz & H. Hafner (Eds.), *Search for the causes of schizophrenia* (Vol. IV, pp. 21–33). Steinkopf.

U.K. Essays. (2013). *Ensuring effective assessment in psychiatry and mental health nursing essay*. UKEssays, November.

Falloon, I. R. (1992). Early intervention for first episodes of schizophrenia: A preliminary exploration. *Psychiatry*, *55*(1), 4–15. www.ncbi.nlm.nih.gov/entrez/query.fcgi?cmd=Retrieve&db=PubMed&dopt=Citation&list_uids=1557469

Fisher, A. G., & Jones, K. B. (2010). *Assessment of motor and process skills, Vol. 1: Development, standardization, and administration manual* (7th ed.). Fort Collins, CO: Three Star Press.

Fjell, A., Thorsen, G. R. B., Friis, S., Johannessen, J. O., Larsen, T. K., Lie, K., Lyse, H., Melle, I., Simonsen, E., Smeby, N. A., Oxnevad, A. L., McFarlane, W. R., Vaglum, P., & McGlashan, T. (2007). Multifamily group treatment in a program for patients with first-episode psychosis: Experiences from the TIPS Project. *Psychiatric Services*, *58*(2), 171–173. doi.org/10.1176/ps.2007.58.2.171

Fusar-Poli, P., Borgwardt, S., Bechdolf, A., Addington, J., Riecher-Rossler, A., Schultze-Lutter, F., Keshavan, M. S., Wood, S., Ruhrmann, S., Seidman, L., Valmaggia, L., Cannon, T., Velthorst, E., DeHaan, L., Cornblatt, B., Bonoldi, I., Birchwood, M., McGlashan, T., Carpenter, W., McGorry, P., Klosterkotter, J., McGuire, P., & Yung, A. R. (2013). The psychosis high-risk state: A comprehensive state-of-the-art review. *JAMA Psychiatry*, *70*(1), 107–120. doi.org/10.1001/jamapsychiatry.2013.269

Fusar-Poli, P., McGorry, P., & Kane, J. (2017). Improving outcomes of first-episode psychosis: An overview. *World Psychiatry*, *16*(3), 251–265. doi.org/28941089

Granö, N., Karjalainen, M., Edlund, V., Saari, E., Itkonen, A., Anto, J., & Roine, M. (2014). Changes in depression, anxiety and hopelessness symptoms during family- and community-oriented intervention for help-seeking adolescents and adolescents at risk of psychosis. *Nordic Journal of Psychiatry*, *68*(2), 93–99. doi.org/10.3109/08039488.2013.768294

Haas, A. P., & Drescher, J. (2014). Impact of sexual orientation and gender identity on suicide risk: Implications for assessment and treatment. *Psychiatric Times*, *31*(12). www.psychiatrictimes.com/view/impact-sexual-orientation-and-gender-identity-suicide-risk-implications-assessment-and-treatment

Hall, R. C. (1995). Global assessment of functioning. A modified scale. *Psychosomatics*, *36*(3), 267–275. doi.org/10.1016/S0033-3182(95)71666-8

Hinojosa-Marqués, L., Tecelli, D. M., & Neus, B. V. (2022). Family environmental factors in at-risk mental states for psychosis. *Clinical Psychology & Psychotherapy*, *29*(2), 424–454. doi.org/10.1002/cpp.2651

Hjorthøj, C., Stürup, A. E., McGrath, J. J., & Nordentoft, M. (2017). Years of potential life lost and life expectancy in schizophrenia: A systematic review and meta-analysis. *The Lancet Psychiatry*, *4*(4), 295–301. doi.org/10.1016/S2215-0366(17)30078-0

Humensky, J. L., Essock, S. M., & Dixon, L. B. (2017). Characteristics associated with the pursuit of work and school among participants in a treatment program for first episode of psychosis. *Psychiatric Rehabilitation Journal*, *40*(1), 108–112. doi .org/10.1037/prj0000256

Joa, I., Johannessen, J. O., Auestad, B., Friis, S., McGlashan, T., Melle, I., Opjordsmoen, S., Simonsen, E., Vaglum, P., & Larsen, T. K. (2008). The key to reducing duration of untreated first psychosis: Information campaigns. *Schizophrenia Bulletin*, *34*(3), 466–472. doi.org/sbm09510.1093.

Joly, B. M., Pukstas, B. K., Elbaum, W. M., & Mittal, P. (2012). Promoting early detection of psychosis: The role of community outreach. *Journal of Public Mental Health*, *11*(4), 195–208.

Judd, C., & Park, B. (1996). Definition and assessment of accuracy in stereotypes. *Psychological Review*, *100*, 109–128.

Kessler, R. C., Birnbaum, H., Demler, O., Falloon, I. R., Gagnon, E., Guyer, M., Gagnon, E., Howes, M. J., Kendler, K. S., Shi, L., Walters, E., & Wu, E. Q. (2005). The prevalence and correlates of nonaffective psychosis in the National Comorbidity Survey Replication (NCS-R). *Biological Psychiatry*, *58*(8), 668–676. doi .org/S0006-3223(05)00495-610.1016

Killackey, E., Kelly, A., Jackson, H. J., Scutella, R., Tseng, Y.-P., & Cotton, S. (2019). Individual placement and support for vocational recovery in first-episode psychosis: Randomised controlled trial. *The British Journal of Psychiatry*, *214*(2), 76–82. doi .org/10.1192/bjp.2018.191

Krstev, H., Carbone, S., Harrigan, S. M., Curry, C., Elkins, K., & McGorry, P. D. (2004). Early intervention in first-episode psychosis – The impact of a community development campaign. *Social Psychiatry and Psychiatric Epidemiology*, *39*(9), 711–719. doi .org/10.1007/s00127-004-0798-5

Lucksted, A., McFarlane, W., Downing, D., & Dixon, L. (2012). Recent developments in family psychoeducation as an evidence-based practice. *Journal of Marital and Family Therapy*, *38*(1), 101–121. doi.org/10.1111/j.1752-0606.2011.00256.x

Luepker, R. V., Murray, D. M., Jacobs, D. R., Jr., Mittelmark, M. B., Bracht, N., & Carlaw, R. (1994). Community education for cardiovascular disease prevention: Risk factor changes in the Minnesota Heart Health Program. *American Journal of Public Health*, *84*(9), 1383–1393. doi.org/10.2105/ajph.84.9.1383

Lynch, S., McFarlane, W. R., Joly, B., Adelsheim, S., Auther, A., Cornblatt, B. A., Migliorati, M., Ragland, J. D., Sale, T., Spring, E., Calkins, R., Carter, C. S., Jaynes, R., Taylor, S. F., & Downing, D. (2016). Early detection, intervention and prevention of psychosis program: Community outreach and early identification at six U.S. sites. *Psychiatric Services*, *67*(5), 510–516. doi.org/10.1176/appi.ps.201300236

McFarlane, W. R. (2002). *Multifamily groups in the treatment of severe psychiatric disorders*. Guilford Press.

McFarlane, W. R. (2010). Integrating the family in the treatment of psychotic disorders. In R. Hagen, D. Turkington, T. Berge, & R. W. Grawe (Eds.), *CBT for psychosis: A symptom-based approach*. Routledge.

McFarlane, W. R., & Cook, W. L. (2007). Family expressed emotion prior to onset of psychosis. *Family Process*, *46*(2), 185–197. doi.org/10.1111/j.1545-5300.2007.00203.x

McFarlane, W. R., Cook, W. L., Downing, D., Verdi, M. B., Woodberry, K. A., & Ruff, A. (2010). Portland identification and early referral: A community-based system for identifying and treating youths at high risk of psychosis. *Psychiatric Services*, *61*(5), 512–515. doi.org/61/5/51210.1176/appi.ps.61.5.512

McFarlane, W. R., Dushay, R. A., Deakins, S. M., Stastny, P., Lukens, E. P., Toran, J., & Link, B. (2000). Employment outcomes in family-aided assertive community treatment. *American Journal of Orthopsychiatry*, *70*(2), 203–214. doi.org/10.1037/h0087819

McFarlane, W. R., Dushay, R., Lukens, E., Stastny, P., Deakins, S., & Link, B. (1999). Work outcomes in family-aided assertive community treatment: Vocational rehabilitation for persons with psychotic disorders. *Epidemiologia e Psichiatria Sociale*, *8*(3), 174–182. doi.org/10.1017/s1121189x00008046

McFarlane, W. R., Dushay, R. A., Stastny, P., Deakins, S. M., & Link, B. (1996). A comparison of two levels of family-aided assertive community treatment. *Psychiatric Services*, *47*(7), 744–750. doi.org/10.1176/ps.47.7.744

McFarlane, W. R., Levin, B., Travis, L., Lucas, F. L., Lynch, S., Verdi, M., Williams, D., Adelsheim, S., Calkins, R., Carter, C. S., Cornblatt, B., Taylor, S. F., Auther, A. M., McFarland, B., Melton, R., Migliorati, M., Niendam, T., Ragland, J. D., Sale, T., Salvador, M., & Spring, E. (2015). Clinical and functional outcomes after 2 years in the early detection and intervention for the prevention of psychosis multisite effectiveness trial. *Schizophrenia Bulletin*, *41*(1), 30–43. doi.org/10.1093/schbul/sbu108

McFarlane, W. R., Link, B., Dushay, R., Marchal, J., & Crilly, J. (1995). Psychoeducational multiple family groups: Four-year relapse outcome in schizophrenia. *Family Process*, *34*(2), 127–144. doi.org/10.1111/j.1545-5300.1995.00127.x

McFarlane, W. R., Lukens, E., Link, B., Dushay, R., Deakins, S. A., Newmark, M., Dunne, E. J., Horen, B., & Toran, J. (1995). Multiple-family groups and psychoeducation in the treatment of schizophrenia. *Archives of General Psychiatry*, *52*(8), 679–687. doi.org/10.1001/archpsyc.1995.03950200069016

McFarlane, W. R., Stastny, P., & Deakins, S. (1992). Family-aided assertive community treatment: A comprehensive rehabilitation and intensive case management approach for persons with schizophrenic disorders. *New Directions for Mental Health Services* (53), 43–54. doi.org/10.1002/yd.23319925306

McFarlane, W. R., Susser, E., McCleary, R., Verdi, M., Lynch, S., Williams, D., & McKeague, I. W. (2014). Reduction in incidence of hospitalizations for psychotic episodes through early identification and intervention. *Psychiatric Services*, *65*(10), 1194–1200. doi.org/10.1176/appi.ps.201300336

McGlashan, T. H., Walsh, B., & Woods, S. W. (2010). *The psychosis risk syndrome*. Oxford University Press.

Melle, I., Johannesen, J. O., Friis, S., Haahr, U., Joa, I., Larsen, T. K., Opjordsmoen, S., Rund, B. R., Simonsen, E., Vaglum, P., & McGlashan, T. (2006). Early detection of the first episode of schizophrenia and suicidal behavior. *American Journal of Psychiatry*, *163*(5), 800–804. doi.org/10.1176/ajp.2006.163.5.800

Miklowitz, D. J., O'Brien, M. P., Schlosser, D. A., Addington, J., Candan, K. A., Marshall, C., Addington, J., Candan, K. A., Marshall, C., Domingues, I., Walsh, B. C., Zinberg, J. L., De Silva, S. D., Friedman-Yakoobian, M., & Cannon, T. D. (2014). Family-focused treatment for adolescents and young adults at high risk for psychosis: Results of a randomized trial. *Journal of the American Academy of*

*Child and Adolescent Psychiatry*, *53*(8), 848–858. doi.org/http://dx.doi.org/10.1016/j.jaac.2014.04.020

Minuchin, S. (1974). *Families and family therapy*. Harvard University Press.

Murphy, T., Krasa, H., Lavigne, G., Frangiosa, T., Palsgrove, A., & Stalters, L. (2021). *Societal costs of schizophrenia and related disorders*. S. a. P. A. Alliance. https://sczaction.org/wp-content/uploads/2021/11/571-012_WhitePaper_Report_FINAL_updated_11.09.21.pdf

NIMH. (2017). *Mental illness*. National Institute of Mental Health

Nordentoft, M., Thorup, A., Petersen, L., Ohlenschlaeger, J., Melau, M., Christensen, T. O., Krarup, G., Jorgensen, P., & Jeppesen, P. (2006). Transition rates from schizotypal disorder to psychotic disorder for first-contact patients included in the OPUS trial. A randomized clinical trial of integrated treatment and standard treatment. *Schizophrenia Research*, *83*(1), 29–40. doi.org/10.1016/j.schres.2006.01.002

Parks, J., Svendsen, D., Singer, P., & Foti, M. E. (2006). *Morbidity and mortality in people with serious mental illness*.

Petersen, L., Nordentoft, M., Jeppesen, P., Ohlenschaeger, J., Thorup, A., Christensen, T. O., Krarup, G., Jorgensen, P., Nordentoft, M., & Jorgensen, P. (2005). Improving 1-year outcome in first-episode psychosis: OPUS trial. *British Journal of Psychiatry. Supplement*, *48*, s98–103. doi.org/10.1192/bjp.187.48.s98

Robertson, I., Ward, T., Ridgeway, V., & Nimmo-Smith, I. (1994). *The test of everyday attention*. Pearson.

Rosenheck, R., Mueser, K. T., Sint, K., Lin, H., Lynde, D. W., Glynn, S. M., Robinson, D. G., Schooler, N. R., Marcy, P., Mohamed, S., & Kane, J. M. (2017). Supported employment and education in comprehensive, integrated care for first episode psychosis: Effects on work, school, and disability income. *Schizophrenia Research*, *182*, 120–128. doi.org/10.1016/j.schres.2016.09.024

Ruff, A., McFarlane, W. R., Downing, D., Cook, W. L., & Woodberry, K. A. (2012). A community outreach and education model for early identification of mental illness in young people. *Adolescent Psychiatry*, *2*(2), 140–145.

Rupp, A., & Keith, S. J. (1993). The costs of schizophrenia. *Psychiatric Clinics of North America*, *16*(2), 413–423.

Stein, L. I., & Test, M. A. (1980). Alternative to mental hospital treatment. I. Conceptual model, treatment program, and clinical evaluation. *Archives of General Psychiatry*, *37*(4), 392–397. doi.org/10.1001/archpsyc.1980.01780170034003

Substance Abuse and Mental Health Services Administration. (2011). *Supported Education: Building Your Program*. HHS Pub. No. SMA-11-4654, Rockville, MD: Center for Mental Health Services, Substance Abuse and Mental Health Services Administration, U.S. Department of Health and Human Services.

Thompson, E., Rakhshan, P., Pitts, S. C., Demro, C., Millman, Z. B., Bussell, K., DeVylder, J., Kline, E., Reeves, G. M., & Schiffman, J. (2019). Family functioning moderates the impact of psychosis-risk symptoms on social and role functioning. *Schizophrenia Research*, *204* (February), 337–342. doi.org/10.1016/j.schres.2018.08.035

van der Gaag, M., Nieman, H., Rietdijk, J., Dragt, S., Ising, H. K., Klaassen, R. M., Smit, F., Bechdolf, A., French, P., Linszen, D. H., Yung, A. R., McGorry, P., & Cuijpers, P. (2013). Preventing a first episode of psychosis: Meta-analysis of randomized controlled prevention trials of 12 month and longer-term follow-ups. *Schizophrenia Research*, *149*(1–3), 56–62. doi.org/http://dx.doi.org/10.1016/j.schres.2013.07.004

Wehman, P., & Moon, M. S. (1988). *Vocational rehabilitation and supported employment*. Paul H. Brookes.

World Health Organization (2004). *Evidence for action: Effectiveness of community-based outreach in preventing HIV/AIDS in injecting drug users*. Geneva: World Health Organization.

Woodberry, K. A., McFarlane, W. R., Giuliano, A. J., Verdi, M. B., Cook, W. L., Faraone, S. V., & Seidman, L. J. (2013). Change in neuropsychological functioning over one year in youth at clinical high risk for psychosis. *Schizophrenia Research*, *146*(1–3), 87–94. doi.org/10.1016/j.schres.2013.01.017

Wu, E. Q., Birnbaum, H. G., Shi, L., Ball, D. E., Kessler, R. C., Moulis, M., & Aggarwal, J. (2005). The economic burden of schizophrenia in the United States in 2002. *Journal of Clinical Psychiatry*, *66*(9), 1122–1129. doi.org/10.4088/jcp.v66n0906

Yung, A. R., McGorry, P. D., McFarlane, C. A., Jackson, H. J., Patton, G. C., & Rakkar, A. (1996). Monitoring and care of young people at incipient risk of psychosis. *Schizophrenia Bulletin*, *22*(2), 283–303. doi.org/10.1093/schbul/22.2.283

# 15 Retirement Transition as a Preventive Intervention Target

Robert K. Conyne

Often when you think you're at the end of something you're at the beginning of something else.

—Fred Rogers, "Mr. Rogers"

For many, life's prolonged second half will be a time to chart a new course.

—Ken Dychtwald, *Age Power*

Retirement transition marks the entrée into retirement. It signifies the dynamic shift from a person's familiar work life to the uncharted experience of retirement. How the transition unfolds contributes strongly to subsequent retirement adjustment.

This chapter will focus on retirement transition as a preventive intervention target, organized by theoretical context and practice. The *Charting Your Personal Future* approach to prevention in retirement transition (Conyne, 2021) will be presented to inform retirement phases and prevention planning.

## 15.1 Theoretical Context: Support for Prevention in Retirement Transition

### 15.1.1 Retirement: Definition, Frequency, and Description

The etymology of the word "retire" derives from the French *re* (back) and *tire* (to draw), synonymous with "retreat" (fall back). It was typically used in a military context, as in "the enemy fled and retired behind the tree line." Applied to working life, one commonly applied conception of retirement involves working less than full time, or not at all, while receiving a retirement pension, social security, and/or drawing from self-funded accounts (Atchley, 1980).

I acknowledge Professor Emeritus Howard Jackson, University of Cincinnati, for his helpful comments on the chapter manuscript draft.

Retirement has become a part of life for millions of Americans, and it continues to expand its reach. The third quarter of 2021 found 50.3% of US adults over age 55 to be retired. Since the coronavirus 19 pandemic and its variants, the ranks of retirees aged 55 and older have grown by 3.5 million, reversing a decline from 2000 in which many members of that age group had chosen to continue working. This choice of remaining working, whether in the same position, a similar one, or in an entirely new direction is becoming increasingly popular among those considering retirement (Silver, 2018). Of those seniors in the 65–74 age group, 66.9% reported being retired in 2021. Between 2008 and 2019, the retired population aged 55+ increased by about 1 million per year (Fry, 2021). Finally, the number of new retirees currently averages around 10,000 per day with census projections reaching 12,000 a day by 2050 (Myers, 2018). Among other consequences, those large numbers foretell a robust continuing opportunity for prevention in retirement transition.

The once predictable pattern associated with retirement is altering although the individual factors affecting retirement (income, health, marital/relationship stability, and social support) remain intact (Donaldson & Muratore, 2010). Retirement is no longer a single event marking the end of paid employment (Wang & Shultz, 2010), but a process that is a function of duration and timing, being socially constructed and connected to social class, race, and gender.

Retirement also is an uncertain process (Wang & Shultz, 2010). While preplanning for it is important, any plan needs to make room for the unpredictable and unknown (Moffatt & Heaven, 2017). The degree of personal control is influential, whether emanating from internal sources (e.g., health condition status) and/or from external ones (e.g., financial circumstances). Those with fewer resources and/or in poorer health are especially subjected to lessened control and to increased constraint in choices available.

Views of retirement vary. In a survey of "Boomers" (those born between 1946 and 1964) conducted by Age Wave and HSBC Bank headquarters in London and Hong Kong, thousands of people in 20 countries that represented two-thirds of the world's population were asked about their views of retirement (Dychtwald & Morison, 2020). Among other areas probed, respondents were given four choices to describe retirement: (a) "a time to wind down"; (b) "a time for rest and relaxation"; (c) "a whole new chapter in life"; and (d) "the beginning of the end."

In the United States, Canada, Sweden, France, Germany, Japan, and China, "a whole new chapter in life" was the preferred option. Most Boomers in those countries view retirement as a time to begin anew. Consequently, other words are appearing to describe retirement as a new chapter in life, such as the term suggested in the Spanish word *jubilación:* retirement defined as a time of joyfulness. The term "*refirement*," a minor play on the word of retirement itself, illustrates one concept that is gaining some traction. It pictures retirement as being infused with novelty, positive engagement, adventure, new energy, zest, innovation, experimentation, and creativity (Blanchard & Shaevitz, 2015).

Perceptions of retirement align with how paid work is conceived. Tangibly, paid work conveys income and status. More subtly, but as beneficially, work provides a pattern for how time is spent, affords a context for social interaction, can enable a professional identity to form, includes routines of regularly reoccurring activities, and allows a way to become involved with others in shared effort (Jahoda, 1982).

Retirement threatens these pivotal factors and, in many cases, erodes or displaces them. It requires that different assumptions about one's "new life chapter" be authored, with adjustments to be made. Indeed, retirement is a period of transition and adaptation from the world of work to another one, yet to be articulated and experienced.

## 15.2 Retirement Transition

Retirement involves a dynamic individual developmental process of transition (Wang, 2007). This transition is a predictable and normative change that is experienced singularly and is subject to flux. It is like other developmental life transitions, such as moving from middle to high school, college graduation, weddings, birth of a child, divorce, and changing jobs.

Retirement also can be a stressful life transition. When it is forced, for instance, challenges can overwhelm the internal and external resources available, sapping retirees' daily energy supply. It may also edge them toward despondency and, in some cases, to depression (Keyes & Haidt, 2003). Whether forced or not, retirement transition can usher in a wide range of significant disruptions, "such as a loss of stable income, detachment from colleagues at work, and an increase in unstructured time" (Leung & Earl, 2012, p. 212). Depending on one's mindset, however, these and other kinds of disruptions may also provide growth prospects.

Retirement transition involves a variety of challenges and opportunities, including those mentioned earlier and others, such as preparing for retirement, redefining roles and role behavior, and making ongoing changes as the structure and significance of paid employment are replaced by other activities (Floyd et al., 1992). How effectively this transition is managed shapes the nature of overall retirement adjustment. More about retirement transition will follow in this chapter.

## 15.3 Retirement Adjustment

Retirement adjustment and aging are inexorably intertwined, with both positive and negative aspects (Cohen, 2008; Hill & Duffy, 2013). An advantageous adjustment to retirement is accelerated when retirees hold a favorable view of aging. Such a perspective can lead to a healthier life, fewer complications medically, and reduced risk of Alzheimer's, not to mention a gain of up to 7.5 years in life longevity (Levy, 2022). In addition, happiness is associated with increasing age, rising from age 50 or so into the 80s. It is remarkable to note that "even those over age ninety were happier than the middle-aged" (Aronson, 2019, p. 255). While increased age confers a range of benefits, the inevitable decline in mental and physical health as one moves into ever more advanced years certainly challenges a positive retirement adjustment and quality of life.

Retirement adjustment is receiving increased attention by researchers. It is understood to mean how positively or negatively retirees assess their retirement transition and its associated changes (Earl et al., 2015). It is influenced by a host of factors beyond the individual ones mentioned earlier, including resources available, activity levels, mastery and control, the presence of positive affect and absence of negative affect, and self-efficacy (Earl et al., 2015; Van Solinge & Henkens, 2008).

Wang (2007) found three general patterns of psychological well-being during retirement transition and adjustment: (a) maintaining levels of well-being throughout, (b) recovering during retirement from a negative preretirement state to a positive level, or (c) having a U-shape experience, in which initial elevated levels bottom out and then rise. Retirement adjustment patterns vary among retirees during the retirement process and are not unidirectional.

A research review and study by Donaldson, Earl and Muratore (2010) found that psychosocial and contextual factors predicted retirement adjustment. The best predictor was how a sense of mastery of retirement conditions, especially how employees exit their work position, mediated the postretirement and adjustment relationship. Possessing choice and control over retirement from work, such as in a phased or gradual retirement, can contribute to retirement adjustment (Calvo et al., 2009; Kim & Moen, 2002).

Research about the effects of preretirement planning showed that preplanning was inconsequential by itself in predicting retirement adjustment and satisfaction. However, preplanning can bolster confidence and set a first direction when moving into the early phases of retirement (Donaldson, Earl & Muratore, 2010). More comprehensive preretirement planning, including psychosocial and contextual factors in addition to the typically included financial ones, might yield more positive results for preplanning effects (Inoue-Smith, 2017).

Postretirement planning, however, was identified as mattering for retirement adjustment (Donaldson, Earl & Muratore, 2010). While creating a retirement plan is good practice, the ability to be adaptive, flexible, and resilient may be more functional throughout the retirement process. A plan created prior to retirement, however comprehensive, needs to evolve consistently with the personal and environmental changes that occur over the course of a retirement that could stretch 30 years or even more (Donaldson et al., 2010; Moffatt & Heaven, 2017).

Even so, anxiety and a sense of loss can manifest themselves when work and its supportive features are over, thereby jeopardizing a positive retirement adjustment. Retirement anxiety can appear from the absence of control. It also can result from the loss of existing friendships and the need to develop new friends and connections. Anxiety can intensify because a familiar life's work has been exchanged in retirement for something that is not yet personally charted, yielding what can be an abrupt and uncomfortable experience. For others, this shift to novelty may be greeted with excitement. How people experience their own retirement is a uniquely personal phenomenon.

## 15.4 Retirement Transition and Prevention: Brief Summation of Studies

A growing body of research exists to specifically support retirement transition prevention. For example, Rodriguez-Monforte et al. (2020) conducted a large review assessing the size and scope of available research evidence of retirement transition interventions aimed at improving well-being, a corollary of prevention. Their analysis included 15 publications containing both experimental designs and systematic reviews. Interventions focused on physical activity, social roles, health education, and psychological adjustment.

Within this large review of studies by Rodriguez-Montforte et al. (2020), one by Vrkljan et al. (2018) reported that group-based approaches provided by trained professionals can promote positive transition and adjustment to retirement, resulting in lowered stress levels. Also, within that same comprehensive review, a study of 21 stakeholders was reported, including recent and prospective retirees, health and social professionals, and policymakers. Results identified support for physical activity and social involvement as being central to a positive retirement transition, and the role of mentor as being a valuable resource. An additional analysis of 11 studies addressing social roles, such as assisting in local schools and kindergartens and serving as mentors of newer organizational employees, showed that such roles can enhance the health and well-being of those executing them (Heaven et al., 2013).

## 15.5 Phases of Retirement: *Charting Your Personal Future* Approach

In general, retirement progresses through overlapping phases. Atchley's (1980) classic six-phase model serves as common reference: preretirement, retirement, disenfranchisement, reorientation, retirement routines, and termination of retirement. Various adaptations of this model have been proposed over the ensuing decades.

The *Charting Your Personal Future* approach to retirement phases is presented next (Conyne, 2021). Its five phases emphasize transition and adjustment. Prevention can occur throughout all retirement phases, and through preretirement planning. During retirement, transition phases two and three, marked by an asterisk (*) below, are most amendable for preventive interventions.

### 15.5.1 Phase 1: Retirement Transition: Freedom/Liberation

The first phase begins just after the retirement party and singing ends, and the newly minted retiree walks out the work door for the last time. It may last for up to three to six months. New retirees often experience a liberation from the structure and routine of their work/career and an invitation to explore what is out there for them, more on their own terms.

For those who experience this sense of freedom, this first phase is colloquially branded the "honeymoon." Finally, new retirees experience time abundance, rather than time constraint. They can feel free from various restrictions, suddenly able to pursue, without fetters, all those things they have been eagerly dreaming about for years. Retirees can read all those books, care for the grandkids, travel to all those amazing places, golf all those courses, catch that elusive big one that has always lurked, put up one's feet and just relax, and/or do absolutely nothing, each and every day. One gets a sense of a honeymoon kind of existence, like living in the fun and sun.

### 15.5.2 Phase 2. *Retirement Transition: "Slough of Despond"

The freedom/liberation phase may continue over time, but in general, honeymoons do not last long. An unanticipated and acute internal (e.g., life-threatening health diagnosis) or external (e.g., loss of home via tornado) or lifestyle event (e.g., divorce) may send what seemed like a smooth-sailing retirement journey suddenly off-course. Such crises call for corrective action to try putting the pieces back together.

Moreover, everyone does not experience a sense of euphoria early in retirement. Some, whose exit into retirement has been forced and not of their own choosing, or who may enter retirement experiencing poor health, weak financial status, or some other lifestyle threat, may experience dread in which retirement feels anything but positive and free. Consistent with Wang's (2007) analysis, this state can continue, if no correction is enacted or, with improvements realized, it can be met with recovery.

In other instances, harsh reality may seep in gradually over a few months, often accompanied by a gathering sense of ennui that can drain energy and purpose. Fortunately, this downward slippage is not guaranteed to occur, but some one-third of retirees do experience it (Bosse et al., 1991; Renner,

2019). This state is what I term the "slough of despond," borrowed from John Bunyan's (2003) usage in his classic, *Pilgrim's Progress.* For retirees experiencing a gradual evolution of despair, which tends to ooze in from three to eighteen months into retirement, the following question becomes relevant: "Is that all there is?" Reading all day, every day may lose some of its luster. Similarly, many other activities, although high on one's "bucket list," can begin to fade due to overexposure. Some sense of variety or balance may become attractive, if not necessary, as an antidote to the despondency that may be experienced by doing the same thing, repetitively.

In addition to preretirement education and planning, this "slough of despond" phase presents a prime target for preventive intervention. This positive potential points to why I became involved with projects aimed at improving retirement transition, particularly as experienced by academics about to retire. This emphasis on the prevention of ill effects and the promotion of healthy ones has dominated my career as a counseling psychologist.

### **15.5.3** Phase 3. *Retirement Transition: Changes

Fortunately, the "slough" need not be permanent and may not even occur for some retirees. Its appearance triggers the need to make necessary changes. If done well, retirees can find themselves transitioning into a positive recalibration of what being retired now means for them. Usually on their own, but sometimes with the help of a counselor, they can reorient and adapt, fashioning a new way that fits better.

Making retirement transitional changes calls for resilience (Reivich & Shatté, 2002), which can be thought of as the capacity to adapt, recover, and bounce back from adversity. Sometimes, this bounce-back of resiliency may stretch above and beyond a return to the status quo, such that capabilities can exceed their previous level. This positive phenomenon is known as antifragility (Taleb, 2012). Transitional adaptations also are a function of mindset (Dweck, 2006) which, simply understood, refers to how one looks at and makes sense of the world. This perspective guides judgment, choices, and behavior. Holding a "growth" mindset in which retirees are open to learning and changing, rather than a "fixed" or closed one, is more amenable to a positive transition.

Drawing from resilience/anti-fragility and a growth mindset, transition changes can be made during this retirement phase in areas such as health care, financial management, lifestyle choices, geographic location, part-time working or volunteering, relaxation, and relationships, among others. Adaptations made in the transition phase stimulate the creation of revised or new roles, responsibilities, routines, relationships, and assumptions (Schlossberg, 2004) that will serve retirees well as they move to next phases.

### 15.5.4 Phase 4. Retirement Adjustment: Guided Gliding

Having made changes, retirees now tend to move more comfortably into a longer period. Depending on circumstances, this period may extend some 15 to 30 years or so, given the trend toward improved quality of life and reduced mortality rates.

In guided gliding, retirees find ways to keep forward momentum. Successful strategies include being open to their experience, monitoring and adjusting as needed, while remaining positively and actively engaged. Doing so can lead to finding purpose and meaning in their lives (Frankl, 2006; Garcia & Miralles, 2016) and, ideally, to having fun! (Note the exclamation point). For most retirees, these are generally enjoyable and satisfying years and decades, though not without challenges, both expected and unexpected.

### 15.5.5 Phase 5. Retirement Adjustment: Reflecting, Reintegrating, Reminiscing, and Reconciling

This final phase typifies the last years of retirement and of life. Retirees still can, and many do, experience overall satisfaction during this third stage of life (Dychtwald & Morison, 2020; Weiss & Bass, 2002). Following childhood and adulthood, this life stage is referred to increasingly as "elderhood" (Aronson, 2019). Reflecting and reintegrating events and experiences from one's retirement and overall life can yield a valuable sense of perspective and wisdom.

Loss can be counted on to occur now, too, due to the inevitable downspiraling of life events. Friends and family members may die, one's own physical and mental health can decline, disabilities might increase, and activities once performed with relative ease and competence can now be threatened or can even become out of reach. The denouement of this last phase of retirement life revolves around coming to terms with one's lessening life and considering one's legacy through reminiscing and reconciling (Newman & Newman, 2018).

## 15.6 Prevention

A set of *Best Practice Guidelines for Prevention in Psychology* (American Psychological Association, 2014) is available to aid researchers and practitioners in pursuing prevention. In fact, the literature on prevention in mental health has burgeoned over the last three decades, mirroring its increased use. The literature shows that preventive interventions in mental health are more efficient and cost-effective than remedial ones because they hold the potential to reach large numbers, stop the spread of problem behavior, and develop strengths and resources (Conyne, 2015; Gullotta & Bloom, 2003; Romano, 2015).

Prevention is intended to reduce the incidence (new cases or rates of development) of dysfunction and/or to promote wellness and effectiveness in a target population (individual through population levels) or setting (organization through community levels). Ideally, it is conducted "before-the-fact," launched prior to the onset of dysfunction or disturbance in a target, or failing that, at the earliest possible opportunity before entrenchment. Preventive interventions are designed to reduce or eliminate deficits and negative conditions while promoting strengths and positive conditions. Approaches used to reach these goals include proactive activities and programs that are aimed at both person-centered enhancement (e.g., increasing competencies) and system-centered change interventions (e.g., policy creation). See Cohen et al. (2010); Conyne (1997); Conyne & Horne (2013); Kenny et al., (2009); Romano & Hage (2000); and Vera (2013) for details.

## 15.7 Practice: Preventive Interventions in Retirement Transition

### 15.7.1 Person-Centered Enhancement Approach

The person-centered enhancement approach is used to identify and/or develop personal strengths and supports to promote psychological well-being, satisfaction, and success while avoiding setbacks. Consistent with prevention, person-centered enhancements are delivered to targeted individuals and groups as close as possible prior to their experiencing troubles and dysfunction (in this case, retirement transition despair).

### 15.7.2 Whole-Person Domain Foundation

Whole-person domains (emotional, physical, environmental, spiritual, social, financial, and intellectual) provide a broad foundation to prevention (Conyne, 2021), informing both person-centered enhancement and system-centered change interventions. One way these domains can be catalyzed is by implementing "therapeutic lifestyle changes" (TLC; Walsh, 2011), which include the following evidence-based activities: exercise, nutrition and diet, time in nature, social relationships, recreation, stress management, religious/spiritual involvement, relaxation, and service to others. The whole-person domain foundation is salient given, for example, that just an alarmingly low 2.7% of the US population lead an overall positive lifestyle, failing in the key areas of diet, exercise, body fat, and nonsmoking (U.S. National Health and Nutrition Study, 2016).

Consistent with earlier research cited on retirement, attention given to social relationships and exercise activities can be especially helpful for retirees, although all other whole-person domains and TLCs are relevant. Reading books, walking, hiking, and joining pickle ball clubs, for instance, provide avenues for social interaction and active involvement. All person-centered enhancement interventions discussed later in this section can, and should, take full advantage of the whole-person perspective in efforts to prevent retirement transition dips.

### 15.7.3 Counseling

It is not uncommon for prospective retirees to report being both excited and hesitant, sometimes even terrified, about the prospect of retirement. Moreover, not everyone enters retirement willingly or eagerly. As mentioned before, whether an exit from work is positive or negative matters in determining the nature of the transition. Counseling can help clients work through these challenges before retirement hits (American Counseling Association, 2022), thus diminishing and sometimes preventing, the size and strength of potential downturns.

### 15.7.4 Mentoring

Those who have traversed a process and succeeded can share their experience with more inexperienced others. Mentoring allows for wisdom to be passed down. It draws from crystallized intelligence, identified in classic research by Cattell (1963). It involves the storage and retrieval of learned information, with increasing access to insight, judgment, and wisdom as one ages.

Mentoring has received support in the prevention literature (e.g., the large review conducted by Rodriguez-Monforte et al. [2020]) as an important means for aiding the retirement transition. An example can be found when older volunteers help in class with kindergarten children (Heaven et al., 2013).

### 15.7.5 Psychoeducational Teaching and Training

Teaching and training from a psychoeducational perspective is a staple of person-centered prevention (Matthews, 2013; Morgan & Vera, 2011). For instance, teaching a course for prospective retirees which translates the retirement transition model, concepts, and strategies into practical application can supply helpful guidance. The course I teach, "Whole-Person Retirement," provides one illustration of such a psychoeducational approach (Communiversity, 2022).

### 15.7.6 Interactive Groups and Workshops

Interactive groups and workshops are a primary method used in preventive interventions (Clanton Harpine, 2011; Conyne & Clanton Harpine, 2010; Conyne & Horne, 2001), and they show signs of being useful in retirement transition preventive interventions (Vrkjian, 2018). Interactive groups and workshops that are focused on topics related to retirement transition, such as psychosocial aspects of retirement planning, can enhance awareness and skills beyond what the more typical workshops based on financial considerations (although important by themselves) can provide.

### 15.7.7 Planning

Planning by itself can exert a preventive effect (Conyne, 2010, 2013). Planning efforts ask prospective retirees to self-assess and to project into the future. Planning can provide focus, mobilize energy and confidence, and ease anxiety, promoting opportunities for a positive transition to occur. The *Charting Your Personal Future* planning approach is presented later in this chapter.

## 15.8 System-Centered Change Interventions

This second class of preventive interventions is concerned with improving the systemic and environmental conditions surrounding people who are passing through a particular transition, such as retirement (Conyne & Cook, 2004; Cook, 2012). Examples of systems include families, organizations, institutions, and communities. In terms of retirement transition, systems often targeted are the organization or work setting from which a retiree will transition, as well as the retiree's own family.

### 15.8.1 Consultation/Collaboration

Providing person-centered enhancement services directly to a target population, discussed earlier, indisputably has merit. Indirect methods, such as consultation (Dougherty, 2013), which may lead to embedding desired content or approaches within the offerings of another party (office, department, provider), can also be of significant benefit. Consultation and collaboration can be used to help another party include important resources within their own repertoire that otherwise would not be present. An example is providing an academic department head with new strategies for assisting faculty who are facing end-of-career decisions.

### 15.8.2 Research/Writing

The transition to retirement area is amendable for research. Developing clarity in defining the concept itself is needed. Exploring how retirement is a viable phenomenon across society or is relevant to only those who are "well-off" requires examination. Examples of other areas for investigation include what retirement transition interventions deliver the most preventive punch and how they can be best delivered.

Writing and scholarly work in this area needs expansion. Translating what is discovered into readable forms and finding ways to target and disseminate the information widely to prospective retirees await further development.

### 15.8.3 Social Media

"Readable forms," mentioned earlier, include but can extend beyond paper to embrace the ethical and appropriate use of social media (American Psychological Association, 2021). Social media provide vehicles to broadly disseminate information in palatable, digital ways to prospective users. The *Charting Your Personal Future* (2021) website contains a range of materials related to retirement and its transition.

The creation of public health messages and campaigns is another method for broad transmission of valuable messages to heighten awareness of lifestyle challenges and approaches. The National Institute of Aging's *Go4Life* campaign (2022), for example, highlights advantages of physical activity over a sedentary lifestyle. Physical activity is a critical area to address, as only 28% of Americans over age 50 report they engage in it regularly (Centers for Disease Control and Prevention, 2022).

### 15.8.4 Screening

Screening is a low-cost prevention procedure that can identify health problems before they become crises (Bell et al., 2017). Organizations specializing in physical and mental health areas can be asked to offer free screening services for prospective and current retirees. At my university, for example, the Emeriti Association's Health and Wellness committee has arranged with the speech and hearing clinic to make available ongoing, gratis diagnostic testing and hearing screening for emeriti.

Extending this approach, tailored screenings can be offered in the context of a national day, week, or month, such as National Senior Health and Fitness Day on the final Wednesday of May each year, National Mental Health Awareness Week in May, or Suicide Prevention Month in September. Fairs or festivals can be organized for a weekend that could hold not only screenings, but also samples of a full range of such services for retirees.

### 15.8.5 Advocacy

Advocacy can promote innovation and change (Pieterse et al., 2013). Proactively bringing one's message to systems that routinely impact retirees can increase possibilities for positive change. For instance, a university's human resources department can be nudged to expand its regularly occurring retirement workshops to integrate psychosocial material within the usual financially oriented approach that is featured. Indeed, a prime, but still undervalued, message in the retirement transition sphere is the critical role played by whole-person and psychosocial dimensions. The imperative task is to advocate for their wider adoption in retirement advising to supplement attention given routinely to financial issues.

## 15.9 Prevention Planning in Retirement Transition: *Charting Your Personal Future* Approach

As discussed, the transition to retirement can strip away familiar roles, routines, responsibilities, and relationships while demanding new assumptions and ways to view one's life (Schlossberg, 2009). It is likely that colleagues who were counted on during one's work or career may no longer be available. Therefore, it is important to get out in front of these potential losses before they occur.

Prevention planning in retirement can help design ways to buffer the losses and to maximize growth opportunities, at least in the short run into retirement. Armed with "pre-thought" in the form of a plan, the confidence of new retirees can be bolstered. Building awareness of the inevitability of future uncertainty is also important, along with the principle that planning is an ongoing process demanding adjustments over time.

The *Charting Your Personal Future* (*CYPF*; Conyne, 2021) approach provides one illustration of how this planning can be accomplished. The *CYPF* planning process (differentiated from its five retirement phases, discussed earlier) consists of a preretirement phase, including steps of *review, dream, plan*; and a *retirement* phase, with a step of *engage*. This approach is adapted from the three-phase retirement decision-making model (Feldman & Beehr, 2011), which involves imagining the possibility of retirement, assessing when it is time to let go of a career or of long-standing jobs, and then enacting concrete plans for retirement.

## 15.10 Pre-retirement Phase Steps

### 15.10.1 Review (Left Brain, Linear)

Future retirees are guided to reflect on their lives to identify what they have done, liked, accomplished, what has worked for them, and what they might like to continue or discontinue. They identify their "psychosocial tool kit": knowledge, skills, abilities, interests, attitudes, values, and experiences that they have developed and used successfully over the decades and which of these might place them in good stead moving forward.

### 15.10.2 Dream (Right Brain, Creative)

Forecasting ahead, prospective retirees let their right brain germinate future possibilities. Sparking flights of fancy is encouraged. What have they always wanted to do? What might make them happy? What accomplishments might they want to make? With what small, comforting things might they get involved? What places around the world, or close to home, might pique their curiosity? The task is to imagine possibilities and ignite their inquisitiveness, something with which many people at this stage of life have little experience. Of course, for those who are continually curious, such as those in creative and investigative lines of work (e.g., artists, university faculty), the capacity to dream may come more naturally.

### 15.10.3 Plan (Left Brain x Right Brain, Integration)

Planning before retirement is important and can contribute to the prevention of stress and despair. As previously reviewed, planning gets one ready; it can build confidence. It sets a course of action during what can be experienced as a stressful time. However, while the notion of planning for retirement is culturally accepted, its practice is paradoxically constrained. Many retirees have not planned at all. This failure sometimes reflects inertia and procrastination. More often, it results from a sudden exit from work due to ill health or bereavement, being "let go" or "pushed out," or as a function of occupational and social class status (Moffatt & Heaven, 2017).

Those approaching retirement are encouraged in this step to synthesize information derived from the review and dream steps and to begin converting this information into a tentative plan of action that is subject to adaptation over time. This plan might be detailed, stipulating goals-methods-dates, or it might be quite general and open-ended. The level of specificity often is a matter of personal preference.

For some, planning may seem too formal an act, being overly restrictive and structured. Two alternatives to planning may be more acceptable in such situations: (a) "thinking through" that is more informal than the structured certainty frequently associated with planning (Moffatt & Heaven, 2017) or (b) creating scenarios, stories about a retirement future that may be "possible," "most likely," the "best case," and the "worst case."

If either of these alternatives sits easier than developing a more detailed plan, then that is what is done. The pivotal point is for prospective retirees to become meaningfully engaged in considering prospects for their lives. Representing the plan as an important but tentative document that is open to revision is emphasized.

## 15.11 Retirement Phase Step

### 15.11.1 Engage: Honeymoon–Transition–Adjustment Phases

The preretirement steps of review, dream, and plan are beneficial by themselves because they can deepen self-awareness and contribute to a mindset for action. Once retirement is engaged, retirees move through the retirement phases discussed earlier, from honeymoon (phase one), through transition (phase two: "slough of despond"), transition (phase three: changes), adjustment (phase four: guided gliding), and adjustment (phase five: reflection). Recall that phases two and three are most suited for retirement transition prevention.

Engaging in retirement means to put the plan (or "thinking through," or scenario) into action and then to monitor how it goes, entirely subject to revision along the way. Emotional highs and lows will become reality; for some, retirement transition will include coping with the "slough of despond." One also can hope that for most retirees, engaging in retirement will be experienced as an enjoyable, happy, and meaningful time.

## 15.12 Retirement from a Social Justice Perspective

Retirement, as noted at the outset of this chapter, is a growing phenomenon. It also is a privilege enjoyed by those fortunate enough to be able to retire and needs to become a topic within social justice prevention (Kenny et al., 2009).

There are many for whom the word "retirement" is unappealing, infeasible, and/or out of reach. For some, retirement is an anathema due to conviction against it or limited resources. As an aggregate, those for whom retirement is a nonstarter either love their work and cannot envision leaving it; are not in any condition to be able to retire due to finances, health, or other conditions; or cannot or will not envision any other kind of life other than the one they have led for all their working lives. Indeed, the number of those unable to retire is weighty; for instance, 59% of Americans report they will need to continue working longer than they had planned, with 36% believing that they never will have the money to retire (Dickler, 2021).

*Social injustice* is inherent in a society in which retirement is not readily available for all. Instead, it is a privilege dependent not only on health status, but also on resource availability (Moffatt & Heaven, 2017). Deficiencies in these areas intensify vulnerability to life's challenges, particularly unplanned ones, and diminish the ability to exercise choice and control. This increased susceptibility to the power of negative life events weakens the ability to retire or, if retired, to sustain it satisfactorily over the long haul (Bardasi et al., 2002; Marmot, 2010).

More attention needs to be devoted to researching, understanding, and aiding those who are in a marginalized position to retire due to financial scarcity, racism, sexism, ageism, and other challenges. Retirement for those at such a cumulative disadvantage (Dannefer, 2003) may be improbable (but not impossible), or at the least, uncertain, fragile, and anxiety-laden (Goodwin & O'Connor, 2014). In fact, a range of life circumstances, including work history and exit from work, a spouse's employment, resources, inequities, and self-employment, all affect conceptions of retirement (Szinovacz & DeViney, 1999).

Advocating for retirement policies that are fair (Pieterse et al., 2013) is laudable, such as seeking to guarantee an adequate income for all retirees and targeting social security benefits to those most vulnerable and impoverished. Retirement is more likely to benefit males than females and people who identify as White than minority group members. Advocacy efforts should be conducted to help broaden gender and racial equity and access to retirement across a wider spectrum of economic bases (Richardson, 2003).

## 15.13 Recommendations for Research and Evaluation

Inconsistency exists in defining and operationalizing the concept of retirement transition itself (Rodriguez-Monforte et al., 2020). Variability in specifying this dependent measure across the limited number of studies currently available weakens the meaning and generalizability of retirement transition results. Therefore, researchers could improve future studies of retirement transition if these factors were conceptualized more clearly and uniformly.

How negative aspects of retirement transition could be prevented deserves examination, such as involuntarily exiting into retirement transition (Shultz & Wang, 2011). However, findings that suggest a positive retirement transition and adjustment show research promise, including a positive exit from work (Calvo et al., 2009), and the contributions of leisure, social, health, and psychosocial factors (Earl et al., 2015).

Gender, race, and retirement (Griffin et al., 2013; Kubicek et al., 2011; Szinovacz & DeViney, 1999) warrant more examination. Those studies that have appeared emphasize men's retirement, even while numbers of women entering retirement are increasing and their life conditions (e.g., comparatively lesser pay, living alone longer following death of a partner) leave them more generally susceptible to vulnerability than men (National Committee to Preserve Social Security & Medicare, 2021). The question of how women experience retirement and its anticipation needs investigation.

In terms of couples, different patterns of retirement exist in which both spouses retire at the same time, one continues to work while the other is retired, or both are working while considering how to retire. This variability calls for incorporating diversity of retirement circumstances within research and practice (Kim & Moen, 2002).

The nature of studies conducted requires expansion as most have been cross-sectional (Kim & Moen, 2002). Additional types of analyses are needed to learn about the process of retirement transition. Longitudinal designs may better show how men, women, and couples experience the relationship between retirement transition and psychological well-being (Schultz & Wang, 2011), and could lend needed direction to prevention efforts.

Finally, research is welcomed on the "post-retirement trajectory" (Shultz & Wang, 2011, p. 177), which, as has been said, might extend to 30 years or more. This ever-emerging reality presents a whole additional prevention research opportunity.

## 15.14 Conclusion

Counseling psychologists and other mental health specialists with a prevention orientation need to expand their foci to include retirement transition. Their well-developed competencies in person-centered and system-centered interventions delivered prior to dysfunction stand these professionals in good stead to be helpful with those who are approaching retirement. Moreover, training programs need to accelerate not only attention to prevention but, also, to prevention with the aging population, many of whom are nearing retirement.

There is urgency in moving in these directions. The aging population is growing quickly along with an increasing number transitioning into retirement. As was pointed out, for too many this transition can be severely challenged; it provides a cogent nexus for prevention.

Furthermore, the trajectory of retirees often occurs with limited or no support being readily available for the important psychosocial factors that accompany retirement transition – the very ones that help define the competencies of many mental health preventionists. Indeed, as discussed throughout this chapter, retirement transition provides a prevention intervention target that eagerly awaits broader adoption by prevention specialists.

## References and Resources

Sources are arranged in three exclusive categories: those especially pertinent to prevention, and to retirement, with the balance serving to support both. Websites and popular movies (not included within text) addressing a retirement theme are provided for additional follow-up.

## Some Particularly Relevant Prevention References


American Psychological Association. (2014). Guidelines for prevention in psychology. *American Psychologist, 69*(3), 285–296. doi.org/10.1037/a0034569.

Cohen, G. (2008). *The mature mind: The positive power of the aging brain*. Basic Books.

Cohen, L., Chavez, V., & Chehimi, S. (Eds.). (2010). *Prevention is primary: Strategies for community well-being*. Jossey-Bass.

Conyne, R. (1997). Educating students in preventive counseling. *Counselor Education and Supervision, 36*, 259–269. doi.org/10.1002/j.1556-6978.1997.tb00394.x

Conyne, R. (2015). *Counseling for wellness and prevention: Helping people become empowered in systems and settings*. Routledge.

Conyne, R., & Horne, A. (Eds.). (2013). *Prevention practice kit: Action guides for mental health professionals*. Sage.

Gullotta, T., & Bloom, M. (Eds.). (2003). *Encyclopedia of primary prevention and health promotion*. Kluwer Academic/Plenum Publishers.

Kenny, M., Horne, A., Orpinas, P., & Reese, L. (Eds.). (2009). *Realizing social justice: The challenge of preventive interventions*. American Psychological Association.

Romano, J. (2015). *Prevention psychology: Enhancing personal and social well-being*. American Psychological Association.

Romano, J., & Hage, S. (2000). Prevention and counseling psychology: Revitalizing commitments for the 21st century. *The Counseling Psychologist, 28*(6), 733–763. doi .org/10.1177/0011000000286001.

Vera, E. (Ed.). (2013). *The Oxford handbook of prevention in counseling psychology*. Oxford University Press.

Walsh, R. (2011). Lifestyle and mental health. *American Psychologist, 66*(7), 579–592. doi.org/10.1037/a0021769


## Some Particularly Relevant Retirement References


Atchley, R. (1980). *The social forces in later life: An introduction to social gerontology* (3rd ed.). Wadsworth.

Blanchard, K., & Shaevitz, M. (2015). *Refire! Don't retire: Make the rest of your life the best of your life*. Polvera Publishing.

Cohen, G., (2005). *The mature mind: The positive power of the aging brain*. Basic Books.

Conyne, R. (2021). *Charting your personal future*. www.chartingyourpersonalfuture.com

Dannefer, D. (2003). Cumulative advantage/disadvantage and the life course: Cross-fertilizing age and social science theory. *Journals of Gerontology: Psychological Sciences and Social Sciences, 58B*(6), S327–337. doi.org/10.1093/geronb/58.6.S327.

Donaldson, T., Earl, J., & Muratore, A. (2010). Extending the integrated model of retirement and adjustment: Incorporating mastery and retirement planning. *Journal of Vocational Behavior, 77*(2), 279–289. doi.org/10.10/vb.2010.03.003.

Dychtwald, K., & Morison, R. (2020). *What retirees want: A holistic view of life's third age*. John Wiley & Sons.

Earl, J., Gerrans, P., & Halim, V. (2015). Active and adjusted: Investigating the contribution of leisure health and psychosocial factors to retirement adjustment. *Leisure Sciences, 37*(4), 354–372. doi.org/10.1080/01490400.2015.1021881

Feldman, D., & Beehr, T. (2011). A three-phase model of retirement decision-making. *American Psychologist, 66*(3), 193–203. doi.org/10.1037/a0022153.

Kim, J., & Moen, P. (2002). Retirement transitions, gender, and psychological well-being: A life-course, ecological model. *Journal of Gerontology: Psychological Sciences*, *57B*(3), 212–222. doi.org/10.1093/geronb/57.3.P212

Kubicek, B., Korunka, C., Raymo, J., & Hoonakker, P. (2011). Psychological well-being in retirement. The effects of personal and gendered contextual resources. *Journal of Occupational Health Psychology*, *16*(2), 230–246. doi.org/10.1037/a0022334

Levy, B. (2022). *Breaking the age code: How your beliefs about aging determines how long and well you live*. William Morrow.

Moen, P., Erickson, W., Agarwal, M., Fields, V., & Todd, L. (2000). *The Cornell retirement and well-being study*. Cornell University Press.

Moffatt, S., & Heaven, B. (2017). 'Planning for uncertainty': Narratives on retirement transition experiences. *Ageing & Society*, *37*(5), 879–898. doi.org/10.1017/S0144686X15001476

Pieterse, A., Hanus, A., & Gale, M. (2013). Advocacy and prevention: Dismantling systems of oppression. In E. Vera (Ed.), *The Oxford handbook of prevention in counselling psychology* (pp. 109–124). Oxford University Press.

Rodriguez-Monforte, M., Fernández-Jané, C., Martin-Arribas, A., Costa-Tutusaus, L., Sitjà Rabert, M., Ramirez-Garcia, K., Vélez, O. C., Kopp, J., Vilaró, J., & Carillo-Alvarez, E. (2020). Interventions across the retirement transition for improving well-being: A scoping review. *International Journal of Environmental Research in Public Health*, *17*(12), 1–20. doi.org/10.3390/ijerph17124341

Schlossberg, N. (2004). *Retire smart, retire happy*. American Psychological Association.

Schlossberg, N. (2009). *Revitalizing retirement*. American Psychological Association.

Shultz, K., & Wang, M. (2011). Psychological perspective on the changing nature of retirement. *American Psychologist*, *66*(3), 170–179. doi.org/10.1037/a0022411. (Special section on retirement).

Silver, M. (2018). *Retirement and its discontents: Why we won't stop working even if we can*. Columbia University Press.

Szinovacz, M., & DeViney, S. (1999). The retiree identity: Gender and race differences. *The Journals of Gerontology*, *548*(4), 207–218. doi.org/10.10931/GERONB/548.4.S207.

Wang, M. (2007). Profiling retirees in the retirement transition and adjustment process: Examining the longitudinal change patterns of retirees' psychological well-being. *Journal of Applied Psychology*, *92*(2), 455–474. doi.org/10.1037/0021-9010.92.2.455.

Wang, M. (Ed.). (2012). *The Oxford handbook of retirement*. Oxford University Press.

Wang, M., & Schultz, K. (2010). Employee retirement: A review and recommendations for future investigation. *Journal of Management*, *36*(1), 172–206. doi.org/10.1177/014920630934957.

## Supportive Chapter References

American Counseling Association (ACA). (2022). *What is professional counseling?* www.counseling.org/aca-community/learn-about-counseling/what-is-counseling/overview

American Psychological Association (APA). (2021). *APA guidelines for the optimal use of social media in professional psychological practice*. www.apa.org/about/policy/guidelines-optimal-use-social-media.pdf

Aronson, L. (2019). *Elderhood: Redefining aging, transforming medicine, reimagining life*. Bloomsbury.

Bardasi, E., Jenkins, S., & Rigg, J. (2002). Retirement and the income of older people: A British perspective. *Aging & Society*, *22*(2), 131–159. doi.org/10.1017/S0144686X02008632

Bell, N., Grad, R., Dickinson, J., Singh, H., Moore, A., Kasperavicius, D., & Kretschmer, K. (2017). Better decision making in preventive health screening. *Canadian Family Physician*, *17*, 525–524.

Bosse, R., Aldwin, C., Levenson, K., & Workman-Daniels, K. (1991). How stressful is retirement? Findings from the normative aging study. *Journal of Gerontology*, *46*(1), 9–14. doi.org/10.1093/geronj/46.1.p9.

Bunyan, J. (2003). *The pilgrim's progress: From this world to that which is to come.* Oxford University Press.

Calvo, E., Haverstick, K., & Sass, S. (2009). Gradual retirement, sense of control, and retirees' happiness. Center for Research at Boston College. *Research on Aging*, *32*(1), 112–135. doi.org/10.1177/0164027508324704

Cattell, R. B. (1963). Theory of fluid and crystallized intelligence: A critical experiment. *Journal of Educational Psychology*, *54*, 1–22. dx.doi.org/10.1037/h0046743

Centers for Disease Control and Prevention. (2022, January 27). *Physical activity.* www.cdc.gov/physicalactivity/data/index.html

Clanton Harpine, E. (2011). *Group-centered prevention programs for at-risk students.* Springer.

Communiversity. (2022). *Whole-person retirement.* www.uc.edu/about/continuing-ed/communiversity/course-catalog/Personal-Development/whole-person-approach-retirement.html

Conyne, R. (2010). *Prevention program development and evaluation: An incidence reduction, culturally relevant approach*. Sage.

Conyne, R. (2013). *Program development and evaluation in prevention*. Sage.

Conyne, R., & Clanton Harpine, E. (Special Issue Eds). (2010). Prevention groups: The shape of things to come. *Group Dynamics: Theory, Research, and Practice*, *14*(3), 193–280. doi.org/10.1037/a0020446.

Conyne, R., & Cook, E. P. (Eds.). (2004). *Ecological counseling: An innovative approach to conceptualizing person-environment interaction*. American Counseling Association.

Conyne, R., & Horne, A. (Special Issue Eds.). (2001). The use of groups for prevention. *Journal for Specialists in Group Work*, *26*(3), 205–292. doi.org/10.1080/01933920108414220

Cook, E. (Ed.). (2012). *Understanding people in context: The ecological perspective in counseling*. American Counseling Association.

Dickler, J. (2021, September 14). *41% of Americans say it's "going to take a miracle" to be ready for retirement, report finds.* www.cnbc.com

Dougherty, A. M. (2013). *Prevention and consultation*. Sage.

Dweck, C. (2006). *Mindset: The new psychology of success*. Random House.

Floyd, F., Haynes, S., Doll, E., Winemiller, D., Lemsky, C., Burgy, T., Werle, M., & Hellman, N. (1992). Assessing retirement satisfaction and perceptions of retirement experiences. *Psychology and Aging*, *7*, 609–621. doi.org/10.1037/0882-7974.7.4.609.

Frankl, V. (2006). *Man's search for meaning*. Beacon Press.

Fry, R. (2021). *Amid the pandemic, a rising share of older U.S. adults are now retired.* Pew Research Center. www.pewresearchcenter.org

Garcia, H., & Miralles, F. (2016). *Ikigai: The Japanese secret to a long and happy life.* Penguin Random House.

Goodwin, J., & O'Connor, H. (2014). Notions of fantasy and reality in the adjustment to retirement. *Anxiety & Society, 34*(4), 569–589. doi.org/10.1017/S0144686X12001122

Griffin, B., Loh, V., & Hesketh, B. (2013). Age, gender, and the retirement process. In M. Wang (Ed.), *The Oxford handbook of retirement* (pp. 354–370). Oxford University Press.

Heaven, B., Brown, L., White, M., Errington, L., Mathers, J., & Moffatt, S. (2013). Supporting well-being in retirement through meaningful social roles: Systematic review of intervention studies. *The Milbank Quarterly 91*(2), 222–287. doi .org/10.1111/milq.12013

Hill, R., & Duffy, M. (2013). Promoting healthy aging in counseling psychology. In E. Vera (Ed.), *The Oxford handbook of prevention in counseling psychology* (pp. 315–329). Oxford University Press.

Inoue-Smith, Y. (2017, Fall). The psychology of retirement: A "Can't Let Go" syndrome. *The Journal of Retirement, 5*(2), 104–110. doi.org/10.3905/jor.2017.5.2.104 10

Jahoda, M. (1982) *Employment and unemployment: Social psychological analysis.* Cambridge University Press.

Keyes, C., & Haidt, T. (Eds.). (2003). *Flourishing: Positive psychology and the life well-lived.* American Psychological Association.

Leung, C., & Earl, J. (2012). Retirement resources inventory: Construction, factor structure and psychometric properties. *Journal of Vocational Behavior, 81*(2), 171–182. doi.org/10.1016/j.jvb.2012.06.00

Marmot, M. (2010). Fair society, healthy lives. *The Marmot Review.* www .instituteofhealthequity.org/projects/fair-society-health-lives-the-marmot-review

Matthews, C. (2013). Teaching prevention: Preparing the next generation of psychologists. In E. Vera (Ed.), *The Oxford handbook of prevention in counseling psychology* (pp. 76–90). Oxford University Press.

Morgan, M., & Vera, E. (2011). Prevention and psychoeducation in counseling psychology. In E. Altmaier & J.-I. Hanson (Eds.), *Handbook of counseling psychology* (pp. 529–544). Oxford University Press.

Myers, K. (2018, November 21). Americans are retiring at an increasing pace. *Yahoo! Finance.* https://finance.yahoo.com/news/americans-retiring-increasing-pace-145837368.html

National Committee to Preserve Social Security & Medicare. (2021, October 28). *Women and retirement: The gender pay gap persists.* www.ncpssm.org

National Institute of Aging. (2022). *Go4Life* from the National Institute of Aging. www.healthinaging.org/tools-and-tips/go4life-national-institute-aging

Newman, B., & Newman, P. (2018). *Development through life: Psychosocial approach* (13th ed). Cengage.

Renner, B. (2019, March 19). *Retirement blues: Average retiree grows bored after just one year, survey finds.* www.studyfinds.org/most-people-grow-bored-retirement-just-one-year/

Reivich, K., & Shatté, A. (2002). *The resilience factor.* Broadway Books.

Richardson, V. (2003). Retirement satisfaction, older adulthood. In T. Gullotta & M. Bloom (Eds.), *Encyclopedia of primary prevention and health promotion* (pp. 900–906). Kluwer Academic/Plenum Publishers.

Taleb, N. N. (2012). *Antifragile: Things that gain from disorder*. Random House.
U.S. National Health and Nutrition Study. (2016). *U.S adults get failing grade in healthy lifestyle behavior.* www.today.oregonstate.edu/archives/2016/mar/us-adults-get-failing-grade-healthy-lifestyle-behavior
Van Solinge, H., & Henkens, K. (2008). Adjustment to and satisfaction with retirement: Two of a kind? *Aging & Society*, *23*(2), 422–434. doi.org/10.1037/0882-7974.23.2.422.
Vrkljan, B., Montpetit, A., Nagile, G., Rapoport, M., & Mazer, B. (2018). Interventions that support major life transitions in older adulthood: A systematic review. *International Psychogeriatrics*, *31*(3), 1–23. doi.org/10.1017/S1041610218000972.
Weiss, R., & Bass, S. (Eds.). (2002). *Challenges of the third age: Meaning and purpose in later life*. Oxford University Press.

## Some Relevant Websites

Age Wave: www.agewave.com
American Association of Retired Persons: www.aarp.org
American Geriatrics Organization: www.americangeriatrics.org
American Psychological Association. *Life Plan for the Life Span*: www.apa.org/pi/aging/lifespan.pdf
Association of Retirement Organizations in Higher Education: www.arohe.org
Center on Aging, Health, and Humanities at George Washington University: https://nursing.gwu.edu/center-aging-health-and-humanities
National Council on Aging: www.ncoa.org
Senior Corps: www.seniorcorps.org
Third Age, Inc.: www.thirdage.com
WebMD: *Ways to stay healthy in retirement.* www.webmd.com/healthy-aging/news/20091016/stay-healthy-in-retirmenet-with-work

## Three Relevant Movies

*About Schmidt* (2002). www.youtube.com/watch?v=hl77NUrbioM (Rent/Buy). From an uninspired life to deciding to start living now before it is too late.
*A Thousand Clowns* (1965). www.youtube.com/watch?v=zpjN97qJ0bk (Free). Spontaneity and "heart" run amok. Delightful (if time bound), the movie can add a dose of improvisation that can be useful in retirement adjustment.
*Lost in America* (1985). www.youtube.com/watch?v=E0bTXgvXqF0 (Rent/Buy). An amusing satire on the American dream.

PART FIVE

# CLOSING

# 16 Future Directions in the Practice of Prevention: Envisioning the Road Ahead

Sally M. Hage and Sean DeMartino

> All you need is the plan, the road map, and the courage to press on to your destination.
>
> —Earl Nightingale, *The Strangest Secret*

The prevention programs and models presented in this book are meant to inspire you, to stimulate your thinking, and to provide, if you will, a road map for you in your own prevention planning and future work. We begin this final chapter by synthesizing some of the lessons learned across the chapters of this book, in order to provide you with a path forward in furthering the development of preventative interventions, policies, research, and training. Following this section, we chart a course for future directions in the field of prevention and health promotion. We offer a blueprint for training, interdisciplinary community collaborations, evaluation and dissemination of evidence, and future practice. These ideas are meant to advance the growth of prevention across and within mental health fields, including psychology, counseling, social work, public health, education, medicine, and more. Ultimately, we call on you, as professional helpers, to be leaders to translate the vision presented in this book into reality (Bennis, 1990).

## 16.1 Components of Successful Prevention Interventions

While each of the interventions and programs presented in this book is unique, a number of common features are important to consider in your own prevention planning, implementation, and evaluation. These elements make for successful prevention efforts and involve, in many ways, envisioning a new paradigm for the mental health fields, one that places prevention at the center of our identities as practitioners, educators, and researchers. In this section, we will explore the following "ingredients" for successful prevention, which include (a) performing community assessment, including strengths, assets, resources, and needs, (b) forming interdisciplinary partnerships with target communities, (c) attending to social and cultural dimensions throughout our prevention work, which includes targeting racial and socioeconomic disparities and promoting social justice, (d) designing comprehensive and multilevel interventions, (e) engaging in thoughtful evaluation of outcomes and disseminating the outcome of your work to the local and larger community so as to inform future practice, research, training, and social policy (Hage & Romano, 2013).

### 16.1.1 Community Assessment

A typical component in the training of mental health professionals is assessment, which typically means utilizing standardized measures and a clinical interview with an individual, followed by a written report that is shared with an individual and/or their family. In contrast, in prevention work the target for assessment is usually a group or community. As noted in the chapter by Reinke and Herman (this volume), the goal in community assessment is to identify the most pressing needs and the resources, assets, and strengths that could be utilized in developing, implementing, and evaluating an intervention.

An example of community-based assessment is found in Chapter 2. Craig-Cook (this volume) urges readers to appraise "organizational capacity," which means assessing the context or setting for its capacity to deliver the evidence-based prevention strategies you have selected. She identifies key community domains for our assessment efforts, including readiness, knowledge, leadership, skills/expertise, staffing, existing prevention programming, the status of community relationships or partnerships, community support, structure/processes, and sustainability.

An additional area for our assessment is risk and protective factors that exist in the target community. These factors occur at the individual, group, community, and societal level. Also, with few exceptions, these factors are not simply two ends of a continuum; for example, while poverty is a risk factor, wealth is not a protective factor (Durlak, 1998). In addition, these factors are embedded and must be viewed within the context of a social and cultural community, where they may operate differently both across and within social and cultural groups (Hage & Romano, 2013). Finally, a multiplier effect appears to exist in which, for example, a child who experiences four or five risk factors (e.g., poverty, peer rejection, poor quality schools, racism, community violence) may experience 20 times the risk of mental health problems than the child who experiences none or one of these risks (Hamby et al., 2021; Rutter, 1979)

In turning to a discussion of the assessment of protective factors or strengths, one important caveat is that no one overarching protective factor typically exists; rather, our goal is to assess for a combination of strengths (e.g., positive racial identity, social capital, faith and spirituality, high-quality schools, caring relationships, a sense of belonging) that, when highlighted, have the potential to buffer risks and enhance the well-being of individuals, families, and communities. A further important point is that a strength-based approach – versus one focused on deficits – which aligns with the social justice approach of this book, has greater potential to attract community partnerships, and, notably, may improve prevention outcomes (Banyard & Hamby, 2022). Finally, we highlight one community resilience assessment framework that offers a resource to prevention work, Tool for Health and Resilience in Vulnerable Environments (THRIVE; Davis et al., 2015), which was developed by the Prevention Institute (www.preventioninstitute.org). The goal of THRIVE is to identify community determinants and assets and to take action to improve health, safety, and health equity.

### 16.1.2 Interdisciplinary Collaborations

> No mass disorder afflicting humankind has ever been brought under control by attempts at treating the individual.
>
> —George Albee (n.d.)

The topic of interdisciplinary collaborations is discussed at length in the later section on future considerations for prevention; hence, it will only be briefly examined here. We begin by emphasizing the importance of organizing our prevention efforts "around communities, instead of around public health problems" (Banyard & Hamby, 2022, p. 212). As noted by Liang et al. (this volume), successful preventative interventions promote effective community collaborations. For example, in their chapter, Liang et al. describe forming partnerships with local school district leaders and community partners, such as teachers, nurses, school psychologists, parents or caregivers, principals, and members of the United Way. These race-centered, trauma-responsive leadership teams developed and implemented effective preventive strategies to promote resilience for all students regardless of trauma history. Another example is found in City Connects, described by Walsh et al. (this volume), which collaborates with numerous community partners (community, university, schools, families) to provide a hub of support for children and to improve long-term outcomes in areas like school readiness, grades, and attendance. A final example is Chandler and Helling's (this volume) *Changing Minds, Changing Lives* curriculum, which has formed partnerships with faculty in numerous departments, athletics, student services, and multicultural affairs to promote psychological health and resiliency through experiential, skill-based courses.

### 16.1.3 Social and Cultural Contextual Dimensions

As noted in the first chapter of this book, social justice work overlaps considerably with prevention. Social justice work can be defined as "professional action designed to change societal values, structure, policies, and practices," such that marginalized groups gain increased access to "tools of self-determination" (Goodman et al., 2004, p. 795). Social justice prevention work uses culturally responsive practices when determining and implementing prevention practices and research. In our prevention work, it is important to address mental health inequities by creating, providing, and evaluating high-quality and culturally responsive interventions with specific marginalized groups, while also demonstrating effectiveness in improving targeted outcomes. Ultimately, the goal of social justice prevention work is overcome and/or mitigate oppressive systems and environments, which "disempower, marginalize, silence, or otherwise subordinate one social group or category, often in order to further empower and/or privilege the oppressor" (https://theantioppressionnetwork.com/what-is-anti-oppression). Two examples of social justice prevention from this book include Vera et al.'s long-term work with schools to build their capacities for identifying and responding to the needs of BIPOC students and Vaughan et al.'s work with Latinx students, which attends to college students' Latinx and gender identities to understand alcohol use.

In their chapter, Tucker et al. (this volume) note that culturally responsive practices begin by our being aware of our biases (e.g., racial, gender, income-related biases) and realizing that others also have biases that may impact access to mental health. Further, Vera et al. (this volume) note that it is also critical for prevention practitioners and researchers to establish a foundational understanding of the cultural worldview (i.e., norms, values, lived experience, understanding of the world) of the community that the intervention will target. Tucker et al. anchor their preventive interventions in a holistic, community-based participatory research (CBPR) approach. Characteristics of a CBPR approach include building on the strengths and resources of members of the community, promoting a long-term collaborative relationship and co-learning among prevention partners, emphasizing the relevance of community-defined problems, and disseminating knowledge gained from the CBPR project to and by all involved partners (Amauchi et al., 2021). Through their Health-Smart Holistic Health Programs, Tucker et al. (this volume) counter the negative health effects of structural barriers, such as poverty and discrimination, which contribute to adverse health conditions that disproportionately impact Black adults and families. Their program involves patients, community member, focus group members, and clinic directors as study partners and tailors the physician training to the cultural preferences and values of the target group.

Similarly, in their chapter, Coard et al. (this volume) address racial health disparities by engaging African American parents to build their efficacy in effective racial–ethnic socialization with their youth with the goal of disrupting the detrimental effects of discrimination and fostering youth well-being. In collaboration with community partners, the Black Parenting Strengths and Strategies (BPSS) program incorporates evidence-based strategies used by parenting and child development specialists, while incorporating the strengths, unique parental strategies, and processes inherent in Black families, with the goal of promoting resilience. This model program promotes racism preparation by emphasizing racial barriers, racial and ethnic pride and commitment to cultural history and heritage, racial equality by emphasizing humanitarianism and multiethnic coexistence, and achievement by emphasizing individual and academic achievement and good work ethic. Additionally, the BPSS model encourages healthy and effective communication regarding race-related issues between Black parents and their children.

### 16.1.4 Comprehensive, Multilevel Intervention

The *Multicultural and Social Justice Counseling Competencies* (MSJCC; Ratts et al., 2016) identify six ecological layers for mental health professional engagement in social justice, and by extension, prevention work (intrapersonal, interpersonal, institutional, community, public policy, international/global). The training and professional work of mental health providers has mostly focused on these first two levels at the intra- and interpersonal levels. More effort is needed to prepare and implement mental health initiative at the institutional, community, and policy levels.

One example of a prevention intervention at the community, policy, and national levels is the Bandana Project, as presented by Conlin Bass in Chapter 9. The Bandana Project that started at a single school in 2016, University of Wisconsin-Madison, is an innovative suicide prevention and mental health program that prepares high school and college students to provide support and referral to peers. Students attach a green bandana to their backpack, signifying they are a safe individual to approach for mental health-related help-seeking tools and resources. Members also work to reduce stigma associated with mental illness.

The Bandana Project intervention, now nationwide, involves the whole community in their preventative efforts using an "it takes a village" model of campus-based mental health prevention. Adopting a model of "it takes a village" provides a possible long-term solution to the college mental health crisis that empowers the community to engage in collective action to better support one another and to improve the well-being of the campus community. Further, a move to a whole campus prevention model addresses the fact that many issues faced by individuals are "reflective of the environmental context" in which they live (p. 17, Glass, 2016).

### 16.1.5 Program Evaluation and Dissemination of Outcomes

A final component highlighted across these chapters is the importance of effective and ongoing program evaluation and dissemination of outcomes. De Lisa La Rue and Maureen Kenny (this volume) highlight the importance of evaluating both individual (person-centered) and systemic (environmental) impact (e.g., systemic racism) in our prevention program evaluation. Because environmental change takes time and is challenging to assess, they recommend including multiple methods and a range of stakeholders over multiple years, with the goal of establishing efficacy, effectiveness, and cost-effectiveness. The final step is to disseminate the findings and evidence widely through numerous methods.

Dissemination in academic settings happens via peer-reviewed journals and professional associations; however, if we are to truly impact the larger community and address health inequities, Fine (2017) argues that we need to be more strategic in our dissemination. For example, legislators may respond to policy briefs or white paper. We may share results to local community groups through newspapers, radio, or pamphlets. Fine notes that participatory public science – creating avenues to engage the larger community in research – is critical to sustaining and engaging a diverse, participatory democracy and to aligning psychological science within human rights struggles.

One example of effective dissemination is Graham-Berman's Kids' Club (KC) and Moms' Empowerment Program (MEP) (this volume). These evidence-based interventions for moms and their children who have been exposed to intimate partner violence have been adopted by 38 states and several countries. Similarly, the PIER Training Model (McFarlane et al., this volume), targeting early intervention for mental illness in youth, has been widely adopted across the Unites States and internationally.

> It is not what you look at that matters; it is what you see.
>
> (Thoreau, 2016)

## 16.2 Future Directions in the Field of Prevention and Health Promotion

### 16.2.1 Training in the Field of Prevention

The previous chapters of this book have demonstrated the effectiveness of prevention practice for a variety of presenting concerns, settings, and age ranges. The field of prevention has been considered important to the field of psychology, yet formal prevention training is limited. Additional work is needed in order to continue advancing the field of prevention science and practice. There have been several calls for the advancement of training mental health professionals in prevention (Rishel, 2014; Romano et al., 2012). Several psychologists have offered frameworks for developing competency in prevention training (Conyne, 1997; Hage et al., 2007; Matthews, 2013; O'Neil & Britner, 2009), (a) which include developing knowledge and skills utilizing prevention theory; (b) recognizing and resolving ethical issues specific to prevention; (c) understanding risk and protective factors; (d) learning how to work with communities and engage in multidisciplinary collaborations; (e) recognizing social and political trends and history; (f) engaging in program development and prevention research and evaluation; (g) competent in systemic level interventions; (h) and utilizing a multicultural and social justice-oriented framework.

Despite the general consensus regarding the types of competencies needed to engage in prevention work, many training programs do not currently offer formal training in prevention in their curriculum. If they do, it is often offered as an elective rather than requirement. Accreditation bodies for training programs often vary in the standards that they hold programs to and will often define curricular requirements for training programs (Romano & Hage, 2000). For example, the profession-wide competencies outlined by the American Psychological Association (APA) as well as the discipline-specific knowledge that doctoral programs are asked to provide trainees do not note any specific competencies or knowledge related to prevention (Commission on Accreditation, 2017). Other organizations, such as the Council for Accreditation of Counseling and Related Education Program (CACREP), the National Association of School Psychology (NASP), and the National Association of Social Work (NASW), only include a brief mention of prevention practice when discussing their competency and accreditation guidelines related to intervention for trainees (CACREP, 2016; CSWE, 2022; NASP, 2020). This void in training standards often puts students in the position of trying to obtain training and experience in prevention indirectly through their practicum and internship experiences. While even a brief mention of prevention in the accreditation standards of several organizations is an encouraging sign forward, further inclusion of prevention training in the accreditation standards across fields will allow greater flexibility for training programs to offer coursework specific to the science and practice of prevention.

Matthews (2013) offered several suggestions for training programs to infuse prevention training throughout curriculum in the absence of accreditation standards focused on prevention. These recommendations include integrating contents into curricula about how prevention fits within the trainee's respective field, education around what makes prevention distinct from traditional therapy services, discussion around the challenges of prevention work, providing opportunities to develop group facilitation and research skills throughout courses and assignments, and expanding opportunities for fieldwork and service learning in prevention. Incorporating prevention training into graduate training programs is an important next step to continue to grow the field of prevention and facilitate the growth of new programming.

Given the tendency for mental health professionals to focus on the practice of psychotherapy, potential educators and supervisors likely do not have formal training or themselves in prevention. The opportunity to engage in continuing education (CE) programs, either through conferences or through journal articles, focused on effectively engaging in prevention science and practice is a necessary next step to help train current mental health professionals in prevention. While it does not yet offer CE credits, the *Journal of Prevention and Health Promotion* that started in 2020 is one example of a resource that current mental health professionals can access to learn more about theory, research, practice, advocacy, and/or training related to prevention and wellness promotion.

> Prevention is better than cure.
>
> —Desiderius Erasmus (n.d.)

### 16.2.2 Need for Structural Changes to Promote Prevention

Despite the growing emphasis on prevention in the field of psychology, certain structural changes are needed to promote the growth of prevention in action. A review of the cost-effectiveness of mental health promotion and prevention from 2008 until 2020 consistently found prevention interventions to be cost-effective or cost saving, with targeted prevention interventions being more likely to be cost-effective compared to universal prevention interventions (Le et al., 2021). Despite this finding, preventative care efforts are frequently undervalued. For example, only 0.5% of the US GDP is devoted to preventative care compared to 10.4% of the US GDP being devoted for curative care (Organization for Economic Cooperation and Development, 2021). The National Health Expenditure (NHS) grew 2.7% in 2021 to $4.3 trillion accounting for 18.3% of the GDP (Centers for Medicare & Medicaid Services, 2021). The focus on curative care has likely been a higher priority for the public due to the more immediate impact that it has for individuals in the short term, while preventative care can be less visible, less personal, and focused on long-term benefits (Jacques & Noel, 2022).

Future efforts to promote prevention should seek to enact structural changes that support the implementation of preventative care. The current medical model of reimbursement typically reimburses for therapy services rather than prevention programming (Vera & Speight, 2003). Mental health professionals that rely on the reimbursement model are limited to the reimbursement codes outlined in the Current Procedural Terminology (CPT)/ Healthcare Common Procedure Coding System (HCPCS) codes (Centers for Medicare & Medicaid Services, 2022). The current psychiatry and psychology Services CPT/HCPCS codes cover curative care services such as various forms of psychotherapy (individual, group, couples, and family) and psychological evaluations, but do not include codes for prevention. This can place an extra burden on mental health professionals interested in engaging in prevention by having to seek other financial supports such as grants on their own time or engage in prevention pro bono while managing full caseloads. One of the challenges of adding CPT/HCPCS codes for prevention services is that the service code is attributed to an individual that received a service that is deemed medically necessary. The idea of preventing a mental health issue prior to the presence of the issue would appear to not fit the criteria for medical necessity. However, the CPT/HCPCS codes do include a set of codes for preventive screen tests and vaccines for physical health issues, suggesting that room may exist in the future for codes for prevention services for psychiatry and psychology services (Centers for Medicare & Medicaid Services, 2022). An additional barrier is that the codes must be assigned to an individual that received the service. Prevention programming often reaches members of a community, making it difficult to assign reimbursement codes to just one or a small group of people.

Researchers face similar challenges that practitioners experience regarding prevention efforts. Researchers in academic settings have been increasingly faced with heightened expectations set by their institutions that create pressure to publish papers, obtain funding, and maintain high teaching loads while often feeling insecure in their job status (Nicholls et al., 2022). Given that the benefits of prevention are often long term in nature, a tension exists for researchers seeking to conduct studies in prevention between the need to complete studies that lead to more frequent presentations and publications compared to their desire for engaging in prevention science that may take longer to publish. Added to this tension is the difficulty that prevention scientists can experience with identifying direct line cause and effect arguments that would show that prevention is beneficial, further compounding the potential challenges to obtaining publications (Israelashvili, 2008). Academic and research institutions that demonstrate support for researchers engaging in prevention science are needed to help foster additional prevention research.

### 16.2.3 Policy Development in Mental Health Training Curricula

Although the roles, training, and identities of mental health professionals differ, members of the field as whole (e.g., counselors, psychologists, social workers, psychiatrists) would benefit from competency-based training on how to engage in prevention as an integral, mandatory, and explicit component of accreditation standards. This policy change in accreditation standards would necessitate educator and faculty efforts to implement policy at the board level. New models for preparing mental health professionals are needed to add to the movement to "move our health system from one based on sickness and disease to one based on wellness and prevention" (National Prevention Council, 2012, p. 2).

To expand prevention activities in the preparation of mental health professionals represents a paradigm shift in our training programs. First, it is necessary to rethink the preferred prerequisites for entrance into our training program. A broad background – particularly in systems change, program evaluation, public health, and social and cultural issues – seems critical to preparing students to enter graduate study in programs incorporating a prevention specialty focus. In addition, the identity of mental health professionals needs to shift, from a primarily remedial individual focus to an ecological approach that views systems change and social justice advocacy as appropriate roles. To accomplish this, graduate education needs to expand prevention learning options. This goal can be accomplished through infusion of prevention-related content into existing courses and through stand-alone courses (Conyne et al., 2008; Matthews & Skowron, 2004).

A prevention perspective can also be integrated into many existing classes. For example, a research methods class could include a focus on needs assessment, program evaluation, and transformative research models. Ethics courses could include ethical challenges of conducting prevention that impact multiple systems, as opposed to a focus on one client. Also, prevention-focused classes that include a specialty track in prevention could be added to the curriculum, such as a class that focuses on micro- and macro-systemic perspectives, a community engagement–participatory focus, and a class on advocacy/social and political systems. Finally, practicum in program development-systems change, in which students engage in advocacy and social policy development or developing intervention with an agency, could be added to the list of practicum offerings across all programs. Such a change necessitates reenvisioning the way clinical hours are counted, so that individual client hours are not the only type of hours that are counted for internship and licensure. Training programs could also encourage students to enroll in prevention courses in other disciplines, thus encouraging interdisciplinary perspectives that are important to prevention.

> The more we are investing in that ounce of prevention the better off we're going to be.
>
> —Barack Obama, Politico

### 16.2.4 Need for Interdisciplinary and Community Collaborations

Mental health professionals engaging in prevention are encouraged to adapt prevention science and research to the social and cultural context of the community that they are working in (American Psychological Association, 2014). This requires mental health professionals to be aware and knowledgeable of the needs and strengths of the populations and communities that they are working within. Promoting mental health and well-being in communities through prevention has been shown to increase community connection, increase levels of social capital in the community, and lead to higher reported value of diversity in the community (Block, 2018). Communities whose members are able to relate to each other more frequently are more economically successful, have better health outcomes, and report higher educational achievement (Prilleltensky, 2012). Engaging in interdisciplinary and community collaborations can help provide opportunities for members of communities to feel empowered, to feel valued, and to add value to the community (Evans & Prilleltensky, 2007).

Collaborations between professionals from different fields are needed in prevention due to the complex and intersecting risk factors that can exist, which require multiple perspectives (Walsh et al., 2009). Attention should be paid to potential challenges to interdisciplinary collaboration, such as finding time and maintaining commitment to the collaboration, with an understanding that it can also lead to increased effectiveness of prevention efforts. One example of what these interdisciplinary collaborations can look like exists in the local area that the authors of this chapter live and work where a resource network of various professionals in the local area, including, but not limited to physical and mental health providers, lawyers, school officials, librarians, housing officials, and members of vocational support agencies, meet monthly to discuss the services offered in the community, strengths and challenges observed in the community, and ways to engage in supporting the community.

Interdisciplinary collaboration with the local community should continue to be emphasized, as local issues require local observations that ultimately understand the unique and subjective experience of the community (Stricker & Trierweiler, 2006). Prevention efforts that fail to incorporate community collaboration often strike a power imbalance and can limit the effectiveness of the efforts (Walsh et al., 2009). Community collaborations with prevention scientists and practitioners should seek to develop a shared vision for prevention, develop supportive messaging about the reasons to promote prevention, collaborate to develop policies and procedures that support prevention, identify meaningful incentives to engage in programming, and review the evaluation of programming (Amaya et al., 2019). Models of engaging in community collaborations, such as "It Takes a Village" (Wolff et al., 2014), can help build interdisciplinary and community collaboration among mental health professionals engaging in prevention.

When possible, interdisciplinary and community collaborations should seek to include trainees, allowing for an overlap of training, research, and programming that support community engagement, advocacy, and empowerment. Doctoral training programs, such as Boston College, the University of Tennessee, and Springfield College, have implemented community projects for first-year doctoral students through coursework to spend 4–6 hours a week working with various organizations and communities to expose students to issues impacting the community at the meso- and macro-levels (Hage et al., 2020). Students engage in prevention through consultation, collaboration, and advocacy with members of the community to address these issues. These collaborations occur in the school setting; public health departments; local court systems; local chapters of the YMCA; nonprofit organizations focused on disrupting incarceration, poverty, and racism; and sexual assault resource agencies. Engaging students in these projects at the onset of their training helps lay the foundation for a professional identity that is aligned with prevention and helps build the skills for engaging in interdisciplinary and community collaborations that can be carried over into their careers.

> Start by doing what's necessary; then do what's possible; and suddenly you are doing the impossible.
>
> ~St. Francis of Assisi

## 16.3 What You Can Do as a Mental Health Professional, Researcher, and Educator

Mrazek and Ritchie (2007) begin their seminal article, *Becoming a Preventionist,* by assuming that a bright new future is just ahead, one in which prevention is as much a part of practice as mental health treatment is now. They envision prevention practice emerging in response to exciting new scientific developments, innovative methods of engaging people and communities, and new outcome evaluation strategies. And while their paper was written more than 17 years ago, Mrazek and Richie's vision of what the future could become, perhaps must become, in the face of overwhelming demand for mental health services is even more relevant today. Concrete steps are necessary to move the field of mental health to include prevention. The first of these steps, while perhaps the hardest, is also the one that is both *most* crucial and most in our control, and that is generating the individual and community "will" to reorient our training, practice, and research to a prevention focus. This mental leap is a necessary first step.

A second step is to position the training environment to be supportive of and to value prevention and social justice. Several studies suggest that changing the culture of training, to be more supportive and to value prevention and social justice, predicts trainees' own commitment to these values in their future practice (Beer et al., 2012; Inman et al., 2015). In addition, students need training and supervision from someone with concrete experience in prevention and community change experience (Goodman et al., 2018), and thus, "training the trainers" in how to engage in prevention work is also critical. Part of this training for educators and students is to learn about and keep abreast of evidence-based preventive research and programming (Mrazek & Ritchie, 2007) A third step is to orient our health-care systems and funding resources (e.g., research grants) to expand support for prevention initiatives. In Weir's (2023) article, she describes a shift toward a mental health primary care model. Just as people are urged to attend an annual wellness exam for their physical well-being, they can also be urged to attend a regular mental health wellness primary care visit with a mental health provider trained in prevention.

> Real change occurs from the bottom up; it occurs person to person, and it almost always occurs in small groups and locales and then bubbles up and aggregates to larger sectors of change.
>
> —Paul Hawken, *Drawdown*

## 16.4 In Closing

If we are to meet the incredible mental health demands of this historic period, our vision of what it means to be a mental health practitioner must expand beyond diagnosing and treating mental health disorders to include innovative prevention, health promotion, and policy/systems interventions. It is clear that prevention has efficacy and utility in the current mental health landscape. Up to this point, it has not been well integrated into the training and practice of mental health practitioners. As a result, new competency models and training curricula that incorporate prevention across the professions, cultivating a preventative mindset, are critically needed. A true prevention mindset is necessary to move from a reactionary approach based on illness to a proactive approach based on fostering strengths and wellness and aimed at averting and reducing human suffering.

## References

Amauchi, J., Gauthier, M., Ghezeljeh, A., Giatti, L., Keats, K., Sholanke, D., Zachari, D., & Gutberlet, J. (2021). The power of community-based participatory research: Ethical and effective ways of researching. *Community Development Journal, 53*(1) 3–20. doi.org/10.1080/15575330.2021.1936102

Amaya, M., Donegan, T., Conner, D., Edwards, J., & Gipson, C. (2019). Creating a culture of wellness: A call to action for higher education, igniting change in academic institutions. *Building Healthy Academic Communities, 3*(2), 27–40. doi.org/10.18061/bhac.v3i2.7117

American Psychological Association. (2014). Guidelines for prevention in psychology. *American Psychologist*, *69*(3), 285–296. doi.org/10.1037/a0034569

Banyard, V., & Hamby, S. (2022). *Strengths-based prevention: Reducing violence and other public health problems*. American Psychological Association. doi .org/10.1037/0000267-000

Beer, A. M., Spanierman, L. B., Greene, J. C., & Todd, N. R. (2012). Counseling psychology trainees' perceptions of training and commitments to social justice. *Journal of Counseling Psychology*, *59*(1), 120–133. doi.org/10.1037/a0026325

Bennis, W. (1990). Managing the dream: Leadership in the 21st century. *Training: The Magazine of Human Resources Development*, *27*(5), 43.

Block, P. (2018). *Community: The structure of belonging*. https://ebookcentral .proquest.com

Centers for Medicare & Medicaid Services. (2021, December 1). *National health expenditure data*. www.cms.gov/Research-Statistics-Data-andSystems/ Statistics-Trends-and-Reports/NationalHealthExpendData

Centers for Medicare & Medicaid Services. (2022, September 21). *Billing and coding: Psychiatry and psychology services*. www.cms.gov/medicare-coverage-database/view/ article.aspx?articleId=57480#:~:text=CPT%20Codes%2090832%2D90838%20 represent,90833%3B%2090836%3B%2090838).

Commission on Accreditation. (2017). *Implementing regulations*. www.apa.org/ed/ accreditation/section-c-soa.pdf

Conyne, R. K. (1997). Educating students in preventive counseling. *Counselor Education and Supervision*, *36*, 259–269.

Conyne, R. K., Newmeyer, M. D., Kenny, M., Romano, J. R., & Matthews, C. (2008). Two key strategies for teaching prevention: Specialized course and infusion. *Journal of Primary Prevention*, *29*, 375–401 (2008). doi.org/10.1007/s10935-008-0146-8

Council for Accreditation of Counseling and Related Education programs. (2016). *2016 CACREP standards*. www.cacrep.org/for-programs/2016-cacrep- standards/

Council on Social Work Education. (2022). *2022 educational policy and accreditation standards*. www.cswe.org/accreditation/standards/2022-epas/

Davis, R., Rivera, D., & Fujie Parks, L. (2015). *Moving from understanding to action on health equity: Social determinants of health frameworks and THRIVE*. Prevention Institute, National Network of Public Health Institutes.

Durlak, J. A. (1998). Common risk and protective factors in successful prevention programs. *American Journal of Orthopsychiatry*, *68*(4), 512–520. doi.org/10.1037/ h0080360

Evans, S. D., & Prilleltensky, I. (2007). Youth and democracy: Participation for personal, relational, and collective well-being. *Journal of Community Psychology*, *35*(6), 681–692. doi-org.springfieldcollege.idm.oclc.org/10.1002/jcop.20172p://www .echoesofincarceration.org/Watch.html

Fine M. (2017). *Just research in contentious times: Widening the methodological imagination*. Teachers College Press.

Glass, G. D. (2016). Introducing a psychotherapy for the collective: A paradigm shift for college mental health. *Change: The Magazine of Higher Learning*, *48*(6), 16–23. doi.org/10.1080/00091383.2016.1247576

Goodman, L. A., Liang, B., Helms, J. E., Latta, R. E., Sparks, E., & Weintraub, S. R. (2004). Training counseling psychologists as social justice agents: Feminist and multicultural principles in action. *The Counseling Psychologist*, *32*, 793–837. doi .org/10.1177/0011000004268802

Goodman, L. A., Wilson, J. M., Helms, J. E., Greenstein, N., & Medzhitova, J. (2018). Becoming an advocate: Processes and outcomes of a relationship-centered advocacy training model. *The Counseling Psychologist*, *46*(2), 122–153. doi.org/10.1177/0011000018757168

Hage, S. M., Miles, J. R., Lewis, J. A., Grzanka, P. R., & Goodman, L. A. (2020). The social justice practicum in counseling psychology training. *Training and Education in Professional Psychology*, *14*(2), 156–166. doi-org.springfieldcollege.idm.oclc.org/10.1037/tep0000299

Hage, S., & Romano, J. L. (2013). *Best practices in prevention*. SAGE Publications. dx.doi.org/10.4135/9781452275581

Hage, S. M., Romano, J. L., Conyne, R. K., Kenny, M., Matthews, C., Schwartz, J. P., & Waldo, M. (2007). Best practice guidelines on prevention practice, research, training, and social advocacy for psychologists. *The Counseling Psychologist*, *35*(4), 493–566. doi.org/10.1177/0011000006291411

Hamby, S., Elm, J. H. L., Howell, K. H., & Merrick, M. T. (2021). Recognizing the cumulative burden of childhood adversities transforms science and practice for trauma and resilience. *American Psychologist*, *76*(2), 230–242. doi.org/10.1037/amp0000763

Inman, A. G., Luu, L. P., Pendse, A. C., & Caskie, G. I. L. (2015). Graduate trainees' social justice supports, beliefs, interest, and commitment. *The Counseling Psychologist*, *43*(6), 879–905. doi.org/10.1177/0011000015578932

Israelashvili, M. (2008). From acquaintance to engagement: Support in confronting primary prevention hassles. *The Journal of Primary Prevention*, *29*(5), 403–412. doi-org.springfieldcollege.idm.oclc.org/10.1007/s10935-008-0147-7

Jacques, O., & Noël, A. (2022). The politics of public health investments. *Social Science & Medicine*, *309*, 1–9. doi-org.springfieldcollege.idm.oclc.org/10.1016/j.socscimed.2022.115272

Kenny, M., Romano, J. R., & Matthews, C. (2008). Two key strategies for teaching prevention: Specialized course and infusion. *Journal of Primary Prevention*, *29*, 375–401 (2008). doi.org/10.1007/s10935-008-0146-8

Le, L. K-D., Esturas, A. C., Mihalopoulos, C., Chiotelis, O., Bucholc, J., Chatterton, M. L., & Engel, L. (2021). Cost-effectiveness evidence of mental health prevention and promotion interventions: A systematic review of economic evaluations. *PLoS Med*, *18*(5). doi.org/10.1371/journal.pmed.1003606

Matthews, C. R. (2013). Teaching prevention: Preparing the next generation of psychologists. In E. M. Vera (Ed.), *The Oxford handbook of prevention in counseling psychology* (pp. 76–90). Oxford University Press.

Matthews, C. R., & Skowron, E. A. (2004). Incorporating prevention into mental health counselor training. *Journal of Mental Health Counseling*, *26*(4), 349–359. doi.org/10.17744/mehc.26.4.xgc40bjahd05l47q

Mrazek, P. J., & Ritchie, G. F. (2007). Becoming a preventionist. *Psychiatric Annals*, *37*(5), 365–370. www.proquest.com/scholarly-journals/becoming-preventionist/docview/217055373/se-2

National Association of School Psychologists. (2020). *NASP 2020 professional standards*. www.nasponline.org/standards-and-certification/nasp-2020-professional-standards-adopted

National Prevention Council. (2012). *National Prevention Council action plan: Implementing the national prevention strategy*. National Prevention Council.

Nicholls, H., Nicholls, M., Tekin, S., Lamb, D., & Billings, J. (2022). The impact of working in academia on researchers' mental health and well-being: A systematic review and qualitative metasynthesis. *PLoS ONE, 17*(5). doi-org.springfieldcollege.idm.oclc.org/10.1371/journal.pone.0268890

Organization for Economic Cooperation and Development. (2021). *Health expenditures and financing*. https://stats.oecd.org/index.aspx?DataSetCode=SHA

O'Neil, J. M., & Britner, P. A. (2009). Training primary preventionists to make a difference in people's lives. In M. E. Kenny, A. M. Horne, P. Orpinas, & L. E. Reese (Eds.), *Realizing social justice: The challenge of preventive interventions* (pp. 141–162). American Psychological Association. doi-org.springfieldcollege.idm.oclc.org/10.1037/11870-007

Prilleltensky, I. (2012). Wellness as fairness. *American Journal of Community Psychology, 49*(1–2), 1–21. doi-org.springfieldcollege.idm.oclc.org/10.1007/s10464-011-9448-8

Ratts, M. J., Singh, A. A., Nassar-McMillan, S., Butler, S. K., & McCullough, J. R. (2016). Multicultural and social justice counseling competencies: Guidelines for the counseling profession. *Journal of Multicultural Counseling and Development, 44*(1), 28–48. doi.org/10.1002/jmcd.12035

Rishel, C. W. (2014). Teaching note – Integrating prevention content into clinical social work practice courses. *Journal of Social Work Education, 50*(4), 752–762.

Romano, J. L., & Hage, S. M. (2000). Prevention and counseling psychology: Revitalizing commitments for the 21st century. *The Counseling Psychologist, 28*, 733–763.

Romano, J. L., Koch, J., & Wong, Y. J. (2012). Prevention in counseling psychology: Promoting education, health, and well-being across the life cycle. In N. A. Fouad, J. A. Carter, & L. M. Subich (Eds.), *APA handbook of counseling psychology, Vol. 1: Theories, research, and methods* (pp. 345–367). American Psychological Association. doi-org.springfieldcollege.idm.oclc.org/10.1037/13754-013

Rutter M. (1979). Protective factors in children's responses to stress and disadvantage. *Annals of the Academy of Medicine, Singapore, 8*(3), 324–338.

Stricker, G., & Trierweiler, S. J. (2006). The local clinical scientist: A bridge between science and practice. *Training and Education in Professional Psychology, S*(1), 37–46. doi.org/10.1037/1931-3918.S.1.37

Thoreau, H. D. (2016). *Walden*. Macmillan Collector's Library.

Vera, E. M., & Speight, S. L. (2003). Multicultural competence, social justice, and counseling psychology: Expanding our roles. *The Counseling Psychologist, 31*(3), 253–272. doi.org/10.1177/0011000003031003001

Walsh, M., DePaul, J., & Park-Taylor, J. (2009). Prevention as a mechanism for promoting positive development in the context of risk: Principles of best practice. In *Realizing social justice: The challenge of preventive interventions* (pp. 57–78). American Psychological Association. doi-org.springfieldcollege.idm.oclc.org/10.1037/11870-003

Weir, K. (2023, January). Psychologists are rebranding the field, expanding the one-to-one therapy approach, *Monitor on Psychology, 54*(1), 87.

Wolff, L. A., Barclay, S. R., & Buning, M. M. (2014). Promoting student well-being on campus: It takes a village. In S. Degges-White & C. Borzumato Gainey (Eds.), *College student mental health counseling: A developmental approach* (pp. 339–353). Springer Publishing Company.

# Index

www.ingramcontent.com/pod-product-compliance
Lightning Source LLC
LaVergne TN
LVHW081939200926
848484LV00009B/2473
* 9 7 8 1 0 0 9 2 4 4 4 8 0 *